Antioxidants in Diabetes Management

OXIDATIVE STRESS AND DISEASE

Series Editors

LESTER PACKER, PH.D.
University of California
Berkeley, California

ENRIQUE CADENAS, M.D., PH.D.
University of Southern California School of Pharmacy
Los Angeles, California

1. Oxidative Stress in Cancer, AIDS, and Neurodegenerative Diseases, *edited by Luc Montagnier, René Olivier, and Catherine Pasquier*
2. Understanding the Process of Aging: The Roles of Mitochondria, Free Radicals, and Antioxidants, *edited by Enrique Cadenas and Lester Packer*
3. Redox Regulation of Cell Signaling and Its Clinical Application, *edited by Lester Packer and Junji Yodoi*
4. Antioxidants in Diabetes Management, *edited by Lester Packer, Peter Rösen, Hans J. Tritschler, George L. King, and Angelo Azzi*
5. Free Radicals in Brain Pathophysiology, *edited by Giuseppe Poli, Enrique Cadenas, and Lester Packer*

Additional Volumes in Preparation

Related Volumes

Vitamin E in Health and Disease: Biochemistry and Clinical Applications, *edited by Lester Packer and Jürgen Fuchs*

Vitamin A in Health and Disease, *edited by Rune Blomhoff*

Free Radicals and Oxidation Phenomena in Biological Systems, *edited by Marcel Roberfroid and Pedro Buc Calderon*

Biothiols in Health and Disease, *edited by Lester Packer and Enrique Cadenas*

Handbook of Antioxidants, *edited by Enrique Cadenas and Lester Packer*

Handbook of Synthetic Antioxidants, *edited by Lester Packer and Enrique Cadenas*

Vitamin C in Health and Disease, *edited by Lester Packer and Jürgen Fuchs*

Lipoic Acid in Health and Disease, *edited by Jürgen Fuchs, Lester Packer, and Guido Zimmer*

Flavonoids in Health and Disease, *edited by Catherine Rice-Evans and Lester Packer*

Antioxidants in Diabetes Management

edited by

LESTER PACKER
University of California
Berkeley, California

PETER RÖSEN
Diabetes Research Institute
Heinrich Heine University
Düsseldorf, Germany

HANS J. TRITSCHLER
ASTA Medica AWD GmbH
Frankfurt, Germany

GEORGE L. KING
Harvard Medical School
Joslin Diabetes Center
Boston, Massachusetts

ANGELO AZZI
University of Bern
Bern, Switzerland

UNESCO—MCBN
Global Network of Molecular & Cell Biology

Oxygen Club of California, '98 World Congress Sponsored Workshop

MARCEL DEKKER, INC. NEW YORK • BASEL

ISBN: 0-8247-8844-3

This book is printed on acid-free paper.

Headquarters
Marcel Dekker, Inc.
270 Madison Avenue, New York, NY 10016
tel: 212-696-9000; fax: 212-685-4540

Eastern Hemisphere Distribution
Marcel Dekker AG
Hutgasse 4, Postfach 812, CH-4001 Basel, Switzerland
tel: 41-61-261-8482; fax: 41-61-261-8896

World Wide Web
http://www.dekker.com

The publisher offers discounts on this book when ordered in bulk quantities. For more information, write to Special Sales/Professional Marketing at the headquarters address above.

Current printing (last digit):
10 9 8 7 6 5 4 3 2 1

PRINTED IN THE UNITED STATES OF AMERICA

Series Introduction

Oxygen is a dangerous friend. Overwhelming evidence indicates that oxidative stress can lead to cell and tissue injury. However, the same free radicals that are generated during oxidative stress are produced during normal metabolism and thus are involved in both human health and disease.

Free radicals are molecules with an odd number of electrons. The odd, or unpaired, electron is highly reactive as it seeks to pair with another free electron.

Free radicals are generated during oxidative metabolism and energy production in the body.

Free radicals are involved in:

- Enzyme-catalyzed reactions
- Electron transport in mitochondria
- Signal transduction and gene expression
- Activation of nuclear transcription factors
- Oxidative damage to molecules, cells, and tissues
- Antimicrobial action of neutrophils and macrophages
- Aging and disease

Normal metabolism is dependent upon oxgyen, a free radical. Through evolution, oxygen was chosen as the terminal electron acceptor for respiration. The two unpaired electrons of oxygen spin in the same direction; thus, oxygen is a biradical, but is not a very dangerous free radical. Other oxygen-derived free radical species, such as superoxide or hydroxyl radicals, formed during metabolism or by ionizing radiation are stronger oxidants and are therefore more dangerous.

In addition to research on the biological effects of these reactive oxygen species, research on reactive nitrogen species has been gathering momentum.

NO, or nitrogen monoxide (nitric oxide), is a free radical generated by NO synthase (NOS). This enzyme modulates physiological responses such as vasodilation or signaling in the brain. However, during inflammation, synthesis of NOS (iNOS) is induced. This iNOS can result in the overproduction of NO, causing damage. More worrisome, however, is the fact that excess NO can react with superoxide to produce the very toxic product peroxynitrite. Oxidation of lipids, proteins, and DNA can result, thereby increasing the likelihood of tissue injury.

Both reactive oxygen and nitrogen species are involved in normal cell regulation in which oxidants and redox status are important in signal transduction. Oxidative stress is increasingly seen as a major upstream component in the signaling cascade involved in inflammatory responses, stimulating adhesion molecule and chemoattractant production. Hydrogen peroxide, which breaks down to produce hydroxyl radicals, can also activate NF-κB, a transcription factor involved in stimulating inflammatory responses. Excess production of these reactive species is toxic, exerting cytostatic effects, causing membrane damage, and activating pathways of cell death (apoptosis and/or necrosis).

Virtually all diseases thus far examined involve free radicals. In most cases, free radicals are secondary to the disease process, but in some instances free radicals are causal. Thus, there is a delicate balance between oxidants and antioxidants in health and disease. Their proper balance is essential for ensuring healthy aging.

The term *oxidative stress* indicates that the antioxidant status of cells and tissues is altered by exposure to oxidants. The redox status is thus dependent upon the degree to which a cell's components are in the oxidized state. In general, the reducing environment inside cells helps to prevent oxidative damage. In this reducing environment, disulfide bonds (S—S) do not spontaneously form because sulfhydryl groups kept in the reduced state (SH) prevent protein misfolding or aggregation. This reducing environment is maintained by oxidative metabolism and by the action of antioxidant enzymes and substances, such as glutathione, thioredoxin, vitamins E and C, and enzymes such as superoxide dismutase (SOD), catalase, and the selenium-dependent glutathione and thioredoxin hydroperoxidases, which serve to remove reactive oxygen species.

Changes in the redox status and depletion of antioxidants occur during oxidative stress. The thiol redox status is a useful index of oxidative stress mainly because metabolism and NADPH-dependent enzymes maintain cell glutathione (GSH) almost completely in its reduced state. Oxidized glutathione (glutathione disulfide, GSSG) accumulates under conditions of oxidant exposure, and this changes the ratio of oxidized to reduced glutathione; and increased ratio indicates oxidative stress. Many tissues contain large amounts of glutathione, 2–4 mM in erythrocytes or neural tissues and up to 8 mM in hepatic tissues. Reactive oxygen and nitrogen species can directly react with glutathione to lower the levels of this substance, the cell's primary preventative antioxidant.

Current hypotheses favor the idea that lowering oxidative stress can have a clinical benefit. Free radicals can be overproduced or the natural antioxidant system defenses weakened, first resulting in oxidative stress, and then leading to oxidative injury and disease. Examples of this process include heart disease and cancer. Oxidation of human low-density lipoproteins is considered the first step in the progression and eventual development of atherosclerosis, leading to cardiovascular disease. Oxidative DNA damage initiates carcinogenesis.

Compelling support for the involvement of free radicals in disease development comes from epidemiological studies showing that an enhanced antioxidant status is associated with reduced risk of several diseases. Vitamin E and prevention of cardiovascular disease is a notable example. Elevated antioxidant status is also associated with decreased incidence of cataracts and cancer, and some recent reports have suggested an inverse correlation between antioxidant status and occurrence of rheumatoid arthritis and diabetes mellitus. Indeed, the number of indications in which antioxidants may be useful in the prevention and/or the treatment of disease is increasing.

Oxidative stress, rather than being the primary cause of disease, is more often a secondary complication in many disorders. Oxidative stress diseases include inflammatory bowel disease, retinal ischemia, cardiovascular disease and restenosis, AIDS, ARDS, and neurodegenerative diseases such as stroke, Parkinson's disease, and Alzheimer's disease. Such indications may prove amenable to antioxidant treatment because there is a clear involvement of oxidative injury in these disorders.

In this new series of books, the importance of oxidative stress in diseases associated with organ systems of the body will be highlighted by exploring the scientific evidence and the medical applications of this knowledge. The series will also highlight the major natural antioxidant enzymes and antioxidant substances such as vitamins E, A, and C, flavonoids, polyphenols, carotenoids, lipoic acid, and other nutrients present in food and beverages.

Oxidative stress is an underlying factor in health and disease. More and more evidence is accumulating that a proper balance between oxidants and antioxidants is involved in maintaining health and longevity, and that altering this balance in favor of oxidants may result in pathological responses causing functional disorders and disease. This series is intended for researchers in the basic biomedical sciences and clinicians. The potential for healthy aging and disease prevention necessitates gaining further knowledge about how oxidants and antioxidants affect biological systems.

Diabetes (both type I and type II) has been found to be associated with indices of oxidative damage. This suggests that oxidative stress is a contributing factor in these disorders. Aging itself is known to involve the deleterious effects of oxygen and glucose, which, albeit essential for energy, may also lead to oxidative stress. Indeed, insulin insufficiency is thought to be one of the underlying factors in accelerating aging. Thus, it is logical that natural antioxidants may have beneficial implications for diabetes management and healthy aging. Vitamin E and lipoic acid are two such substances receiving attention in this regard. Therefore, *Antioxidants in Diabetes Management* is an appropriate addition to the entire series, Oxidant Stress and Disease, since this volume provides a comprehensive and up-to-date evaluation of the role of oxidants and antioxidants in diabetes. Chapters focusing on biochemistry, molecular biology, cell and organ physiology, as well as human clinical studies of diabetes management, are included.

Lester Packer
Enrique Cadenas

Preface

Diabetes and its complications present a serious medical and socioeconomic problem. Diabetes mellitus is a chronic derangement of insulin action and carbohydrate metabolism. Its major distinguishing diagnostic feature is hyperglycemia, in which blood glucose rises above 200 mg/dL within 2 h of ingestion of 75 g oral glucose. There are two major classifications: insulin-dependent diabetes (IDDM, also known as type I or juvenile-onset diabetes), which accounts for about 20% of cases, and non-insulin-dependent diabetes (NIDDM, also known as type II or adult-onset diabetes), which accounts for the rest. IDDM is characterized by lack of insulin secretion, whereas NIDDM patients generally exhibit normal or elevated insulin levels but their peripheral tissues lack insulin sensitivity. NIDDM presently affects 30 to 50% of the elderly and is also characterized by the loss of insulin-triggered glucose uptake from the bloodstream to the insulin-sensitive tissues, thus leading to elevated blood glucose levels.

The management of diabetes has changed significantly in the past half century. Diabetic coma due to uncontrolled hyperglycemia was the medical challenge 50 years ago, but with greater availability of increasingly effective insulin (e.g., recombinant human insulin), the focus of medical care has shifted toward the management of diabetic complications. Polyneuropathy, one of the most common of these, occurs in 50% of those patients who have had diabetes for 25 or more years, and leads to pain and decreased mobility and function. Nephropathy and retinopathy are also common complications, which can result in kidney dysfunction and blindness, respectively. The major cause of death among diabetic patients, cardiovascular disease, is two to four times more common in diabetic than in nondiabetic populations. In addition, peripheral vascular disease and neuropathy can cause ischemia and, in some cases, gangrene of the lower limbs leading to amputation.

The medical and socioeconomic impact of these complications is enormous: diabetes is the leading cause of adult blindness, dialysis, kidney transplantation, and foot amputations. Diabetes afflicts approximately 6% of the population and is expected to rise to over 10%. Globally, there will be about 150 million diabetic patients by the year 2000, and 215 million by the year 2015. In the United States alone, the cost of diabetes mellitus and its complications increased from $20 billion in 1987 to $90 billion in 1997.

The current strategy to combat diabetes focuses on increasingly stringent control of hyperglycemia to prevent or modify the onset and progression of the disease and it complications. The Diabetes Control and Complication Trial (DCCT) demonstrated that intensified insulin treatment with an improvement in blood sugar control in type I diabetic patients reduced the rate of development and progression of some diabetic micro- and neurovascular complications. This clinical study supported the hypothesis that hyperglycemia is a major risk factor in the development of diabetic complications. Research over the last 10 years has shown that there are direct, potentially damaging, effects of diabetic hyperglycemia, including glucose-induced vascular abnormalities that are relevant to many diabetic complications. Cardiovascular risk, however, was not diminished by the intensified insulin treatment used in the study.

Only a minority of diabetic patients can achieve this kind of strict blood sugar control over several years in order to reach the preventive effects of hypoglycemia therapy on late diabetic complications. This is especially true for type II diabetic patients. The UKPDS study has shown that only 30% of type II diabetic patients can achieve the required glycemic control levels necessary to prevent late diabetic complications after 3 years and only 10% can do so after 9 years. Because of the therapeutic limitations of hypoglycemic therapy in practice, further interventional strategies must be developed.

Recent research indicates another promising area for inquiry and therapy—glucose (AGE)-induced vascular abnormalities, which are of relevance for all or most diabetic complications. Impaired microcirculation, capillary hypoxia, and ischemia syndrome are present in most diabetic complications. In addition to elevated blood glucose levels, increased production of reactive oxygen species (free radicals), which are known to exhibit direct tissue-damaging properties, may contribute to a number of diabetic complications and to the development of insulin resistance itself. These deleterious species can be neutralized by endogenous and exogenous antioxidants such as vitamin E, vitamin C, and thioctic (lipoic) acid. Compared to control subjects, NIDDM patients have lower plasma antioxidant vitamins (E and C) and double the lipid hydroperoxides (a measure of oxidative damage). IDDM patients also have low serum total antioxidant activity.

Increased oxidative stress in diabetic patients appears to be related to the underlying metabolic abnormalities, and is also an early stage in the disease pathology that may contribute to the development of complications. The impaired microcirculation, capillary hypoxia, and ischemia syndrome present in most diabetic complications are associated with the production of reactive oxygen species. In addition to control of blood sugar, control of oxidative stress offers another avenue for the treatment of the disease.

This volume summarizes the current knowledge of the pathogenic role of oxidative stress in the onset and progression of diabetes and its complications, and presents results of studies aimed at modulating oxidatively induced complications through the use of antioxidants. Chapters in this volume focus on (1) basic research on oxidative stress in the development of diabetes and diabetic complications; (2) studies aimed at specific complications such as cardiovascular disease and polyneuropathy; and (3) clinical trials of antioxidants in diabetic subjects.

An overall understanding of free radical pathology and its modulation by antioxidants is central to basic research into the relationships between diabetes, oxidative stress, and antioxidants. The concept of oxidative stress and antioxidant protection is explored with emphasis on the potential synergistic effects of an interlinked antioxidant network. The significance of oxidative stress markers in diabetes, and the evidence for and against an oxidative component in the genesis of diabetes is an ongoing controversy. Oxidative stress appears to play a role not only in complications arising from the disease, but in the development of insulin resistance in NIDDM. The possibility of its modulation by the antioxidant α-lipoic acid is explored. A related report focuses on oxidative stress and antioxidant treatment in animal models of both IDDM and NIDDM. The nonobese diabetic mouse model is often used in diabetic research, providing the basis for respective inquiries on basic research into diabetic mechanisms and prevention of NIDDM by antioxidant therapy.

Recently, much interest has been expressed in the possible interactions of oxidative stress induced by diabetes and cell signaling molecules in the development of diabetic complications. Studies concentrate on the tissue-damaging effects of free radicals, and also on oxidative-stress-sensitive molecular factors such as IRS-I, PI-3, PKC, and NF-κB, which are known to contribute to insulin resistance and diabetic complications. All of these molecular factors are redox-sensitive, which means that an imbalance between oxidative stress and antioxidant dysfunction can convert them to pathogenic factors. If one accepts the concept of oxidative stress described here as an important risk factor for diabetes and its complications, one has to consider the possible therapeutic value of antioxidants in treating this disorder. Research is presented in this volume that examines, in particular, the relationship between oxidative stress, NF-κB activation, and late diabetic complications, as well as the effects of α-tocopherol (vitamin E) on protein kinase C and its implications for diabetes.

Polyneuropathy, one of the most common, painful, and disabling complications of diabetes, also comes into focus. The hypothesis that ischemic reperfusion, a mechanism that induces oxidative stress, is the primary cause of diabetic polyneuropathy is explored, as is the potential for treatment with antioxidants in synergistic combination with essential fatty acids. This concept is further examined in an experimental model of polyneuropathy, using a thioctic acid (α-lipoic acid)–gamma-linolenic acid conjugate for protection.

As mentioned, cardiovascular complications represent the most common cause of death among diabetics, as well as the most frequent reason for limb amputation. Potential mechanisms for antioxidant intervention are discussed. Myocardial infarction is a leading cause of death among diabetics, and oxidation of low-density lipoprotein (LDL) is now a well-established causal factor in this pathology. One chapter links protein kinase C activation with the development of diabetic vascular complications and also suggests a role for vitamin E in their prevention. Another way in which oxidative stress may be involved in vascular complications, especially microangiopathy, is explored by one group through effects on cell adhesion molecules and the related potentially protective effect of antioxidants. Antioxidant vitamins, especially vitamin E, may reduce LDL oxidation in diabetes.

The ultimate goal of research on oxidative stress and diabetes is to introduce new therapeutic possibilities and to establish the efficacy of various therapeutic regimens. Therefore, several contributions to this volume relate to clinical trials of therapeutic effects of antioxidants such as vitamin E and lipoic acid. These include an overview of clinical trials of antioxidants to reduce isulin resistance, an evaluation of the clinical evidence on antioxidants in the treatment of diabetic polyneuropathy, and a report on the clinical status of antioxidants in the treatment of diabetic vascular abnormalities. Thus, research in oxidative stress, antioxidants, and diabetes may be achieving progress in attacking the basic mechanisms of the disease and in ameliorating some of its most common complications.

The medical and socioeconomic burden of diabetes and its complications requires a successful therapeutic concept. We hope that this selection of preclinical and clinical studies will stimulate scientific discussion of the possible pathogenic role of oxidative stress in diabetes and its complications, and will help to illustrate the therapeutic potential of antioxidants for treatment of the disease.

This volume is the result of two recent workshops, ‘‘Oxidative Stress in Diabetes and Its Complications: Implications of Antioxidant Treatment,'' held in Leipzig, as a satellite of the German Diabetes Association annual meeting and in Santa Barbara at the Oxygen Club of California World Congress. We would like to acknowledge the support of the following sponsors: UNESCO-MCBN (Global Network for Molecular and Cell Biology), the American Diabetes Association, the Henkel Nutrition and Health Group, and ASTA Medica AWD GmbH.

Lester Packer
Peter Rösen
Hans J. Tritschler
George L. King
Angelo Azzi

Contents

Series Introduction (Lester Packer and Enrique Cadenas) *iii*
Preface *vii*
Contributors *xvii*

1. Oxidative Stress and Antioxidants: The Antioxidant Network, α-Lipoic Acid, and Diabetes 1
Lester Packer

2. Oxidative Stress in Diabetes: Why Does Hyperglycemia Induce the Formation of Reactive Oxygen Species? 17
Peter Rösen, Xueliang Du, and Guang-Zhi Sui

3. Oxidative Stress Markers in Human Disease: Application to Diabetes and to Evaluation of the Effects of Antioxidants 33
Barry Halliwell

4. Plasma Lipid Hydroperoxide and Vitamin E Profiles in Patients with Diabetes Mellitus 53
Jaffar Nourooz-Zadeh

5. Concentrations of Antioxidative Vitamins in Plasma and Low-Density Lipoprotein of Diabetic Patients 65
Wolfgang Leonhardt

6. Oxidative Stress in Diabetes 77
John W. Baynes and Suzanne R. Thorpe

7. Antioxidative Defense in Diabetic Peripheral Nerve: Effects of DL-α-Lipoic Acid, Aldose Reductase Inhibitor, and Sorbitol Dehydrogenase Inhibitor 93
Irina G. Obrosova, Douglas A. Greene, and Hans-Jochen Lang

8. Pathways of Glucose-Mediated Oxidative Stress in Diabetic Neuropathy 111
Douglas A. Greene, Irina G. Obrosova, Martin J. Stevens, and Eva L. Feldman

9. Experimental Diabetic Neuropathy: Oxidative Stress and Antioxidant Therapy 121
Hans J. Tritschler, James D. Schmelzer, Yutaka Kishi, Yoshiyuki Mitsui, Masaaki Nagamatsu, Kim K. Nickander, Paula J. Zollman, and Phillip A. Low

10. Antioxidants in the Treatment of Diabetic Polyneuropathy: Synergy with Essential Fatty Acids 129
Norman E. Cameron and Mary A. Cotter

11. A Thioctic Acid–Gamma-Linolenic Acid Conjugate Protects Neurotrophic Support in Experimental Diabetic Neuropathy 155
Luke Hounsom and David R. Tomlinson

12. Clinical Trials of α-Lipoic Acid in Diabetic Polyneuropathy and Cardiac Autonomic Neuropathy 173
Dan Ziegler

13. Oxidative Stress, NF-κB Activation, and Late Diabetic Complications 185
Peter P. Nawroth, Valentin Borcea, Angelika Bierhaus, Martina Joswig, Stephan Schiekofer, and Hans J. Tritschler

14. Role of Oxidative Stress and Antioxidants on Adhesion Molecules and Diabetic Microangiopathy 205
Klaus Kusterer, Jörg Bojunga, Gerald Bayer, Thomas Konrad, Eva Haak, Thomas Haak, Klaus H. Usadel and Hans J. Tritschler

15. Molecular Basis of α-Tocopherol Action and Its Protective Role Against Diabetic Complications 219
Angelo Azzi, Roberta Ricciarelli, Sophie Clément, and Nesrin Özer

16. Protein Kinase C Activation, Development of Diabetic Vascular Complications, and Role of Vitamin E in Preventing These Abnormalities 241
Sven-Erik Bursell and George L. King

17. Oxidative Stress and Pancreatic β-Cell Destruction in Insulin-Dependent Diabetes Mellitus 265
Mizuo Hotta, Eiji Yamato, and Jun-ichi Miyazaki

18. Interrelationship Between Oxidative Stress and Insulin Resistance 275
Karen Yaworsky, Romel Somwar, and Amira Klip

19. Oxidative Stress and Antioxidant Treatment: Effects on Muscle Glucose Transport in Animal Models of Type 1 and Type 2 Diabetes 303
Erik J. Henriksen

20. Oxidative Stress and Insulin Action: A Role for Antioxidants? 319
Stephan Jacob, Rainer Lehmann, Kristian Rett, and Hans-Ulrich Häring

Index *339*

Contributors

Angelo Azzi, M.D. Institute of Biochemistry and Molecular Biology, University of Bern, Bern, Switzerland

Gerald Bayer University of Frankfurt, Frankfurt, Germany

John W. Baynes, Ph.D. Department of Chemistry and Biochemistry, University of South Carolina, Columbia, South Carolina

Angelika Bierhaus University of Heidelberg, Heidelberg, Germany

Jörg Bojunga University of Frankfurt, Frankfurt, Germany

Valentin Borcea University of Heidelberg, Heidelberg, Germany

Sven-Erik Bursell Harvard Medical School, Beetham Eye Institute Eye Research, Boston, Massachusetts

Norman E. Cameron, D.Phil. Institute of Medical Sciences, University of Aberdeen, Aberdeen, Scotland

Sophie Clément, Ph.D. Institute of Biochemistry and Molecular Biology, University of Bern, Bern, Switzerland

Mary A. Cotter, Ph.D. Department of Biomedical Sciences, University of Aberdeen, Aberdeen, Scotland

Xueliang Du, Ph.D. Department of Clinical Biochemistry, Diabetes Research Institute, Heinrich-Heine-University, Düsseldorf, Germany

Eva L. Feldman University of Michigan Medical Center, Ann Arbor, Michigan

Douglas A. Greene Division of Endocrinology and Metabolism, University of Michigan Medical Center, Ann Arbor, Michigan

Eva Haak University of Frankfurt, Frankfurt, Germany

Thomas Haak University of Frankfurt, Frankfurt, Germany

Barry Halliwell Department of Biochemistry, National University of Singapore, Singapore

Hans-Ulrich Häring, M.D. Department of Endocrinology, Metabolism, and Pathobiochemistry, University of Tübingen, Tübingen, Germany

Erik J. Henriksen, Ph.D. Department of Physiology, University of Arizona, Tucson, Arizona

Mizuo Hotta, M.D., Ph.D. Department of Nutrition and Physiological Chemistry, Osaka University Medical School, Osaka, Japan

Luke Hounsom, B.Sc. (Hons) Department of Pharmacology, Queen Mary and Westfield College, London, England

Stephan Jacob, M.D. Department of Endocrinology, Metabolism, and Pathobiochemistry, University of Tübingen, Tübingen, Germany

Martina Joswig University of Heidelberg, Heidelberg, Germany

George L. King Joslin Diabetes Center, Harvard Medical School, Boston, Massachusetts

Yutaka Kishi Department of Neurology, Mayo Foundation, Rochester, Minnesota

Amira Klip, Ph.D. Cell Biology Programme, The Hospital for Sick Children and University of Toronto, Toronto, Ontario, Canada

Thomas Konrad University of Frankfurt, Frankfurt, Germany

Klaus Kusterer University of Frankfurt, Frankfurt, Germany

Hans-Jochen Lang Hoechst Marion Roussel, Frankfurt, Germany

Rainer Lehmann, Ph.D. Department of Endocrinology, Metabolism, and Pathobiochemistry, University of Tübingen, Tübingen, Germany

Wolfgang Leonhardt Technical University, Dresden, Germany

Phillip A. Low Department of Neurology, Mayo Foundation, Rochester, Minnesota

Yoshiyuki Mitsui Department of Neurology, Mayo Foundation, Rochester, Minnesota

Jun-ichi Miyazaki, M.D., Ph.D. Professor, Department of Nutrition and Physiological Chemistry, Osaka University Medical School, Osaka, Japan

Masaaki Nagamatsu Department of Neurology, Mayo Foundation, Rochester, Minnesota

Peter P. Nawroth Department of Internal Medicine I, University of Heidelberg, Heidelberg, Germany

Kim K. Nickander Department of Neurology, Mayo Foundation, Rochester, Minnesota

Jaffar Nourooz-Zadeh, Ph.D. Department of Medicine, University College London, London, England

Irina G. Obrosova Division of Endocrinology and Metabolism, University of Michigan Medical Center, Ann Arbor, Michigan

Nesrin Özer, Ph.D. Department of Biochemistry, Marmara University, Istanbul, Turkey

Lester Packer, Ph.D. Department of Molecular and Cell Biology, University of California, Berkeley, California

Kristian Rett, M.D. Department of Endocrinology, Metabolism, and Pathobiochemistry, University of Tübingen, Tübingen, Germany

Roberta Ricciarelli, Ph.D. Institute of Biochemistry and Molecular Biology, University of Bern, Bern, Switzerland

Peter Rösen, Prof.Dr. Department of Clinical Biochemistry, Diabetes Research Institute, Heinrich-Heine-University, Düsseldorf, Germany

Stephan Schiekofer University of Heidelberg, Heidelberg, Germany

James D. Schmelzer Department of Neurology, Mayo Foundation, Rochester, Minnesota

Romel Somwar The Hospital for Sick Children and University of Toronto, Toronto, Ontario, Canada

Martin J. Stevens University of Michigan Medical Center, Ann Arbor, Michigan

Guang-Zhi Sui, Ph.D. Department of Clinical Biochemistry, Diabetes Research Institute, Heinrich-Heine-University, Düsseldorf, Germany

Suzanne R. Thorpe Department of Chemistry and Biochemistry, University of South Carolina, Columbia, South Carolina

David R. Tomlinson, Ph.D., D.Sc. University of Manchester, Manchester, England

Hans J. Tritschler ASTA Medica Aktiengesellschaft, Frankfurt, Germany

Klaus H. Usadel University of Frankfurt, Frankfurt, Germany

Eiji Yamato, M.D., Ph.D. Associate Professor, Department of Nutrition and Physiological Chemistry, Osaka University Medical School, Osaka, Japan

Karen Yaworsky The Hospital for Sick Children and University of Toronto, Toronto, Ontario, Canada

Dan Ziegler, M.D. Professor, Diabetes Research Institute, Heinrich Heine University, Düsseldorf, Germany

Paula J. Zollman Department of Neurology, Mayo Foundation, Rochester, Minnesota

1

Oxidative Stress and Antioxidants: The Antioxidant Network, α-Lipoic Acid, and Diabetes

Lester Packer
University of California, Berkeley, California

In this introductory chapter, oxidative stress in diabetes and implications of antioxidant treatment are considered. It is thought that free radicals may play a major role in aging and disease. Free radicals arise from radiation, environmental chemicals, cigarette smoke, and various other environmental sources. In addition, all through our life, we have a fire burning inside of us—our own body metabolism, which generates free radicals. Finally, many environmental substances (as well as drugs and alcohol) are metabolized in our body, generating free radicals through cytochrome P450-mediated oxidations. Many free radicals can be cytotoxic.

However, free radical reactions are also essential. They are essential for enzymes and for host defense mechanisms such as neutrophils, macrophages, and other cells of the immune system. Free radicals are important in the activation of transcription factors and in cell signal transduction and gene expression. But if free radicals are overproduced, they also can create oxidative stress and damage to molecules, cells, and tissues.

So what, then, is oxidative stress? Oxidative stress is an upset in the balance between oxidants and antioxidants. It was defined by Helmut Sies (1) in the following way: ''Oxidative stress is a change in the pro-oxidant/antioxidant balance in the favor of the former, potentially leading to biological damage.'' The result is molecular damage products, which are markers of oxidative stress.

I. DEFINITION OF AN ANTIOXIDANT

What is an *antioxidant*? To find a definition, we went to the dictionary. Dorland's Medical Dictionary reports (2), ''An antioxidant is one of many widely used synthetic or natural substances added to a product to prevent or delay deterioration by action of oxygen in the air.'' Examples of such products to which antioxidants may be added are rubber, paint, vegetable oils, and so on. But there are many other definitions of an antioxidant. For example, Halliwell and Gutteridge (3) defined an antioxidant as ''any substance that, when present at low concentrations compared to those of an oxidizable substrate, significantly delays or inhibits oxidation of that substrate.'' Another definition of an antioxidant (and the one I favor) is that of a *metabolic antioxidant* (4,5): ''An antioxidant is a substance which protects biological tissues from free radical damage, which is able to be recycled or regenerated by biological reductants.'' Thus, metabolic antioxidants have something similar to a catalytic activity, as long as they are connected, directly or indirectly, to biological reductants.

So what, then, is the antioxidant network? If antioxidants can be recycled and regenerated, then there must be some sort of coordinated network connecting them to one another and to cellular metabolic processes. The antioxidant network consists of a series of proteins and substances that provide these connections.

Among the proteins that are most important in antioxidant defense are superoxide dismutases to remove superoxide; enzymes that catalyze the removal of hydroperoxides; reduced thioredoxin; and a number of proteins, like transferrin and ceruloplasmin, that bind transition metals like iron and copper in such a way that they are not able to catalyze free radical reactions. Another vital antioxidant enzyme is methionine sulfoxide reductase, which repairs sulfhydryl groups of methionine residues, thus protecting cysteine residues (which are critical for biological protection against oxidation). The group of antioxidant substances, all of which are phytonutrients, is rather small: vitamin C, also known as ascorbate; vitamin E, a family of eight compounds—four tocopherols and four tocotrienols; carotenes, of which 500 different varieties may exist in nature; and flavonoids and polyphenols, of which there may be 4000–5000 different varieties. Of course, few of the carotenoids and flavonoids are common in the diet. α-Lipoic acid is another antioxidant compound naturally occurring in foods and also produced by the body. Others are metals that are covalently bound to the antioxidant defense proteins to assist with the proteins' catalytic functions.

Lipoic acid is a good example of a metabolic antioxidant. It is an analogue of octanoic acid and has a dithiolane ring in its oxidized form, but the ring can be broken by reduction to form dihydrolipoic acid. Both lipoic acid and dihydrolipoic acid have unique antioxidant profiles (6). The reduced form of lipoate has somewhat more antioxidant properties than the oxidized form in that the reduced form can scavenge superoxide and peroxyl radicals. Lipoic acid was found some years ago, in work from Helmut Sies's laboratory, to be taken up by the fatty acid carrier in isolated mammalian hepatocytes (7). Thus, lipoic acid can readily be taken up by cells. Three different enzymes have been identified as contributing to the reduction of lipoic acid so far: glutathione reductase (8,9) and thioredoxin reductase (10), which are NADPH-dependent enzymes, and the more abundant lipoamide dehydrogenase, an NADH-dependent enzyme. Lipoamide dehydrogenase is the E-3 component common to the α-keto acid dehydrogenase complexes that exist only in the mitochondria of animal cells. After reduction, lipoic acid can be released to the extracellular compartment, so there can be a cycle of lipoic acid reduction inside the cell, its release to the outside where it is oxidized, its reuptake into cells as the oxidized form, and its reduction again, as the cycle continues (11).

II. THE ANTIOXIDANT NETWORK

The antioxidant network is composed of redox-sensitive antioxidant substances. I like to say that the hub of the antioxidant network is vitamin C. The antioxidant network usually gets activated by vitamin E (12). After vitamin E is oxidized by oxidants or lipid free radicals, then the vitamin E free radical is formed, which in turn activates vitamin C to regenerate vitamin E nonenzymatically. Vitamin C itself becomes a radical, the vitamin C radical, in this process. Glutathione, with the aid of enzymes, can reduce the vitamin C radical (or dehydroascorbate, the completely reduced form of vitamin C). The oxidized glutathione thus produced can be reduced through enzymatic reactions that draw on cellular reducing power. There are also substances that we can obtain in our diet or that we can supplement—like flavonoids, polyphenols, and lipoic acid—that can also act in the antioxidant network (13,14). An example of how the antioxidant network works with respect to vitamin C, vitamin E, and thiol antioxidants is shown in Figure 1.

If vitamin E is made into a radical by reacting with a lipid peroxyl radical, the chromanol of vitamin E becomes a chromanoxyl radical and a lipid hydroperoxide forms. If this process is induced in human low-density

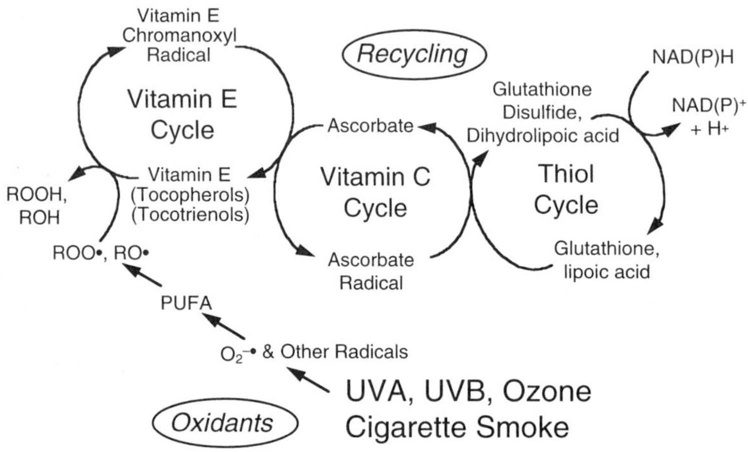

Figure 1 Oxidative stress activates network antioxidants.

lipoproteins, there is enough vitamin E present in these lipoproteins to follow these reactions by detecting the electron spin resonance (ESR) signal of the vitamin E radical. Once vitamin E is made into a radical, it is more reactive, of course. It can react with itself or other radicals in a chain-breaking reaction. It is a slowly reacting radical because the free electron is delocalized around the chromanol ring of vitamin E. Thus, it exists for a sufficient time for ascorbic acid to react with most of the vitamin E radicals and convert them back to vitamin E, thus sparing vitamin E (15,16). When ascorbic acid does that, it becomes an ascorbyl radical (Fig. 2). The vitamin C radical can be regenerated by glutathione with the aid of enzymes or nonenzymatically by lipoic acid or certain flavonoids.

Lipoic acid is unique in this regard because it has a redox potential (−320 mV) that is even lower (17) than the glutathione system (−280 mV); thus, in its reduced form, it can nonenzymatically regenerate vitamin C, which in turn can regenerate vitamin E.

A dramatic example of this effect was recently observed by Podda et al. (18). When animals were placed on a vitamin E-deficient diet, they lost weight and eventually died. But when 1.65 g lipoic acid/kg of diet was fed to these animals, they did not develop the symptoms of vitamin E deficiency—weight loss and motor discoordination. Hence, lipoic acid was obviously able to take over some functions of vitamin E in these animals, presumably either

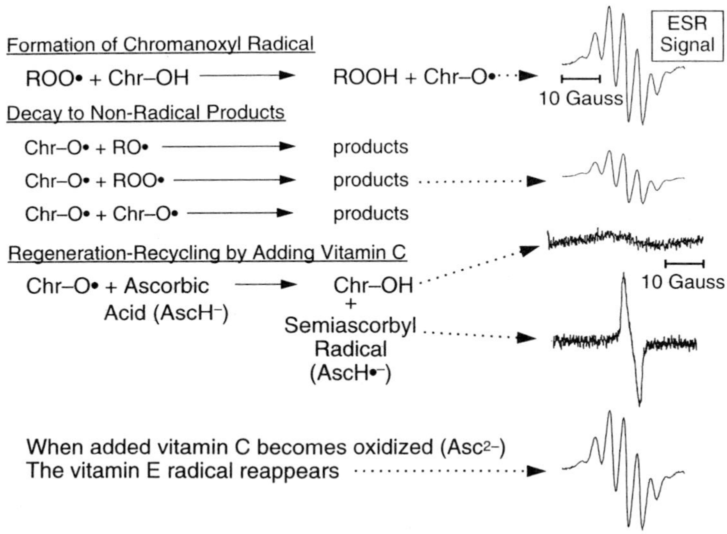

Figure 2 Vitamin E radical reactions during lipid peroxidation.

through regenerating vitamin E as described above or through directly substituting for vitamin E as an antioxidant, or some combination of both.

The vitamin E radical slowly decomposes as a result of reacting with itself or with other radicals. When ascorbic acid is added to a system in which vitamin E radical is being generated, the vitamin E radical disappears as it is reduced back to vitamin E by reaction with ascorbate and the semiascorbyl radical appears. But the vitamin E radical eventually returns as the the semiascorbyl radical disappears. From this experiment, the time that it takes for the vitamin E radical to reappear, or the lag period, can be determined. The time of the lag period is directly related to the vitamin C concentration. However, if dihydrolipoic acid is added to the reaction mixture, as well as vitamin C, and the same experiment is performed, one now observes that it takes a much longer time for the vitamin E radical to return. In this experiment, the lag period time is directly related to the concentration of the reduced lipoic acid. Reduced lipoic acid recycles the vitamin C radical (13). There are other ways in which lipoic acid can react with, and thus recycle, other antioxidants. After lipoic acid is reduced, it can regenerate oxidized thioredoxin, glutathione disulfide, or dehydroascorbate. Also, reduced lipoic acid has been reported to regenerate the semiquinone of ubiquinone (coenzyme Q10) in membranes (H.

Nohl Laboratory, Vienna). Thus, the entire antioxidant defense system can be affected by the presence of reduced lipoic acid.

III. OXIDATIVE STRESS, THE ANTIOXIDANT NETWORK, AND DIABETES

Why are oxidative stress, antioxidants, and the antioxidant network important in diabetes? Hyperglycemia causes, as a result of stimulation of the sorbitol dehydrogenase pathway, accumulation of NADH and an increase in the lactate/pyruvate ratio. This is accompanied by decreased glycolysis, increased reactive oxygen species formation, increased protein kinase C activity, and decreased Na^+/K^+ ATPase, among other effects, as shown in Figure 3. It is reasoned that the reductive imbalance that occurs in hyperglycemia, and which may also occur in ischemia/hypoxia injury (20–22), might be reversed by

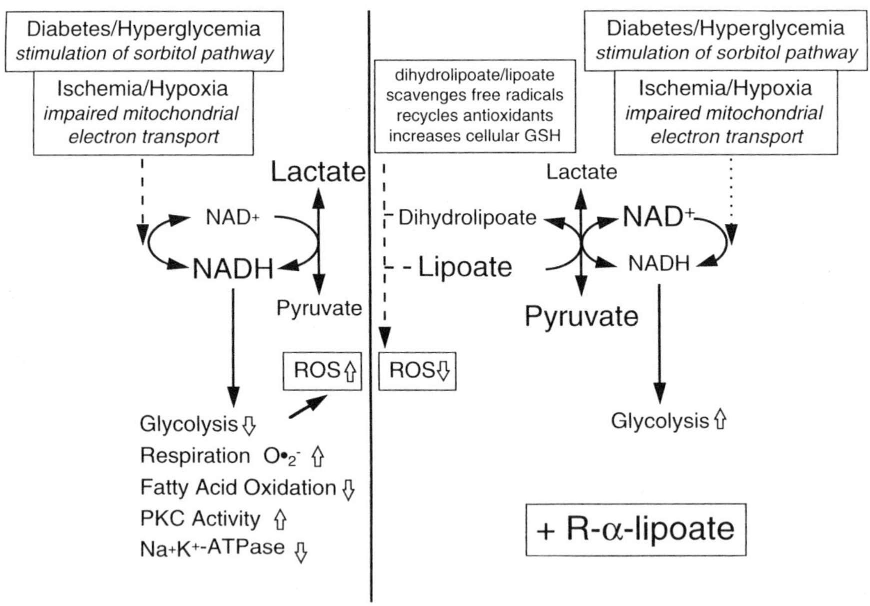

Figure 3 Proposed mechanism of lipoate-mediated reversal of the reductive imbalance in hyperglycemia.

lipoic acid. Roy et al. (19) performed experiments to study if lipoic acid could affect the metabolic situation in hyperglycemia.

If R-lipoic acid is added to cells, it should, as a result of its reduction by mitochondrial dihydrolipoamide dehydrogenase activity, reverse the reductive imbalance in hyperglycemia and perhaps normalize the imbalance of overproduction of NADH and change the NADH/NAD^+ ratio toward normal. Using human T lymphocytes as a model system, we performed experiments to determine if this was the case (19). Indeed, treating these human T cells with R-lipoic acid (but not S-lipoic acid) normalized the redox status (Fig. 4).

Lipoate treatment caused the NADH/NAD^+ ratio to be reversed in hyperglycemia; the ATP/ADP ratio, which had fallen, was increased, and the imbalance of the pyruvate/lactate ratio was also reversed. Furthermore, the uptake of glucose by these cells was stimulated. With lipoic acid treatment, even at 100-μM concentrations, significant increases in the uptake of glucose by these cells were observed (19).

Of course, one may wish to know how relevant these observations from a cellular system are to diabetes. We have proposed two models to link the ideas presented above and the possible therapeutic effects of lipoic acid in diabetes:

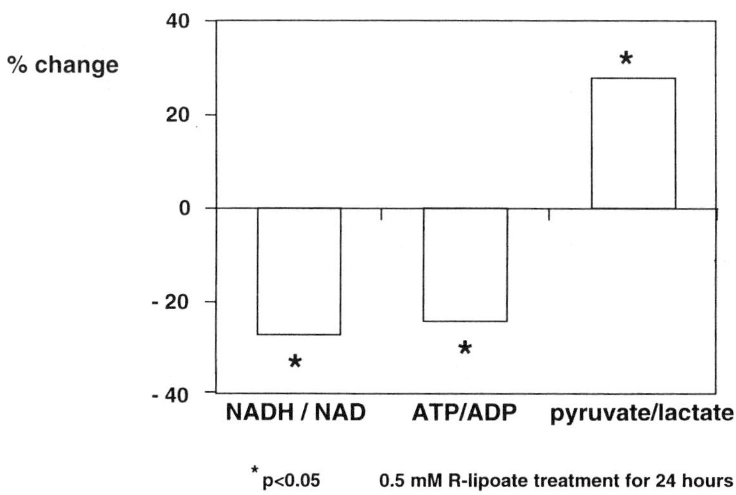

Figure 4 Effect of R-lipoate treatment on redox status and ATP/ADP ratio in Wurzburg T cells.

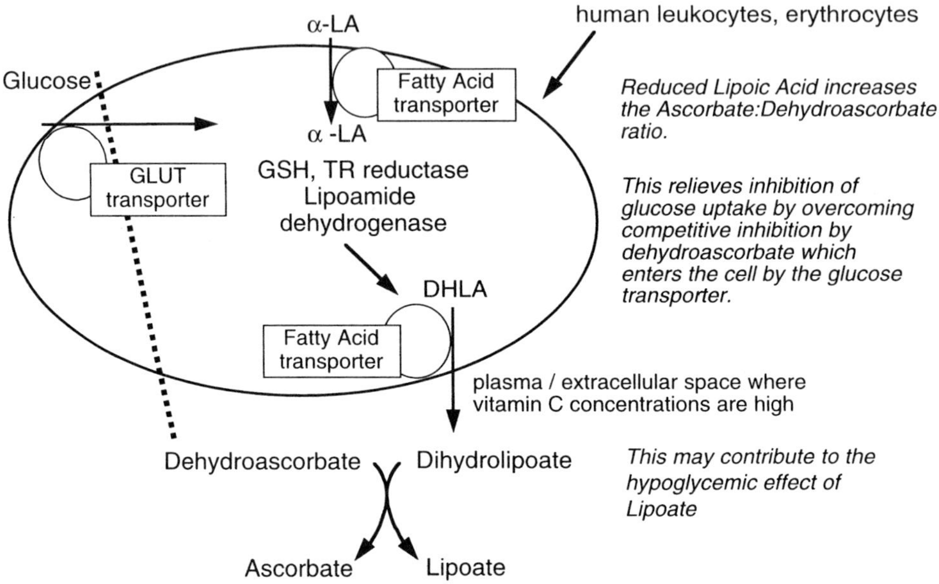

Figure 5 Proposed mechanism whereby α-lipoic acid stimulates glucose uptake.

1. Lipoic acid, when it became reduced, would be exported from the cells as dihydrolipoic acid; this in turn could regenerate vitamin C radicals or dehydroascorbate, because vitamin C in the plasma becomes oxidized after reacting with radicals that are produced by neutrophils or other cells of the immune system. This maintains plasma ascorbate in its reduced form. This is important because dehydroascorbate competes with glucose for uptake by the ''fast track'' glucose (GLUT) transport system present in most cells. Hence, the inhibition of glucose uptake by dehydroascorbate would be overcome (23), as shown schematically in Figure 5.
2. There also may be a direct effect of lipoate on the uptake of glucose by the glucose (GLUT) transport system and thus an effect on the insulin-dependent stimulation of glucose uptake. It was of interest to investigate some of those parameters using the skeletal muscle-derived L6 myotube cell culture system. When L6 myoblasts differentiate into myotubes, they gain the ability to take up glucose. Amira Klip's laboratory has reported extensively on this system

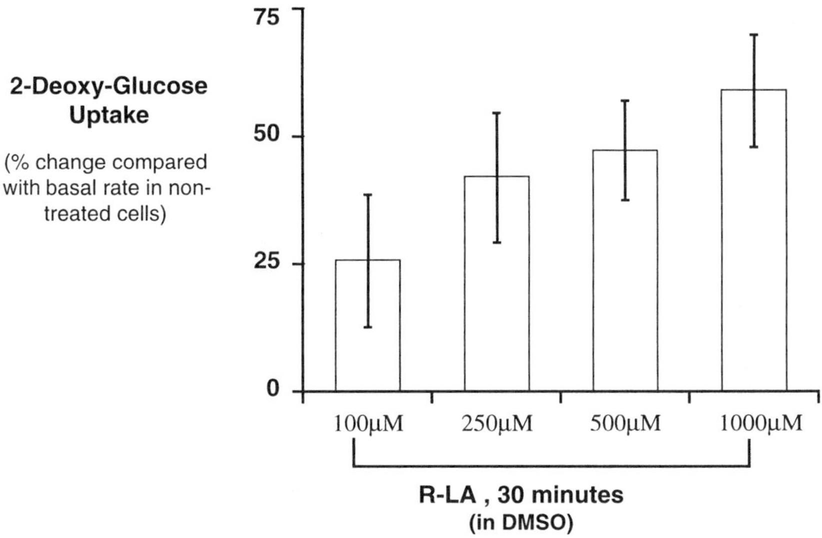

Figure 6 Dose-dependent effect of lipoate on glucose uptake by skeletal muscle L6 myotubes. (From Sen CK, Khanna S, Loukianoff S, Roy S, Packer L, unpublished data.)

(24,25). Using similar conditions, my colleagues Chandan Sen, Savita Khanna, Sonia Loukianoff, and Sashwati Roy have measured the cellular uptake of deoxy-*d*-glucose from a buffer system by following the uptake of the radiolabeled deoxy-glucose. A dose-dependent effect of lipoate on glucose uptake by L6 myotubes showed that under our conditions, even 100 μM lipoic acid was sufficient to markedly stimulate glucose uptake. At higher concentrations, it continuously increased glucose uptake in a dose-dependent manner (Fig. 6).

In further experiments, pretreatment with 250 μM lipoic acid for 30 min was used; after such treatment, a 30–40% stimulation of glucose uptake was usually observed. This is about the same extent of stimulation that has been observed under the same conditions with insulin treatment. If insulin and lipoic acid are added together, an additive, not a synergistic effect, is observed as has been reported previously (24,25).

It was of interest to determine whether the effect of lipoic acid on stimulating glucose uptake was due to the fatty acid molecular structure of lipoic acid. Octanoic acid, an analogue of lipoic acid, had no effect on glucose uptake stimulated by 250 μM lipoic acid, indicating that the fatty acid structure is not the cause of the stimulation.

Lipoic acid is a thiol antioxidant. Hence, it was of interest to know whether other thiol antioxidants or thiol reagents can mimic the effect of lipoic acid, one of which is the ability to increase glutathione levels or maintain levels under oxidative stress conditions (26,27). Therefore, we tested pyrrolidine dithiocarbamate (PDTC) (28), a thiol reagent, which upregulates glutathione levels in cells; diamide, which oxidizes thiol residues; and thioredoxin, which can reduce thiol residues. None of these reagents or treatments had any stimulatory effects on the lipoate-induced uptake of glucose by L6 myotubes. Next we wanted to determine if the intracellular glutathione level, which is the cell's primary preventive antioxidant, was important for glucose uptake. To find out whether modulations in the internal glutathione level was responsible for promoting glucose uptake, we treated the L6 myotubes with the inhibitor of a glutathione synthesis, butamine sulfoxamine (BSO) (29). This reagent inhibits cell glutathione synthesis. After treating cells for 24 h with BSO, glutathione levels in cells fall to very low levels. The effect of lipoic acid in stimulating glucose uptake in the presence of BSO was unchanged. So modulation of the internal glutathione level is not responsible for the stimulation of glucose uptake by lipoic acid. Confirming this, PDTC, the thiol reagent known to upregulate glutathione, also does not prevent lipoic acid from stimulating glucose uptake.

What was regulating the lipoate-dependent glucose uptake? Because calcium is an important factor in cell regulation (30), we investigated the effect of calcium-binding reagents. Two types of calcium chelators were used: EGTA, which is membrane impermeable, and the esterified form of EGTA, which is known to permeate to the inside of cells. Both reagents, when added to the L6 myotubes, inhibited the lipoic acid-stimulated glucose uptake. Further evidence was obtained from the effects of calcium channel blockers like verapamil and nifedipine; both of these reagents inhibited lipoic acid-stimulated glucose uptake. To prove that one of the effects of lipoic acid was stimulating calcium uptake, we directly followed the uptake of radiolabeled ^{45}C by L6 myotubes. After 30 min, 250 μM lipoic acid markedly stimulated (~30%) $^{45}Ca^{2+}$ uptake.

It is known that a ryanodine-sensitive receptor is involved in calcium entry. Indeed, 25 μM ryanodine inhibited the lipoic acid-stimulated uptake of glucose. Moreover, by adding 250 μM 4-chloro-*m*-cresol, it was possible to mimic the effect of lipoic acid. 4-Chloro-*m*-cresol is known to stimulate the ryanodine receptor (31,32). Stimulating the ryanodine gives almost the same effect as the lipoic acid, suggesting that this receptor is involved.

IV. LIPOATE- AND INSULIN-DEPENDENT CELL SIGNALING PATHWAYS

Insulin activates numerous metabolic and mitogenic effects by first binding to its specific transmembrane glycoprotein receptor, which has intrinsic tyrosine kinase activity. Tyrosine phosphorylation of various other substrates, particularly the insulin receptor substrate (IRS) proteins, then induces formation of a network of docking proteins that mediate insulin action of gene expression involved in its anabolic and catabolic effects (33).

From the results of the present study, it would appear that the action of lipoate in stimulating glucose uptake may also be through protein kinase activation, likely mediated by transient increases in cytosolic calcium, which is essential for the Wortmanin-sensitive, PI-3 kinase-dependent, lipoate-stimulated glucose uptake in the L6 myotube system (24,25). After upregulation of glucose transport after mobilizing GLUT transporters from the cytosolic to the plasma membrane domain, lipoate, like insulin, may recruit a broad array of kinases in target cells to activate its numerous metabolic actions.

V. LIPOIC ACID, DIABETIC POLYNEUROPATHY, AND DIABETES

Lipoic acid has been used successfully as a therapeutic agent in the treatment of diabetic polyneuropathy both in animal models and in human clinical trials (34–36). Diabetes is considered as an oxidative stress disease; evidence indicates that both insulin-dependent and noninsulin-dependent diabetes exhibit molecular markers indicative of oxidative stress. Thus, it could be anticipated that one of the most potent metabolic antioxidants known in biological systems, free α-lipoic acid, should be effective in treating diabetic complications. In particular, R-lipoic acid is recognized by the mitochondrial lipoamide dehydrogenase that reduces it to dihydrolipoate, a powerful reductant that is capable of direct scavenging of radicals, regenerating vitamins E and C, increasing the potency of the entire redox antioxidant network, upregulating cellular levels of glutathione, affecting important cell regulatory activities such as nuclear factor-κB transcriptional activation, regulating free cytosolic calcium, and re-

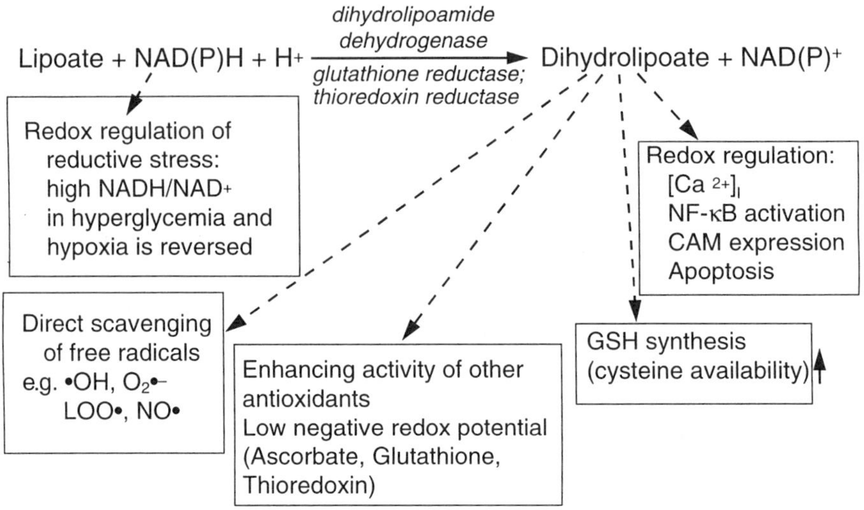

Figure 7 Redox regulation of cell functions by α-lipoate: biochemical and molecular aspects. (From Ref. 37.)

versing the reductive imbalance in diabetes resulting from hyperglycemic conditions. These various effects of lipoic acid have been described previously (37) and are shown schematically in Figure 7. These properties may have therapeutic effects in oxidative stress diseases and aging.

Importantly, lipoic acid has also been demonstrated, at higher concentrations, to have hypoglycemic effects. It exhibits effects on glucose disposal, an important function of skeletal muscle, as demonstrated in animal models by Henriksen et al. (38) and in human clinical studies. It is therefore to be expected that lipoic acid somehow has a profound effect on the mechanism of glucose uptake and disposal and in regulating the glucose-dependent metabolic changes that ensue. The evidence, summarized in this chapter, provides new and interesting findings relevant to these questions.

The many molecular effects of lipoate and dihydrolipoate on receptor-mediated activity, cell signaling, transcriptional activation, and gene expression remain to be elucidated. Important among these considerations for diabetes is how it modulates insulin-dependent cell signaling system pathways.

Because the effects of insulin and lipoate in the L6 myotube experiments are additive, it is reasonable to suggest that the pathways of insulin-stimulated glucose uptake and utilization and that of lipoate-stimulated glucose uptake differ from one another. Lipoate may affect protein kinases and phosphatases, which will modulate phosphorylation systems, and at some point may have common actions with the insulin-signaling pathways. These pathways remain to be elucidated, particularly the mechanism whereby lipoate stimulates calcium-dependent signaling pathways related to glucose transport.

VI. SUMMARY

Oxidative stress, antioxidants, and the antioxidant network can be relevant to diabetes because diabetes appears to involve oxidative stress. One antioxidant that may have particular relevance to diabetes is lipoic acid. Reduced lipoic acid powers the antioxidant network after being taken up by cells. Lipoic acid reverses the reductive imbalance that occurs in hyperglycemia. Plausible mechanisms for this effect are as follows. First, cell reduction of lipoic acid is released into the extracellular space and maintains reduced plasma ascorbate. It can thus relieve the competitive inhibition of glucose uptake by dehydroascorbate. Second, lipoic acid stimulates glucose uptake in skeletal muscle (the main tissue responsible for glucose disposal). In L6 myotubes, used as a model system for glucose disposal, this stimulation apparently occurred by a calcium-dependent mechanism.

REFERENCES

1. Sies H, ed. Oxidative Stress: Oxidants and Antioxidants. London: Academic Press, 1991.
2. Dorland's Illustrated Medical Dictionary. 25th ed. Philadelphia: W.B. Saunders, 1974:111.
3. Halliwell B, Gutteridge JMC. Free Radicals in Biology and Medicine. Oxford: Clarendon Press, 1985.
4. Packer L, Tritschler HJ. Alpha-lipoic acid—the metabolic antioxidant. Free Rad Biol Med 1996; 20:625–626.
5. Packer L, Roy S, Sen CK. Alpha-lipoic acid: metabolic antioxidant and potential redox modulator of transcription. Adv Pharmacol 1996; 38:79–101.
6. Packer L, Witt EH, Tritschler HJ. Alpha-lipoic acid as a biological antioxidant. Free Rad Biol Med 1995; 19:227–250.
7. Peinado J, Sies H, Akerboom TP. Hepatic lipoate uptake. Arch Biochem Biophys 1989; 273:389–395.
8. Haramaki N, Han D, Handelman GJ, Tritschler H-J, Packer L. Cytosolic and mitochondrial systems for NADH and NADPH dependent reduction of α-lipoic acid. Free Rad Biol Med 1997; 22:535–542.

9. Pick U, Haramaki N, Constantinescu A, Handelman GJ, Tritschler H-J, Packer L. Glutathione reductase and lipoamide dehydrogenase have opposite stereospecificities for α-lipoic acid enantiomers. Biochem Biophys Res Commun 1995; 206:724–730.
10. Marcocci L, Flohé L, Packer L. Evidence for a functional relevance of the selenocysteine residue in mammalian thioredoxin reductase. BioFactors 1997; 6:351–358.
11. Handelman GJ, Han D, Tritschler H-J, Packer L. Alpha-lipoic acid reduction by mammalian cells to the dithiol form, and release into the culture medium. Biochem Pharmacol 1994; 47:1725–1730.
12. Packer L. Vitamin E is nature's master antioxidant. Sci Am Sci Med 1994; 1: 54–63.
13. Packer L. Antioxidant defenses in biological systems: an overview. In: Packer L, Traber M, Xin W, eds. Proceedings of the International Symposium on Natural Antioxidants: Molecular Mechanisms and Health Effects. Champaign: AOCS Press, 1996:9–23.
14. Packer L, Witt EH, Tritschler HJ. Antioxidant properties and clinical implications of alpha-lipoic acid and dihydrolipoic acid. In: Cadenas E, Packer L, eds. Handbook of Antioxidants. Vol. 3. New York: Marcel Dekker, 1996:545–591.
15. Kagan VE, Serbinova EA, Forte T, Scita G, Packer L. Recycling of vitamin E in human low density lipoproteins. J Lipid Res 1992; 33:385–397.
16. Kagan VE, Shvedova A, Serbinova E, Khan S, Swanson C, Powell R, Packer L. Dihydrolipoic acid—a universal antioxidant both in the membrane and in the aqueous phase. Reduction of peroxyl, ascorbyl and chromanoxyl radicals. Biochem Pharmacol 1992; 44:1637–1649.
17. Jocelyn PC. The standard redox potential of cysteine-cystine from the thiol-disulphide exchange reaction with gluatathione and lipoic acid. Eur J Biochem 1967; 2:327–331.
18. Podda M, Tritschler, H-J, Ulrich H, and Packer L. Alpha-lipoic acid supplementation prevents symptoms of vitamin E deficiency. Biochem Biophys Res Commun 1994; 204:98–104.
19. Roy S, Sen CK, Tritschler H-J, Packer L. Modulation of cellular reducing equivalent homeostasis by α-lipoic acid: mechanisms and implications for diabetes and ischemic injury. Biochem Pharmacol 1997; 53:393–399.
20. Williamson JR, Chang K, Frangos M, Hasan KS, Ido Y, Kawamura T, Nyengaard JR, van den Enden M, Kilo C, Tilton RG. Hypoglycemic pseudohypoxia and diabetic complications. Diabetes 1993; 42:801–813.
21. Dawson TL, Gotes GJ, Nieminen AL, Herman B, Lemasters JJ. Mitochondria as a source of reactive oxygen species during reactive stress in rat hepatocytes. Am J Physiol 1993; 264:C961–C967.
22. Jaeschke H, Kleinwaechter C, Wendel A. NADH-dependent reductive stress and territin-bound iron in allyl alcohol induced lipid peroxidation in vivo: the protective effect of vitamin E. Chem Biol Interact 1992; 81:57–68.
23. Packer L. The role of anti-oxidative treatment in diabetes mellitus. Diabetologia 1993; 36:1212–1213.

24. Estrada E, Ewart HS, Tsakiridis T, Volchuk A, Ramlal T, Tritschler H, Klip A. Stimulation of glucose uptake by the natural coenzyme α-lipoic acid/thioctic acid: participation of element of the insulin signaling pathway. Diabetes 1996; 45:1798–1804.
25. Han D, Handelman G, Marcocci L, Sen CK, Roy S, Kobuchi H, Tritschler H-J, Flohé L, Packer L. Lipoic acid increases *de novo* synthesis of cellular glutathione by improving cystine utilization. BioFactors 1997; 6:321–338.
26. Panigrahi M, Sadguna Y, Shivakumar BR, Kolluri VR, Roy S, Packer L, Ravindranath V. Alpha-lipoic acid protects against reperfusion injury following cerebral ischemia in rats. Brain Res 1996; 717:184–188.
27. Packer L, Tritschler JJ, Wessel K. Neuroprotection by the metabolic antioxidant α-lipoic acid. Free Rad Biol Med 1997; 22:359–378.
28. Sen CK, Khanna S, Reznick A, Roy S, Packer L. Glutathione regulation of tumor necrosis factor-α-induced NF-κB activation in skeletal muscle-derived L6 cells. Biochem Biophys Res Commun 1997; 237:645–649.
29. Maitra I, Serbinova E, Trischler H, Packer L. Alpha-lipoic acid prevents buthionine sulfoximine-induced cataract formation in newborn rats. Free Rad Biol Med 1995; 18:823–829.
30. Sen CK, Packer L. Antioxidant regulation of gene transcription. FASEB J 1996; 10:709–720.
31. Herrmannfrank A, Richter M, Sarkozi S, Mohr U, Lehmann-Horn F. 4-Chloro-*m*-cresol, a potent and specific activator of the skeletal muscle ryanodine receptor. Biochim Biophys Acta 1996; 1289:31–40.
32. Zorzato F, Scutari E, Tegazzin V, Clementi E, Treves S. Chlorocresol: an activator of ryanodine receptor-mediated Ca^{2+} release. Mol Pharmacol 1993; 44:1192–1201.
33. Avruch J. Insulin signal transduction through protein kinase cascades. Mol Cell Biochem 1998; 182:31–48.
34. Ziegler D, Hanefeid M, Ruhnau KJ, Meißner HP, Lobisch M, Schutte K, Gries FA. Treatment of symptomatic diabetic peripheral neuropathy with the antioxidant α-lipoic acid. Diabetologia 1995; 38:1425–1433.
35. Strodter D, Lehmann E, Lehmann U, Tritschler H-J, Bretzel RG, Rederlin K. The influence of thioctic acid on metabolism and function of diabetic heart. Diabetes Res Clin Pract 1995; 29:19–26.
36. Ziegler D, Gries FA. Alpha-lipoic acid in the treatment of diabetic peripheral and cardiac autonomic neuropathy. Diabetes 1997; 46(suppl 2):62–66.
37. Roy S, Packer L. Redox regulation of cell functions by α-lipoate: biochemical and molecular aspects. BioFactors 1998; 7:263–267.
38. Henriksen E, Jacob S, Streeper R, Fogt D, Hokama J, Tritschler H. Stimulation by alpha-lipoic acid of glucose transport activity in skeletal muscle of lean and obese Zucker rats. Life Sci 1997; 61:805–812.

2

Oxidative Stress in Diabetes: Why Does Hyperglycemia Induce the Formation of Reactive Oxygen Species?

Peter Rösen, Xueliang Du, and Guang-Zhi Sui
Diabetes Research Institute, Heinrich-Heine-University, Düsseldorf, Germany

There is much evidence that the formation of various markers of oxidative stress are increased in diabetes: In the plasma of diabetic patients the concentrations of lipid hydroperoxides, isoprostanes, malonic dialdehyde, and oxidized lipoproteins are elevated (1–6). The intracellular levels of antioxidants such as tocopherol and glutathione are reduced, whereas the enzymatic activity of antioxidative acting enzymes is at least partly increased (7–12). Similarly, there are many reports about the consequences of an imbalance between pro- and antioxidant actions in the cells (''oxidative stress'') and the importance of disturbances in the intracellular antioxidant network for the development of vascular complications in hypertensive or hypercholesterolemic patients. Such a pathophysiological link between oxidative stress and vascular complications is in line with many experimental observations, with large epidemiological studies, and to a lesser extent with recent clinical investigations (13–22). There is increasing evidence that the generation of reactive oxygen intermediates is also of major importance for the development of vascular complications in diabetes (23–29). However, neither the mechanisms that specifically lead to the generation of reactive oxygen intermediates (ROI) in hyperglycemic states nor the cascade of reactions linking the formation of ROI with the pathophysiological event are well understood.

Here we present evidence that the vasculature is an important source for the formation of reactive oxygen species; that high glucose activates an endothelial NADPH-oxidase and thereby causes the release of superoxide anions; that the superoxide anions are able to react with nitric oxide, leading to the formation of peroxynitrite; and that the formation of peroxynitrite is responsible for the impaired endothelium-dependent vasodilatation and variety of cytotoxic effects on the vasculature observed in hyperglycemia, such as activation of the nuclear transcription factor kappa-B (NF-κB) and induction of a apoptosis.

In addition, peroxynitrite has been shown to accelerate the oxidation of low-density lipoproteins and to activate metalloproteinases. Thus, it is intriguing to suggest that the generation of ROI induced by hyperglycemia is one of the major causes for the transformation of endothelium into a proinflammatory and thrombogenic state as observed in diabetes. We assume that this endothelial activation or dysfunction is the basis for the enhancement of atherosclerosis and the development of other vascular complications in diabetes and may contribute to a destabilization of established plaques that has been shown to be one of the most decisive events for induction of myocardial infarction, angina pectoris, and cardiac death (30,31).

I. IS THE VASCULATURE A SOURCE FOR ROIs?

We have already shown (29) that the endothelium-dependent increase in coronary flow is disturbed in isolated perfused hearts of diabetic rats. The dose–response curve for the increased coronary flow in response to 5-hydroxytryptamin is shifted to higher concentrations in diabetes, whereas the maximum coronary flow is not altered under these conditions. This defect could be prevented in vivo by treatment of the animals with high concentrations of vitamin E (1000 U/kg/day) and, more interestingly, under the aspect of mechanisms, by the addition of superoxide dismutase to the perfusion medium (Fig. 1). This observation suggests that the vasculature of diabetic rats releases superoxide anions spontaneously and continuously into the perfusion medium and that the generated superoxide anions are the cause for the disturbed endothelium-dependent flow regulation. We assume that nitric oxide (NO) as the main mediator of endothelium-dependent vasodilatation becomes inactivated by the simultaneously released superoxide anions.

$$2\ \mathrm{ONOO^-} \xleftarrow[2\ \mathrm{NO}]{} 2\ \mathrm{O_2}^- \xrightarrow[2\mathrm{H^+}]{\mathrm{SOD}} \mathrm{H_2O_2} + \mathrm{O_2}$$

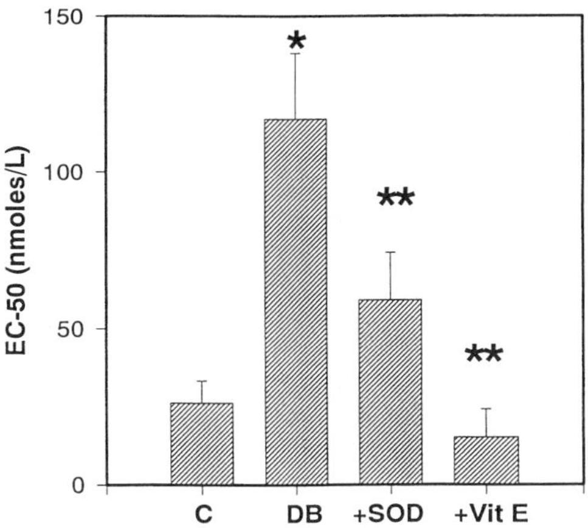

Figure 1 Impairment of the endothelium-dependent increase in coronary flow and its prevention by superoxide dismutase (SOD) and vitamin E. Diabetes was induced in rats by streptozotocin. After a diabetes duration of 16 weeks, the stimulation of coronary flow by 5-hydroxytryptamin was measured in the isolated heart preparation as described (29). The half-maximal concentration ($EC\text{-}_{50}$) was determined and represents a measure for the sensitivity of endothelium to dilate the coronary vasculature. As can be seen, in diabetes (DB), the sensitivity of endothelium is impaired as compared with healthy controls (C), but perfusion with SOD (50 μU/mL) or pretreatment of the animals with α-tocopherol (1000 U/kg body weight) were able to improve or to restore the endothelium-dependent vasodilatation in diabetes. (From Ref. 23.)

Such an interaction between superoxide anions with NO has already been described. In a diffusion controlled reaction, both compounds react with each other under the formation of peroxynitrite (32–34).

Direct evidence for this conclusion is derived from experiments using isolated aortas from streptozotocin diabetic rats. This model enables us to directly measure the formation of superoxide anions by standard techniques as the reduction of cytochrome *c* (35). When aortas from diabetic and control animals were perfused under normoglycemic conditions, vessels from diabetic rats released significantly more superoxide anions than those from controls. In addition, the generation of superoxide anions was stimulated in both types of aortas by hyperglycemic buffers (10–30 mM glucose). The increased generation of superoxide anions could be totally reduced to control values when the endothelium was removed from the intact aortas by mechanical disruption (Rösen 1998, unpublished data). It is interesting to note that an endothelial production of ROI has also been reported for vessels isolated from hypercholesterolemic and hypertonic animals (13–15). Thus, the stimulus for activation of endothelium is different in these various pathophysiological conditions, but the consequences seem to be comparable.

These experimental observations lead to the conclusion that endothelium is an important source of ROI and identify hyperglycemia as a stimulus for the formation of superoxide anions. Furthermore, the disturbed endothelium-dependent vasomotion in diabetes is an immediate pathophysiological consequence of the release of superoxide anions by the vasculature.

II. WHICH MECHANISMS CONTRIBUTE TO THE ENDOTHELIAL FORMATION OF SUPEROXIDE ANIONS IN DIABETES?

To study the mechanisms of ROI generation induced by hyperglycemia in more detail, we used human umbilical vein endothelial cells (HUVECs). To identify the generation of ROI, HUVECs were loaded with dichlorodihydrofluorescin ester (DCF) (36), which is taken up by the cells and then rapidly hydrolyzed. DCF reacts with superoxide anions but presumably also other ROI under the emission of fluorescence light so that the formation of ROI can be determined in a time- and concentration-dependent manner.

Incubation of DCF-loaded cells with increasing concentrations of glucose (5–30 mM) leads to a time- and glucose-dependent increase in fluorescence (Fig. 2). A comparable increase in fluorescence was also observed if the cells were incubated with 3-*O*-methyl-D-glucose (30 mM), a glucose derivative, which is taken by the cells but not metabolized by glycolysis. These data indicate that the formation of ROI is dependent on high glucose in the culture medium but not on the synthesis of diacyl-glycerol and a glucose-dependent activation of protein kinase C. In line with this conclusion, we did not observe an alteration in DCF fluorescence by treating the cells with an inhibitor bisindolylmaleimide (BIM) or activator phorbol 12-myristate 13-acetate (PhA) of protein kinase C (23).

The formation of ROI by endothelial cells incubated with high glucose was completely inhibited by antioxidants (α-tocopherol 10 μg/mL and thioctic acid 0.5 μM) and by diphenyliodonium (DPI, 1 μM), a selective inhibitor of flavoprotein containing NAD(P)H oxidases (37). The inhibitory effect of DPI is consistent with the assumption that NAD(P)H oxidases are the major source of ROI in HUVECs cultivated in hyperglycemic glucose. DPI was also reported to inhibit the NADH-dependent production of superoxide anions in bovine coronary endothelial (38).

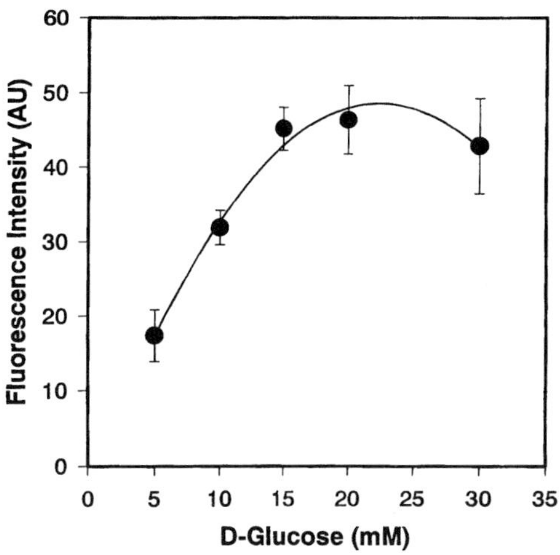

Figure 2 Increase in the formation of ROIs by human endothelial cells in dependence of glucose. HUVECs were preloaded with the DCF (1 μM) and dichlorodihydrofluorescin (10 μM) for 45 min. After washing, the cells were incubated with D-glucose (5–30 mM). For control, cells were incubated with mannitol and L-glucose (25 + 5 mM). After a 15-min incubation (37°C), the fluorescence intensity as a parameter of the ROI generation was analyzed by fluorescent microscopy and quantified.

Although cyclooxygenases and lipoxygenases may also be sources of superoxide anion generation in endothelium (35,38), our data do not link these enzymes to the production of superoxide anions induced by hyperglycemia, because indomethacin and nordihydroguaretic acid did not inhibit the release of superoxide anions. Similar observations have already been reported for porcine endothelial cells (35).

Surprisingly, the DCF fluorescence was also prevented by inhibitors of NO synthase (L-nitroarginine, 100 μM) and a chelator of intracellular calcium 1,2-bis (2-Aminoprenoxy)ethane-N,N,N′,N′-tetraacetic acid (BAPTA). These observations indicate that the mobilization of intracellular calcium and an activation of NO synthesis are necessary steps for the formation of DCF fluorescence by hypoglycemia. In line with this conclusion, the release of nitrite (as parameter of NO synthesis) by HUVECs was stimulated by glucose (Fig. 3).

Thus, under hyperglycemic conditions, both NAD(P)H oxidase and NO synthase become activated, and both steps are a precondition for the formation of DCF fluorescence by HUVECs in hyperglycemia. This synergistic actions of NAD(P)H oxidase and NO synthase suggest that DCF fluorescence does not

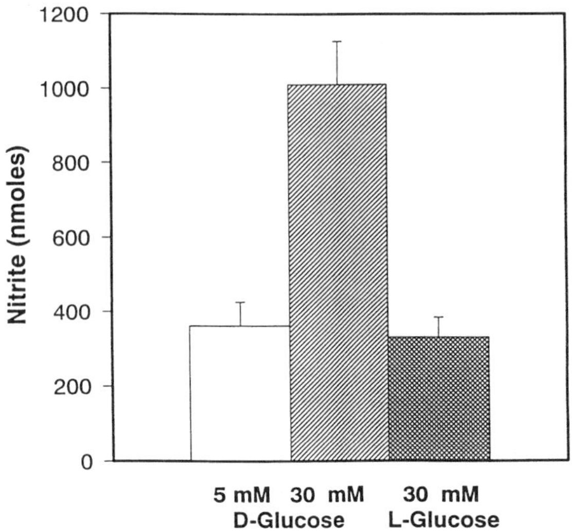

Figure 3 Glucose stimulates the formation of NO by human endothelial cells. HUVECs were incubated with glucose (5–30 mM) for 24 h. The formation of nitrite in the supernatant was analyzed by the Gries reaction. For control, cells were incubated with L-glucose (25 + 5 mM).

specifically reflect the generation of superoxide anions but rather the reaction product of both NO and superoxide anions, presumably peroxynitrite.

Because peroxynitrite has been reported to react with tyrosine residues in proteins, leading to the formation of *o*-nitrotyrosylated proteins, *o*-nitrotyrosylation has been suggested as a long-term parameter for an enhanced formation of peroxynitrite and oxidative stress (32–34). Demonstration of nitrotyrosylated proteins in the vasculature would represent direct evidence of a preceding formation of peroxynitrite and oxidative stress. Endothelial cells were therefore incubated with high glucose and the proteins were extracted, separated by gel electrophoresis, and stained by an antibody specifically recognizing *o*-nitrotyrosylated proteins. As expected, hyperglycemia results in a dose-dependent formation of *o*-nitrotyrosylated proteins (data not shown).

There are at least two other pathways that might contribute to the generation of ROI. Giardino et al. (39) showed that the intracellular formation of advanced glycation endproducts (AGE) products is closely associated with the generation of ROI determined by DCF fluorescence and lipid peroxidation. Inhibition of lipid peroxidation also prevented the formation of AGE products,

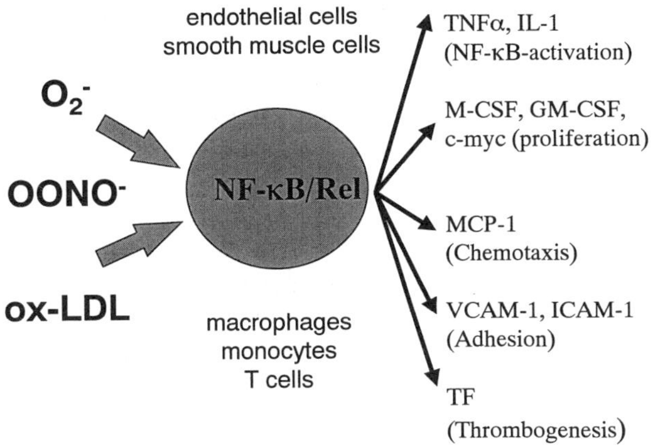

Figure 4 NF-κB-mediated pathways leading to a thrombogenic transformation of the vessel wall.

suggesting that the ROI generation is necessary for the synthesis of AGE products. On the other hand, there is some evidence that endothelium starts to produce ROI as soon as the receptor for AGE products becomes occupied (40,41). Although the exact intracellular signaling is not yet known, there is some evidence that binding of AGE products to its receptors causes an activation of NADPH oxidases (41). This AGE-mediated production of ROI is prevented by antioxidants and inhibitors of NADPH oxidases but not inhibitors of NO synthases, cyclo- and lipoxygenases, or xanthin oxidase.

Thus, the available evidence suggests that activation of NADPH oxidase by glucose or AGE is a key step for the generation of ROI by endothelium. Whether the generated ROI are transformed to peroxynitrite depends on the type of cell and the concomitant reactions. If, as in HUVECs, NO-synthase becomes activated simultaneously, peroxynitrite may be formed and represent the key mediator for the subsequent transformation of endothelium. In the absence of NO synthase activation or insufficient amounts of NO, superoxide anions may directly act as signal mediators and exert the deleterious cytotoxic effects of hyperglycemia and AGE on endothelium and other vascular cells.

There are two open questions. What are the mechanisms for the hyperglycemia-mediated increase in intracellular calcium? The formation of vascular endothelial growth factor (VEGF) as a consequence of the generation of superoxide anions is one interesting mechanism, especially because it has been shown that AGE are able to induce the expression of VEGF (42). Do changes in the cytosolic NADH/NAD ratio contribute to the formation of ROI in addition to the activation of NADPH oxidases? It has been suggested that the NADH/NADPH ratio is elevated in diabetes because more glucose is metabolized by the sorbitol pathway and that the increased NADH/NAD ratio causes the formation of superoxide anions by various mechanisms (43). We do not believe that this mechanism is working in endothelium, because the formation of ROI was not inhibited by inhibitors of the sorbitol dehydrogenase, either in HUVEC or in porcine endothelial cells (35).

In summary, there is good evidence that the vasculature and more specifically the endothelium is one important source for the generation of ROIs. The formation of ROIs is specifically related to the diabetic state because it is stimulated by glucose and advanced glycation end products in a dose-dependent manner. It is interesting to note that similar observations have been reported for the vasculature in hypertension and hypercholesterolemia, suggesting that the initial processes and stimuli might be different, but that the three pathophysiological conditions finally result in an enhanced oxidative stress.

III. WHAT ARE THE CONSEQUENCES OF OXIDANT STRESS IN DIABETES?

There is a lot of evidence that ROI and especially peroxynitrite are involved in activation of transcription factors such as NF-κB. NF-κB is responsible for a variety of reactions contributing to the thrombogenic transformation of endothelium (Fig. 4), (44–48): release of tumor necrosis factor α and interleukin 1β (proinflammatory), release of growth factors (M-CSF [monocyte colony stimulating factor], GM-CSF [granulocyte-monocyte colony stimulating factor], c-*myc*), activation of the monocyte chemoattractant protein MCP-1 (chemotaxis); expression of adhesion proteins (VCAM-1 [vascular cell adhesion molecule-1], ICAM-1 [intercellular adhesion molecule-1]); and expression of tissue factor (thrombogenesis).

We used two different approaches to test whether hyperglycemia causes an activation of NF-κB: the electromobility shift assay (EMSA), measuring the DNA-binding activity of nuclear proteins to an NF-κB-specific oligonucleotide (48), and a histochemical approach using a fluorescence-labeled antibody coupled to the NF-κB-specific oligonucleotide (49). Using both methods we can show that hyperglycemia causes a dose- and time-dependent activation of NF-κB. The maximum of activation by high glucose is achieved after 4 h; after 10–12 h NF-κB is again completely inactivated (Fig. 5). This activation is inhibited by antioxidants (tocopherol 10 μg/mL, thioctic acid 0.5 μM) and

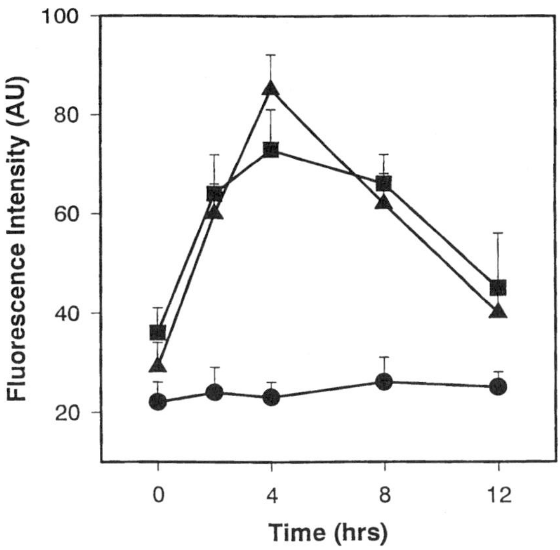

Figure 5 Time dependence of NF-κB activation by hyperglycemia in human endothelial cells. HUVECs were incubated with low glucose (5 mM), high glucose (30 mM), and 3-*O*-methyl-D-glucose (3-OMG, 25 + 5 mM glucose). After a 2-, 4-, 6-, and 12-h incubation (37 °C), the cells were fixed with paraformaldehyde and stained by the specific fluorescein isothiocyanate (FITC)-labeled consensus sequence for NF-κB as described. Osmotic controls (25 mM mannitol + 5 mM glucose) did not show staining above the background. ●, Controls; ■, high glucose; ▲, 3-OMG.

by the NO synthase inhibitor L-nitroarginine (100 μM), whereas the modulation of protein kinase C was without any influence. These data suggest that the short-term activation of NF-κB by hyperglycemia is caused by peroxynitrite. It is an open question whether the recently reported long-term activation of NF-κB by AGE products (48) was caused by a similar mechanism. In any case, hyperglycemia seems to cause an activation of NF-κB by different signaling cascades: High glucose leads to a short-term activation, which might be important for the transformation of immediate and short-term variations in blood glucose into vascular reactions. Such a mechanism would also explain why not only the long-term elevation of blood glucose is cytotoxic for the vessel wall but also the spikes in blood glucose that are often observed even in patients with an overall near normoglycemic metabolic control. Activation of NF-κB by AGE products, on the other hand, would induce a long-term modulation of vascular functions and might be especially of importance for angiogenesis.

In addition to activation of NF-κB, the formation of peroxynitrite may have several other consequences that may contribute to the development of vascular complications in diabetes. First, the induction of apoptosis. We have recently reported (50) that high glucose induces the programmed cell death in HUVECs. This process was inhibited by antioxidants (thioctic acid and tocopherol), but also by inhibitors of NO synthases. The underlying mechanism is not yet fully understood at this time, but there are several lines of evidence that the induction of apoptosis is independent of the activation of NF-κB. The induction of apoptosis can be understood as an indicator of damage of endothelium by high glucose, as an attempt of the vasculature to get rid of damaged endothelial cells. Such a loss of endothelium would be associated with induction of angiogenesis, a process typically observed in the eye and the kidney of many diabetic patients (51,52). On the other hand, loss of endothelium would lead to an exposition of thrombogenic structures (subendothelial matrix) to the bloodstream and thereby cause an increased thrombotic risk.

Another consequence is the oxidation of low-density lipoproteins. It has been reported that peroxynitrite is a strong prooxidant and accelerates the oxidation of low-density lipoproteins (53). Because oxidized low-density lipoproteins are themselves cytotoxic for endothelium, the formation of peroxynitrite would reinforce the oxidant stress by constituting a deleterious vicious cycle. Finally, the activation of metalloproteinases has been reported to become activated by peroxynitrite in vivo and in vitro (54). Such an activation of metalloproteinases at the edge of an atherosclerotic plaque is assumed to cause a destabilization of the plaque, enhance plaque rupture, and finally a thrombotic event that is the most common cause for myocardial infarction, angina pectoris, and cardiac death (30,31).

IV. CONCLUSIONS

Taken together, there is good evidence that short- and long-term hyperglycemia cause an activation of NADPH oxidase and the formation of ROI. The endothelium has been demonstrated as one of the major sources of ROI generation. Experimental data from in vitro and in vivo studies clearly show that these ROIs are able to induce a thrombogenic transformation of the vessel wall and to be the cause for the endothelial dysfunction observed in diabetes but also in hypertension and hypercholesterolemia. Whether these cytotoxic effects are exerted by superoxide anions directly or are mediated by peroxynitrite depends on the local environment and the type of vasculature regarded. Our current knowledge is summarized in the hypothesis shown

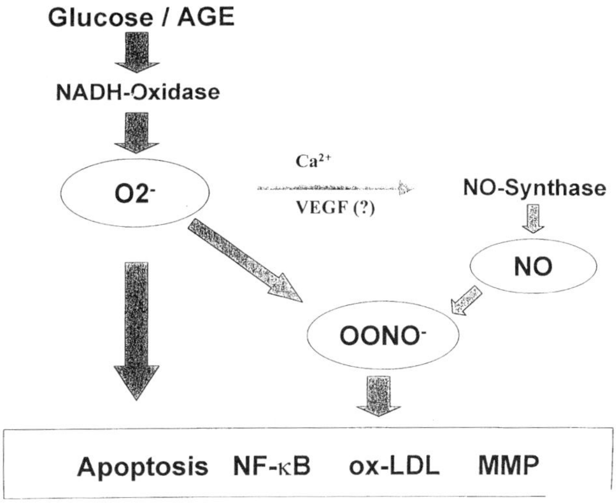

Figure 6 Current hypothesis: formation of ROI by hyperglycemia and the effects of ROI on the vessel wall as cause for the development of vascular complications in diabetes.

in Fig. 6. It is important to recognize that the consequences of these ROI-induced vascular dysfunctions might be different depending on the size of the vasculature affected: In small vessels the oxidative stress induced by hyperglycemia might be one important factor for the stimulation of proliferation of endothelium and the formation of new partially malfunctional vessels and thereby contribute to the development of small vessel disease (retinopathy, nephropathy). In coronary vasculature, the generation of ROI might be more important for the destabilization of atherosclerotic plaques, causing an increased cardiac risk in diabetic patients. The reestablishment of the antioxidative network might therefore be a useful approach to protect the vasculature in diabetes.

ACKNOWLEDGMENTS

Supported by the Ministerium für Frauen, Familie und Gesundheit der Bundesrepublik Deutschland, and the Wissenschaftsministerium des Landes NRW; the Deutsche Forschungsgemeinschaft, Bonn; and the ''Klinische Zellbiologie und Biophysik'' e.V., Düsseldorf.

REFERENCES

1. Nourooz-Zadeh J, Tajaddini-Sarmadi J, McCarthy S, Betteridge DJ, Wolff SP. Elevated levels of authentic plasma hydroperoxides in NIDDM. Diabetes 1995; 44:1054–1058.
2. Nishigaka I, Hagihara M, Tsunekawa H, Maseki M, Yagi K. Lipid peroxide levels of serum lipoprotein fractions of diabetic patients. Biochem Med 1981; 25:373–378.
3. Gopaul NK, Anggard EE, Mallet AI, Betteridge DJ, Wolff SP, Nourooz-Zadeh J. Plasma 8-epi-PGF$_{2\alpha}$ levels are elevated in individuals with NIDDM. FEBS Lett 1995; 368:225–229.
4. Davi G, Mezzetti A, Vitacolonna E, Costantini F, Pennese E, Falco A, Ciabattoni G, Patrono C, Consoli A. In vivo formation of 8-epiprostaglandin F$_{2\alpha}$ in diabetes mellitus. Effects of tight control and vitamin E supplementation. Diabetes 1997; 46(suppl 1):13A.
5. Jain SK, McVie R, Duett J, Herbst JJ. Erythrocyte membrane lipid peroxidation and glycosylated hemoglobin in diabetes. Diabetes 1989; 38:1539–1543.
6. Bellomo G, Maggi E, Polli M, Agosta FG, Bollati P, Finardi G. Autoantibodies against oxidatively modified low density lipoproteins in NIDDM. Diabetes 1991; 44:60–66.
7. Nourooz-Zadeh J, Halliwell B, Tritschler HJ, Betteridge DJ. Decreased lipid standardised plasma α-tocopherol in non-insulin-dependent diabetes mellitus. Diabetes 1997; 6(suppl 2):20–23.
8. Leonhardt W, Hanefeld M, Lattke P, Jarob W. Vitamin E Mangel und Oxidierbarkeit der Low-Density-Lipoproteine bei Typ I und Typ II Diabetes: Einfluβ der Qualilät der Stoffwechselkontrolle. Diabetes 1997; 6(suppl 2):24–28.
9. Simon-Schnass I, Rosak C, Tritschler HJ, Roesen P. Alpha-Tocopherolaufnahme und -zufuhr bei Typ II Diabetikern. Diabetes 1997; 6(suppl 2):16–19.
10. Maxwell SR, Thomason H, Sandler D, Leguen C, Baxter MA, Thorpe GH, Jones AF, Barnett AH. Antioxidant status in patients with uncomplicated insulin-dependent and non-insulin-dependent diabetes mellitus. Eur J Clin Invest 1997; 27:484–490.
11. Kashiwagi A, Asahina T, Ikebuchi M, Tanaka Y, Takagi Y, Nishio Y, Kikkawa R, Shigeta Y. Abnormal glutathione metabolism and increased cytotoxicity caused by H_2O_2 in human umbilical vein endothelial cells cultured in high glucose. Diabetologia 1994; 37:264–269.
12. Bellomo G, Maggi E, Palladini G, Perugini, Seccia M. Oxidation of low density lipoproteins and vitamin E status in non insulin dependent diabetes mellitus (NIDDM). Diabetes 1997; 6(suppl 2): 29–33.
13. Minor RL, Myers PR, Guerra R, Bates JN, Harrison DG. Diet-induced atherosclerosis increases the release of vascular relaxing factor. J Clin Invest 1990; 86:2109–2116.
14. Ohara Y, Peterson TE, Harrison DG. Hypercholesterolemia increases endothelial superoxide anion production. J Clin Invest 1993; 91:2546–2551.

15. Harrison DG. Endothelial function and oxidant stress. Clin Cardiol 1997; 20(suppl 2):II-11–II-17.
16. Riemersma RA, Wood DA, Macintyre CC, Elton RA, Gey KF, Oliver MF. Risk of angina pectoris and plasma concentrations of vitamins A, C and E and carotene. Lancet 1991; 337:1–5.
17. Gey KF, Puska P, Jordan P, Moser UK. Inverse correlation between plasma vitamin E and mortality from ischaemic heart disease in crosscultural epidemiology. Am J Clin Nutr 1991; 53:326S–334S.
18. Stampfer MJ, Hennekens CH, Marrison JE, Colditz GA, Rosner B, Willet WC. Vitamin E consumption and the risk of coronary disease in woman. N Engl J Med 1993; 328:1444–1449.
19. Rimm EB, Stampfer MJ, Ascherio A, Giovannuci E, Colditz GA, Willet WC. Vitamin E consumption and the risk of coronary heart disease in men. N Engl J Med 1993; 328:1450–1456.
20. Stephens NG, Parsons A, Schofield PM, Kelly F, Cheeseman K, Mitchinson M, Brown MI. Randomised controlled trial of vitamin E in patients with coronary disease: Cambridge Heart Antioxidant Study (CHAOS). Lancet 1996; 347:781–786.
21. Hodis HN, Mack WJ, LaBree L, Cashin-Hemphill L, Sevanian A, Johnson R, Azen SP. Serial coronary angiographic evidence that antioxidant vitamin intake reduced progression of coronary artery atherosclerosis. JAMA 1995; 273:1849–1854.
22. DeMaio SJ, King SB, Lembo NJ, Roubin GS, Hearn JA, Bliagavan HN, Sgoutas DS. Vitamin E supplementation, plasma lipids and incidence of restenosis after percutaneous transluminal coronary angioplasty (PTCA). J Am Coll Nutr 1992; 11:68–73.
23. Rösen P, Du XL, Tschöpe D. Role of oxygen derived radicals for vascular dysfunction in the diabetic heart: prevention by α-tocopherol? Mol Cell Biol 1998; 188:103–111.
24. Roesen P, Tchoepe D. Vitamin E and diabetes. Fat Sci Technol 1991; 11:425–431.
25. Lyons TJ. Oxidised low density lipoproteins: a role in the pathogenesis of atherosclerosis in diabetes? Diabetes Med 1991; 8:411–419.
26. Pieper GM, Gross GJ. Oxygen free radicals abolish endothelium dependent relaxation in diabetic rat aorta. Am J Phyiol 1988; 255:H825–H833.
27. Tesfamariam B. Free radicals in diabetic endothelial cell dysfunction. Free Rad Biol Med 1994; 16:383–391.
28. Cohen RA. Dysfunction of vascular endothelium in diabetes mellitus. Circulation 1993; 87(suppl V):V67–V76.
29. Rösen P, Ballhausen Th, Bloch W, Addicks K. Endothelial relaxation is disturbed in the diabetic rat by oxidative stress: the influence of tocopherol as antioxidant. Diabetologia 1995; 38:1157–1168.
30. Falk E, Shah PK, Fuster V. Coronary plaque disruption. Circulation 1995; 92: 657–671.

31. Constantinides P. Plaque hemorrhages, their genesis and therir role in supraplaque thrombosis and atherogenesis. In: Glagov S, Newman WPI, Schaffer SA, eds. Pathobiology of the Human Atherosclerotic Plaque. New York: Springer-Verlag, 1989:392–412.
32. Huie RE, Padmaja S. The reaction of NO with superoxide. Free Rad Res Commun 1993; 18:195–199.
33. Beckman JS, Koppenol WH. Nitric oxide, superoxide, and peroxynitrite: the good, the bad, and the ugly. Am J Physiol 1996; 271:C1424–C1437.
34. Beckman JS, Ye YZ, Anderson PG, Chen J, Accavitti MA, Tarpey MM, White CR. Extensive nitration of protein tyrosines in human atherosclerosis detected by immunohistochemistry. Biol Chem Hoppe-Seyler 1994; 375:81–88.
35. Graier WF, Simecek S, Kukovetz WR, Kostner DM. High D-glucose-induced changes in endothelial Ca^{2+}/EDRF signalling are due to generation of superoxide anions. Diabetes 1996; 45:1386–1396.
36. Possel H, Noack H, Augustin W, Keilhoff G, Wolf G. 2,7-Dihydrodichloro-fluorescein diacetate as a fluorescent marker for peroxinitrite formation. FEBS Lett 1997; 416:175–178.
37. Cross AR, Jones OTG. Enzymatic mechanisms of superoxide production. Biochim Biophys Acta 1991; 1057:291–298.
38. Mohazzab-H KM, Kaminski PM, Wolin MS. NADH oxidoreductase is a major source of superoxide anion in bovine coronary artery endothelium. Am J Physiol 1994; 266:H2568–H2572.
39. Giardino I, Edelstein D, Brownlee M. BCL-2 expression or antioxidants prevent hyperglycemia induced formation of intracellular advanced glycation endproducts in bovine endothelial cells. J Clin Invest 1996; 97:1422–1428.
40. Yan SI, Schmidt AM, Anderson GM, Zhang J, Brett J, Zou YS, Pinsky D, Stern D. Enhanced cellular oxidant stress by the interaction of advanced glycation end products with their receptors/binding proteins. J Biol Chem 1994; 269:9889–9897.
41. Chappey O, Dosquet C, Wautier MP, Wautier JL. Advanced glycation end products, oxidant stress and vascular lesions. Eur J Clin Invest 1997; 27:97–108.
42. Tilton RG, Kawamura T, Chang KC, Ido Y, Bjercke RJ, Stephan CC, Brock TA, Williamson JR. Vascular dysfunction induced by elevated glucose levels in rats is mediated by vascular endothelial growth actor. J Clin Invest 1997; 99: 2192–2202.
43. Williamson JR, Chang K, Frangos M, Hasan KS, Ido Y, Kawamuea T, Nyengaaard JR, van den Enden M, Kilo C, Tilton RG. Hyperglycemic pseudohypoxia and diabetic complications. Diabetes 1993; 42:1497–1505.
44. Brand K, Page S, Rogler G, Bartch A, Brandl R, Knuechel R, Page M, Kaltschmidt C, Baeuerle PA, Neumeier D. Activated transcription factor-kappa B is present in atherosclerosis lesion. J Clin Invest 1996; 97:1715–1722.
45. Lenardo MJ, Baltimore D. NF-κB: a pleiotropic mediator of inducible and tissue-specific gene control. Cell 1989; 58:227–229.

46. Baeuerle PA. The inducible transcription factor NF-κB: regulation by distinct protein subunits. Biochim Biophys Acta 1991; 1972:63–80.
47. Powis G, Gasdaska JR, Baker A. Redox signaling and the control of cell growth and death. In: Sies H, ed. Antioxidants in Disease: Mechanisms and Therapy. New York: Academic Press, 1997:329–359.
48. Bierhaus A, Chevion S, Chevion M, Hofmann M, Quehenberger P, Illmer T, Luther T, Berentshtein E, Tritschler H, Müller M, Wahl P, Ziegler R, Nawroth P. Advanced glycation end product-induced activation of NF-κB is suppressed by α-lipoic acid in cultured endothelial cells. Diabetes 1997; 46:1481–1490.
49. Du XL, Stockklauser-Färber K, Rösen P. Generation of reactive oxygen intermediates, activation of NF-κB, and induction of apoptosis in human endothelial cells by glucose: role of nitric oxide? Free Rad Res Med Biol, in press.
50. Du X, Guang-Zhi Sui, Stockklauser K, Weiβ J, Zink S, Schwippert B, Qi-Xia Wu, Tschöpe D, Rösen P. Induction of apoptosis by high proinsulin and glucose in cultured human umbilical vein endothelial cells is mediated by reactive oxygen species. Diabetologia 1998; 41:249–256.
51. Klein R. Retinopathy and other ocular complications in diabetes. In: Porte D, Sherwin RS, eds. Ellenberg & Rifkin's Diabetes Mellitus. Stamford: Appleton & Lange, 1997:931–970.
52. DeFronzo RA. Diabetic renal disease. In: Porte D, Sherwin RS, eds. Ellenberg & Rifkin's Diabetes Mellitus. Stamford: Appleton & Lange, 1997:971–1008.
53. Hogg N, Darley-Usmar VM, Wilson MT, Moncada S. The oxidation of α-tocopherol in human low density lipoproteins by the simultaneous generation of superoxide amd nitric oxide. FEBS Lett 1993; 326:199–203.
54. Rajagopalan S, Meng XP, Ramasamy S, Harrison DG, Galis ZS. Reactive oxygen species produced by macrophage-derived foam cells regulate the activity of vascular matrix metalloproteinases in vitro. J Clin Invest 1996; 98:2572–2579.

3
Oxidative Stress Markers in Human Disease: Application to Diabetes and to Evaluation of the Effects of Antioxidants

Barry Halliwell
National University of Singapore, Singapore

The biomedical literature contains multiple claims that "free radicals" and other "reactive species" are involved in different human diseases. They have been implicated in over 100 disorders, ranging from rheumatoid arthritis, hemorrhagic shock, and ulcerative colitis to gastrointestinal damage by *Helicobacter pylori* and acquired immunodeficiency syndrome (reviewed in Refs. 1–4). Indeed, their importance in diabetes is widely proposed (5,6). This wide range of disorders implies that free radicals are not something esoteric but that their increased formation accompanies tissue injury in most or all human diseases (1–8), for the reasons summarized in Figure 1. Sometimes they make a significant contribution to the disease pathology; at other times they may not (7,8). Reasons for such differences are summarized in Figure 2. Establishing the real importance of reactive oxygen, nitrogen, and chlorine species (ROS/RNS/RCS) requires specific assays for their formation and the damage that they do in vivo. The lack of such assays in the past has impeded progress in our understanding of the role played by reactive species in normal physiology and in human disease. Thus, as summarized in Table 1, demonstrating that reactive species are important in diabetes (or indeed any other disease) involves much more than a mere demonstration of their formation. Table 2 lists some of the reactive species to be considered.

INJURY

Infection

Radiation

Exogenous toxins

Elevated levels of endogenous toxins, e.g.,glycoxidation

Exercise to excess

Freezing

Trauma

Heat

Ischemia/reperfusion

→

- Phagocyte recruitment and activation (makes $O_2^{\cdot -}$, H_2O_2, $NO^{\cdot}$, HOCl).
- Arachidonic acid release, enzymic peroxide formation (by activation of lipoxygenase, cyclooxygenase enzymes). Decomposition of peroxides to peroxyl/alkoxyl radicals can spread damage to other lipids/proteins.
- Metal ion release from storage sites (Fe^{2+}, Cu), stimulating conversion of H_2O_2 (and perhaps HOCl) to $OH^{\cdot}$ and lipid peroxide breakdown to $RO_2^{\cdot}$/$RO^{\cdot}$.
- Heme protein release (myoglobin, hemoglobin, cytochromes); heme proteins react with peroxides to stimulate free-radical damage and (if peroxide is in excess) to release Fe and haem, which can decompose peroxides to $RO_2^{\cdot}$ and $RO^{\cdot}$.
- Interference with antioxidant defence systems, (e.g. GSH loss from cells).
- Conversion of xanthine dehydrogenase to oxidase in certain tissues, possible release of oxidase from damaged cells to cause systemic damage, increased hypoxanthine levels due to disrupted energy metabolism.
- Mitochondrial damage, increased leakage of electrons to form $O_2^{\cdot -}$, H_2O_2.
- Raised intracellular Ca^{2+}, stimulating calpains, Ca^{2+}-dependent nucleases and Ca^{2+}/calmodulin-dependent nitric oxide synthase, giving more $NO^{\cdot}$ and increased risk of $ONOO^-$ formation.

→ **OXIDATIVE STRESS**

Figure 1 Some reasons why tissue injury causes oxidative stress.

I. OXIDATIVE STRESS IN DISEASE: DOES IT MATTER?

The term *oxidative stress* is widely used in the literature but rarely defined. In essence, it refers to the situation of a *serious imbalance* between production of ROS/RNS/RCS and antioxidant defense. Sies, who introduced the term from the title of the book he edited in 1985, introduced a somewhat vague definition in 1991 in the introduction to the second edition (9) as a disturbance in the pro-oxidant–antioxidant balance in favor of the former, leading to potential damage.

In principle, oxidative stress can result from two mechanisms:

1. Diminished antioxidants, for example, mutations affecting antioxidant defense enzymes (such as CuZnSOD, MnSOD, and glutathione peroxidase) or toxins that deplete such defenses. For example, many xenobiotics are metabolized by conjugation with GSH; high doses can deplete GSH and cause

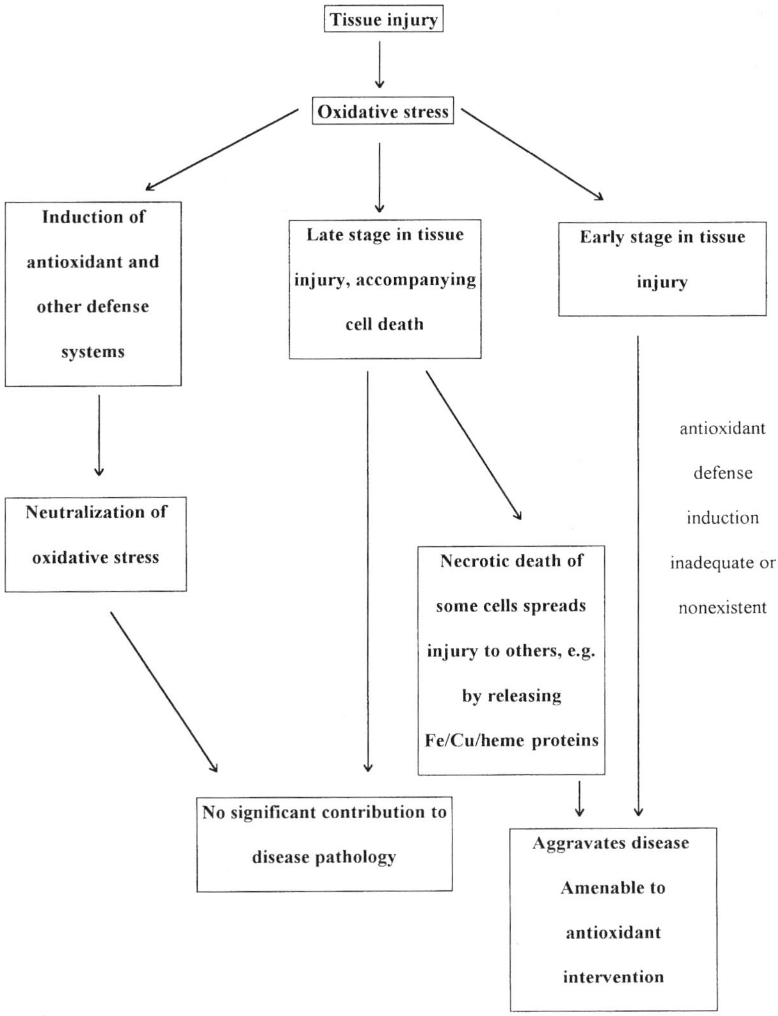

Figure 2 Why reactive species may be important or not important in human disease.

Table 1 Criteria for Implicating Reactive Oxygen/Nitrogen/Chlorine Species or Any Other Agent as a Significant Mechanism of Tissue Injury in Human Disease

1. The agent should always be present at the site of injury.
2. Its time course of formation should be consistent with the time course of tissue injury.
3. Direct application of the agent to the tissue at concentrations within the range found in vivo should reproduce most or all of the damage observed.
4. Removing the agent or inhibiting its formation should diminish the injury to an extent related to the degree of removal of the agent or inhibition of its formation.

oxidative stress even if the xenobiotic is not itself a generator of ROS or RNS. Depletions of dietary antioxidants and other essential dietary constituents can also lead to oxidative stress.

2. Increased production of ROS/RNS/RCS, for example, by exposure to elevated O_2, the presence of toxins that are themselves reactive species (e.g., $NO_2^{\bullet}$) or are metabolized to generate ROS/RNS/RCS, or excessive activation of ''natural'' ROS/RNS/RCS-producing systems (e.g., inappropriate activation of phagocytic cells in chronic inflammatory diseases, such as rheumatoid arthritis and ulcerative colitis).

Mechanism 2 is usually thought to be more relevant to human diseases and is frequently the target of attempted therapeutic intervention but rarely is much attention paid to the antioxidant nutritional status of sick patients (e.g., Ref. 10). For example, calculations show that diabetic patients on fat-restricted diets may sometimes have a suboptimal intake of vitamin E (11). Prolonged oxidative stress can lead to depletion of essential antioxidants. For example, subnormal plasma ascorbate levels are well known in diabetics (12,13). There are conflicting views on whether diabetic patients show depleted plasma vitamin E levels, but data of Nourooz-Zadeh et al. (14) show a clear decrease in lipid standardized α-tocopherol levels in diabetic patients (Table 3), although there is considerable variability between patients, as indicated by the ranges in Table 3. It is possible that variations in dietary intake can account for some of the different results reported in the literature.

In principle, the onset of oxidative stress can result in adaptation, tissue injury, or cell death. *Adaptation*, most often by upregulation of defense systems, may completely protect against damage; protect against damage, but not completely; or ''overprotect,'' for example, the cell is then resistant to higher levels of oxidative stress imposed subsequently. As an example of not completely protecting against damage, if adult rats are gradually acclimatized to

Table 2 Reactive Species

Radicals	Nonradicals
ROS	
Superoxide, $O_2^{\bullet -}$	Hydrogen peroxide, H_2O_2
Hydroxyl, $OH^{\bullet}$	Hypochlorous acid, HOCl
Peroxyl, $RO_2^{\bullet}$	Hypobromous acid, HOBr
Alkoxyl, $RO^{\bullet}$	Ozone, O_3
Hydroperoxyl, $HO_2^{\bullet}$	Singlet oxygen, $^1\Delta g$
RNS	
Nitric oxide (nitrogen monoxide), $NO^{\bullet}$	Nitrous acid, HNO_2
Nitrogen dioxide, $NO_2^{\bullet}$	Nitrosyl cation, NO^+
	Nitroxyl anion, NO^-
	Dinitrogen tetroxide, N_2O_4
	Dinitrogen trioxide, N_2O_3
	Peroxynitrite, $ONOO^-$
	Peroxynitrous acid, ONOOH
	Nitronium (nitryl) cation, NO_2^+ (e.g., as nitryl chloride, NO_2Cl)
	Alkyl peroxynitrites, ROONO
RCS	
Atomic chlorine, $Cl^{\bullet}$	Hypochlorous acid, HOCl
	Chlorine Cl_2
	Nitronium (nitryl) chloride, NO_2Cl

ROS is a collective term that includes both oxygen radicals and certain nonradicals that are oxidizing agents and/or are easily converted into radicals (HOCl, O_3, $ONOO^-$, $^1O_2$, H_2O_2). RNS is also a collective term including nitric oxide and nitrogen dioxide radicals and such nonradicals as HNO_2 and N_2O_4. $ONOO^-$ is often classified as both an RNS and an ROS. ''Reactive'' is not always an appropriate term: H_2O_2, $NO^{\bullet}$, and $O_2^{\bullet -}$ react quickly with few molecules, whereas $OH^{\bullet}$ reacts quickly with almost everything. $RO_2^{\bullet}$, $RO^{\bullet}$, HOCl, $NO_2^{\bullet}$, $ONOO^-$, and O_3 have intermediate reactivities. HOCl and NO_2Cl can also be classified as ''reactive chlorine species,'' HOBr as a ''reactive bromine species.''

elevated O_2, they can tolerate pure O_2 for much longer than control rats, apparently due to increased synthesis of antioxidant defense enzymes and of GSH in the lung. However, the damage is merely slowed, not prevented (15). As an example of overprotection, treatment of *Escherichia coli* with low levels of H_2O_2 increases transcription of genes regulated by the oxyR protein and renders the bacteria resistant to higher H_2O_2 levels (16). However, few examples of this type of ''overadaptation'' have been reported in animals.

Oxidative stress can cause *tissue injury* to all molecular targets: DNA, proteins, and lipids (lipid peroxidation). Often, it is not clear which is the first

Table 3 Parameters of Oxidative Stress in Healthy and Diabetic (NIDDM) Subjects

Variables	Healthy	NIDDM	p
Total cholesterol (mmol/L)	5.0 ± 1.1	6.0 ± 1.3	<0.002
Fasting glucose (mmol/L)	4.9 ± 0.4	12.1 ± 5.1	<0.0005
HbA_1 (%)	—	11.0 ± 2.4	—
ROOH* (μmol/L)	4.1 ± 2.2	9.4 ± 3.3	<0.0005
α-Tocopherol (μmol/L)	23.8 ± 8.3 (10.6–47.0)	19.6 ± 7.5 (8.6–44.3)	<0.05
α-Tocopherol/cholesterol μmol/L/mmol/L	5.1 ± 2.3 (1.9–13.0)	3.3 ± 1.0 (1.5–6.2)	<0.0005
ROOH/α-tocopherol/cholesterol	0.9 ± 0.6 (0.1–2.7)	3.2 ± 1.6 (0.7–8.3)	<0.0005

Values are means ± SD, with ranges in parentheses.
*Measured by FOX assay.
Source: Ref. 14.

point of attack, because injury mechanisms are interrelated in a complex way (1,17). Indeed, depending on the tissue under study and the type of reactive species causing the insult, the primary cellular target of oxidative stress can vary (18). For example, DNA is an important early target of damage when H_2O_2 is added to many mammalian cells; increased DNA damage occurs before detectable lipid peroxidation or oxidative protein damage (19).

Cell death can result from multiple different insults (20). Excessive activation of poly (ADP ribose) polymerase can so deplete intracellular NAD^+/NADH levels that the cell cannot make ATP and dies. This effect has sometimes been called a *suicide response*; because DNA repair is not completely efficient, a cell with extensively damaged DNA may ''commit suicide'' to avoid the risk of becoming an initiated cell. Cells can die from rupture of membrane blebs occurring as a result of uncontrolled increases in intracellular ''free'' Ca^{2+} concentrations (20).

Cell death can be described by essentially two mechanisms, necrosis and apoptosis; both can result from oxidative stress (20). It is increasingly realized, however, that cell death can sometimes have features of both processes. In essence, during necrotic cell death, the cell swells and ruptures, releasing its contents into the surrounding area and affecting adjacent cells. Contents can include antioxidants such as catalase or GSH and pro-oxidants such as copper and iron ions (Fig. 1). Hence, even if a cell dies by mechanisms not involving oxidative stress, necrotic cell death can impose oxidative stress on the surrounding tissues (Figs. 1 and 2). In apoptosis, the cell's own intrinsic ''suicide mechanism'' is activated; apoptosing cells do not release their contents and so apoptosis does not, in general, cause disruption to surrounding cells. Apoptotic cell death may be accelerated by oxidative stress, and added antioxidants often delay or prevent apoptosis induced by a range of insults (20–22). The caspases essential to apoptosis have active site cysteine residues, and so they can be inhibited by ROS/RNS/RCS at high levels (23,24). Hence, oxidative stress can induce apoptosis, but high levels of such stress can halt the apoptotic process and cause cells to die by necrosis (23).

II. NEED FOR "BIOMARKERS"

To assess the importance of oxidative damage in human disease, accurate methods to measure it are essential. Before clinical trials of putative ''antioxidant agents'' take place, it is important to establish whether or not the planned treatment really can decrease oxidative damage in vivo. In principle, one can measure markers of oxidative damage in humans and examine how they are affected by intake of putative therapeutic antioxidants. The optimal dosage could then be determined. The same approach can be used to show not only that an antioxidant drug really is acting as an antioxidant in vivo but also to study nutritional antioxidants (25). It is important to assess all major molecular targets of damage by ROS/RNS/RCS (DNA, proteins, lipids) because an antioxidant that protects one target may fail to protect (or even exacerbate injury to) another (25). Hence, measurements of oxidative damage must accompany clinical tests of the effects of antioxidants (Fig. 3) to show that they actually did or did not affect the ROS/RNS/RCS.

III. WHAT BIOMARKERS ARE AVAILABLE?

A. DNA

Reactive species-mediated DNA damage can lead to cell death and, even worse, might produce initiated cells and thus facilitate cancer development (26–28). The chemistry of DNA damage by several reactive species has been well characterized in vitro (29–38), although further studies are needed with

SPECIFIC MARKERS
show that oxidative damage has occurred

LIPID
peroxides
oxysterols
chlorinated/nitrated lipids
LOOH
MDA-HPLC
other aldehydes
isoprostanes

DNA
oxidized bases in cells and urine
nitrated/deaminated bases in cells and urine
aldehyde-base adducts in cells and urine

PROTEIN
-SH oxidation
carbonyls
aldehyde adducts
oxidized tyr, trp, his, met, lys, leu, ileu, val
nitrated/chlorinated tyrosine, trp
protein peroxides/hydroxides

ANTIOXIDANT DEPLETION
Does not prove oxidative damage, only that the defence system is working

Total AOX potential (multiple methods, e.g. TRAP, FRAP, $ABTS^{\cdot+}$, ORAC)
Depletion of specific AOX,
Measurement of AOX-derived species (e.g. ascorbate radical, urate oxidation products)

INDUCTION OF AOX ENZYMES
Does not prove oxidative damage, only that the defence system is working

ROS/RNS/RCS TRAPPING
ROS/RNS/RCS formation does not imply their importance. If they are important and the traps are efficient, the traps should be protective. For example, L-phe, used as a trap for $OH^{\cdot}$, protected against myocardial stunning at the same time as it detected $OH^{\cdot}$ [25].

PBN/other spin traps
Aromatic probes (e.g. salicylate, phenylalanine)
other detectors.

Figure 3 Some biomarkers of oxidative stress used to study human disease. (Based on Ref. 25.)

$RO_2^{\bullet}$, $RO^{\bullet}$, and O_3. Nitric oxide ($NO^{\bullet}$), probably via products derived from it ($NO_2^{\bullet}$, HNO_2, $ONOO^-$, N_2O_3, etc.) can cause nitrosation and deamination of amino groups on DNA bases (34,39,40).

Whereas $O_2^{\bullet-}$ and H_2O_2 appear not to react with DNA bases, $OH^{\bullet}$ generates a multiplicity of products from all four DNA bases (31). By contrast, $^1O_2$ appears selective for attack upon guanine (32,33). The most common base lesion, and the one most often measured as an index of oxidative DNA damage, is the nucleoside 8-hydroxy-2′-deoxyguanosine (8OHdG) (38). Measurement of 8OHdG alone can give misleading results under certain circumstances (reviewed in Ref. 40), although it is still widely used. In principle, there are two types of measurement of oxidative DNA damage. *Steady-state damage* can be measured when DNA is isolated from human cells and tissues and analyzed for base damage products; it presumably reflects the balance between damage and DNA repair. Hence, a rise in steady-state oxidative DNA damage could be due to increased damage and/or decreased repair. It is worth mentioning that the measurement of baseline levels of oxidatively modified DNA bases does not provide information as to whether this damage is in active genes or quiescent DNA.

However, it is important also to have an index of total DNA damage in the human body (i.e., the ''input'' side of the steady-state equation). The most common approach has been to assess the ''output'' side (i.e., trying to estimate the rate of repair of oxidized DNA). This is usually achieved by measuring urinary excretion of DNA base damage products. Several DNA base damage products are excreted in human urine, including 8OHdG, 8-hydroxyguanine, 8-hydroxyadenine, and 7-methyl-8-hydroxy-guanine (39,41,42), but the one most exploited is 8OHdG, usually measured by a method involving high-performance liquid chromatography (HPLC) with electrochemical detection (38). For example, in one study of 169 humans, the average 8OHdG excretion was 200–300 pmol/kg per 24 h, corresponding to 140–200 oxidative modifications of guanine per cell per day (42,43). Furthermore, smokers excrete 50% more 8OHdG than nonsmokers on average, suggestive of a mean 50% increased rate of oxidative DNA damage from smoking (42). Gas chromatography-mass spectroscopy (GC-MS) has also been used to measure 8OHdG in urine, and the limit of detection was 1.8 pmol, corresponding to a level of 8OHdG in urine of 35 nM (44).

The validity of these urinary measurements of oxidative DNA damage must be considered. The level of 8OHdG in urine is presumably unaffected by the diet because nucleosides are thought not to be absorbed from the gut. However, this question, and the question as to whether any 8OHdG is metabolized to other products in humans, has not been rigorously addressed in the literature. In addition, it is possible that some or all of the 8OHdG excreted in urine may arise not from DNA but from dGTP in the DNA precursor pool of nucleotides. An enzyme has been described that hydrolyzes dGTP containing oxidized guanine, presumably to prevent its incorporation into DNA (45).

1. Relevance to Diabetes

Both steady-state levels of 8OHdG in blood monocytes (46) and urinary excretion of 8OHdG (47) have been reported as elevated in diabetic patients. Gas chromatography/mass spectrometry has recently shown elevated levels of a wide range of base oxidation products in DNA from white blood cells of diabetic patients. The pattern of base damage was diagnostic of increased $OH^{\bullet}$ formation in vivo (48).

B. Lipid Peroxidation

Lipid peroxidation is important in vivo for several reasons, in particular because it contributes to the development of atherosclerosis (49–51), a process known to be accelerated in diabetic patients (6). Lipid peroxides and other end products of the peroxidation process may be toxic to vascular endothelium in diabetics (6,52). Many assays are available to measure lipid peroxidation, but the simpler ones, such as the TBA test and diene conjugation, are notoriously unreliable when applied to human tissues and body fluids (reviewed in Ref. 53), although the TBA test can be improved by linking it to HPLC and adding antioxidants with the TBA reagents to prevent peroxidation during the assay procedure (54). Levels of lipid peroxides in human plasma, as measured by reliable analytical methods (54–59), seem to be low, usually $<0.1\ \mu M$. Human body fluids also contain low levels of F_2-isoprostanes, compounds isomeric to prostaglandins that are thought to arise by free radical oxidation of phospholipids containing arachidonic acid (60). It has been suggested that one of the F_2-isoprostanes, 8-epiPGF$_2\alpha$, can be generated by cyclooxygenase in human platelets (61), although this does not appear to be a significant contributor to total body production of 8-epiPGF$_2\alpha$ (62). Isoprostanes appear to exist in human plasma largely esterified to phospholipids rather than "free," and sensitive assays to measure them have been described (60–65). Families of F_3- and F_4-isoprostanes, derived from eicosapentaenoic and docosahexaenoic acids, respectively, have recently been described (66).

1. Relevance to Diabetes

There seems to be general agreement that lipid peroxidation is elevated in diabetes, although its relationship to disease progression is uncertain. Some investigators have reported an association between plasma or serum TBA-reactive substances (TBARS) or diene conjugates and diabetic complications, whereas others have not (67–70). However, TBARS and diene conjugation assays should be interpreted with caution (53). MacRury et al. (70) compared different methods (conjugated dienes, TBARS, and chemiluminescence) of assessing free radical activities in diabetic subjects. In each case, diabetes was associated with elevated levels of different indirect measurements of lipid peroxidation. However, they did not find a relationship between diabetic complications and plasma measures of oxidative stress. More convincingly, elevated levels of plasma 8-epi $PGF_2\alpha$ have been reported in diabetics, although its association with disease progression was not discussed (71). Another study, using the ferrous oxidation with xylenol orange (FOX) assay to measure lipid peroxides, found higher lipid-standardized peroxides in plasma from diabetic patients (Table 3). This elevated level was not influenced by sex, age, smoking habit, or diabetic complications and was taken to suggest that the elevated levels of plasma hydroperoxide in patients are associated with the diabetes itself rather than consequent tissue injury (e.g., nephropathy, neuropathy). The reliability of the FOX assay as a measure of lipid peroxides in human plasma remains to be established, however. As Table 3 indicates, ''basal'' peroxide levels in plasma from healthy subjects seem higher than the 0.1 μM or less measured by more chemically robust assays (see above).

2. *Measuring ''Total'' Lipid Peroxidation in the Human Body*

Peroxide levels in body fluids or tissues represent a balance between peroxide formation and peroxide metabolism or decomposition (i.e., they are essentially a ''steady-state'' measurement). Can some measure of total body lipid peroxidation be obtained?

This has most often been attempted by measuring hydrocarbon gases (ethane, pentane) in exhaled air (72) and urinary excretion of MDA (more properly called TBA-reactive material) (73). The latter assay is probably confounded by diet: Most lipid-related TBARS appearing in urine seems to arise from lipid peroxides or aldehydes in ingested food, which are presumably largely generated during cooking (74,75). For example, Brown et al. (75) showed that a diet rich in cooked meat promoted urinary TBARS excretion, to an extent depending on the temperature at which the meat was cooked. Hence, urinary TBARS is not a suitable assay to assess whole body lipid peroxidation, although it could theoretically be used to look at effects of antioxidant supplementation of people on a controlled diet (74). In any case, HPLC must be used to separate the real $(TBA)_2MDA$ adduct; much TBARS in urine is not even lipid derived (76) or arises from aldehydes other than MDA (77).

Breath excretion of ethane and pentane, minor end products of lipid peroxidation, is difficult [but not impossible (78)] to measure in humans because of the problem of contamination of the atmosphere by these gases, leading to their partitioning into body fat stores (79). Particular problems with pentane include the fact that it is metabolized by cytochromes P450 (78,80) and that GC columns frequently used to separate ''pentane'' for measurement can fail to separate it from isoprene, a hydrocarbon also excreted in exhaled air (79,81,82). Indeed, the levels of excreted real pentane seem close to zero in most humans (79,81,82). Perhaps further evaluation of the technique of hydrocarbon gas exhalation should focus on ethane (72), but in general the technique would seem difficult to use reliably in human studies except where subjects are confined to controlled environments, breathing air of minimal hydrocarbon content. The possible effect of dietary changes on hydrocarbon gas production by gut flora is another potential confounding factor.

Isoprostanes and their metabolites can be measured in human urine (60,62,64), and this may prove to be a valuable assay of whole body lipid peroxidation if a confounding effect of diet can be ruled out.

C. Protein Damage

Damage to proteins may be important in vivo both in its own right [affecting the function of receptors, enzymes, transport proteins, etc., and perhaps generating new antigens that provoke immune responses (83)] and also because it can contribute to secondary damage to other biomolecules (e.g., by inactivation of antioxidant defense enzymes or repair enzymes). Attack of various RNS ($ONOO^-$, $NO_2^{\bullet}$, NO_2Cl, and possibly some other species) upon tyrosine (both free and within proteins) leads to production of 3-nitrotyrosine, which can be measured immunologically or by HPLC or GC-MS techniques (reviewed in Refs. 84 and 85). RCS can produce chlorinated products (e.g., 3-chlorotyrosine), and these have been detected in human atherosclerotic lesions (50).

The chemical reactions resulting from attack of ROS/RNS/RCS on proteins are complex. Free radical attack can generate protein peroxides, which may decompose to generate free radicals (reviewed in Ref. 86). Several assays to measure damage to specific amino acid residues in proteins by ROS/RNS/RCS have been developed. They include assays of L-DOPA (produced by tyrosine hydroxylation), valine hydroxides (produced from valine hydroperoxides), tryptophan hydroxylation and ring-opening products, 8-oxohistidine, dityrosine, and *ortho*- and *meta*-tyrosines, products of attack of $OH^{\bullet}$ upon phenylalanine (86). The levels of any one (or, preferably, of more than one) of these products in proteins could in principle be used to assess the balance between oxidative protein damage and the removal of damaged proteins. The only products exploited to date have been the hydroxylated phenylalanines. For example, levels of *ortho*- tyrosine and dityrosine in human lens proteins have been reported in relation to age (87). These products were also measured in hair from "Alpine Man," *Homo tirolensis* (88).

1. Carbonyl Assay

More use has been made of the carbonyl assay, a general assay of oxidative protein damage (89), to assess steady-state levels of such damage in human tissues and body fluids. The carbonyl assay is based on the ability of several ROS to attack amino acid residues in proteins (particularly histidine, arginine, lysine, and proline) to produce carbonyl functions that can be measured after reaction with 2,4-dinitrophenylhydrazine (89,90). The carbonyl assay has become widely used, and many laboratories have developed individual protocols for it. Sometimes the assay procedures used in a particular laboratory are not specified precisely in published papers and often differ from those used originally by the group of Stadtman et al. This point is important because there is a considerable variation in the "baseline" levels of protein carbonyls in certain human tissues, depending on how the assay is performed (reviewed in Ref. 91). By contrast, most groups seem to obtain broadly comparable values for protein carbonyls in human plasma, of <1 nmol/mg protein, so plasma protein carbonyls should be a useful assay of oxidative protein damage. However, protein glycation and covalent binding of certain aldehyde end products of lipid peroxidation to proteins can also generate carbonyls (89).

2. Relevance to Diabetes

Glycoxidation seems to play an important role in the vascular endothelial dysfunction detected in diabetic patients (92,93) and perhaps in the nephropathy (94). Elevated glucose may cause increased generation of $O_2^{\bullet -}$ by endothelium, antagonizing the action of $NO^{\bullet}$ and perhaps forming peroxynitrite, $ONOO^{-}$ (92,93). All these effects should be amenable to treatment by appropriate antioxidants (92).

IV. CONCLUSION

Despite the arguments that can be raised about the validity of some individual biomarkers, the sum of evidence from biomarkers reporting oxidative damage shows that such damage is increased in diabetes, affecting DNA, lipids, and proteins (glycoxidation), supporting the concept of increased oxidative stress in diabetes. Indeed, the newly introduced drug troglitazone may exert some of its protective effects by its antioxidant capacity (95). Further work is required using modern biomarkers to evaluate the extent to which agents beneficial in the treatment of diabetes, including lipoic acid (see other chapters in this volume), act by suppressing oxidative stress. Another exciting area is the prevention of the teratogenic effects of hyperglycemia: Studies in rats have shown that vitamin E (96) and overexpression of CuZnSOD (97) can be beneficial.

REFERENCES

1. Halliwell B, Gutteridge JMC. Free Radicals in Biology and Medicine. 3rd ed. Oxford, England: Clarendon Press, 1999.
2. Halliwell B, Cross CE. Reactive oxygen species, antioxidants and acquired immunodeficiency syndrome. Arch Intern Med 1991; 157:29–31.
3. Parks DA. Oxygen radicals: mediators of gastrointestinal pathophysiology. Gut 1989; 30:293–298.
4. Southorn PA. Free radicals in medicine. II. Involvement in human disease. Mayo Clin Proc 1988; 63:390–408.
5. Jones AF, Winkles JW, Jennings PE, et al. Serum antioxidant activity in diabetes mellitus. Diabetes Res 1988; 7:89–92.
6. Tesfamariam B. Free radicals in diabetic endothelial cell dysfunction. Free Rad Biol Med 1994; 16:383–391.
7. Halliwell B, Gutteridge JMC. Lipid peroxidation, oxygen radicals, cell damage and antioxidant therapy. Lancet 1984; 1:1396–1398.
8. Halliwell B, Cross CE, Gutteridge JMC. Free radicals, antioxidants and human disease: where are we now? J Lab Clin Med 1992; 119:598–620.
9. Sies H. ed. Oxidative Stress: Oxidants and Antioxidants. New York: Academic Press, 1991.
10. Scorah CJ, Downing C, Piripitsi A, Gallivan L, Al-Hazaa AH, Sanderson MJ, Bodenham A. Total vitamin C, ascorbic acid, and dehydroascorbic acid concentrations in plasma of critically ill patients. Am J Clin Nutr 1996; 63:760–765.
11. Rosak C, Simon-Schnass I, Rösen P, Tritscher HJ, Halliwell B. Possible dietary induced α-tocopherol deficiency in type II diabetic patients. In preparation.
12. Sinclair AJ, Lunec J. Free radicals, oxidative stress and diabetes mellitus. In: Winyard P, Blake DR, eds. Immunopharmacology of Free Radical Species. London: Academic Press, 1995:183–198.
13. Maxwell SRJ, Thomason H, Sandler D, Leguen C, Baxter MA, Thorpe GHG, Jones AF, Barnett AH. Antioxidant status in patients with uncomplicated insulin-

dependent and non-insulin-dependent diabetes mellitus. Eur J Clin Invest 1997; 27:484–490.

14. Nourooz-Zadeh J, Rahimi A, Tajaddini-Sarmadi J, Tritschler H, Rosen P, Halliwell B, Betteridge DJ. Relationship between plasma measures of oxidative stress and metabolic control in NIDDM. Diabetologia 1997; 40:647–653.
15. Kinnula VL, Crapo JD, Raivio KO. Generation and disposal of reactive oxygen metabolites in the lung. Lab Invest 1995; 73:3–19.
16. Kullik I, Stevens J, Teledano MB, Storz G. Mutational analysis of the redox-sensitive transcriptional regulator oxyR: regions important for DNA binding and multimerization. J Bacteriol 1995; 177:1285–1291.
17. Hyslop PA, Hinshaw DB, Halsey WA Jr, et al. Mechanisms of oxidant-mediated cell injury. The glycolytic and mitochondrial pathways of ADP phosphorylation are major intracellular targets inactivated by hydrogen peroxide. J Biol Chem 1988; 263:1665–1675.
18. Halliwell B. Antioxidant characterization: methodology and mechanisms. Biochem Pharmacol 1995; 49:1341–1348.
19. Spencer JPE, Jenner A, Chimel K, Aruoma OI, Cross CE, Wu R, Halliwell B. DNA strand breakage and base modification induced by hydrogen peroxide treatment of human respiratory tract epithelial cells. FEBS Lett 1995; 374:233–236.
20. Nicotera P, Orrenius S. Molecular mechanisms of toxic cell death: an overview. Methods Toxicol 1994; 1B:23–28.
21. Kohno T, Yamada Y, Hata T, Mori H, Yamamura M, Tomonaga M, Urata Y, Goto S, Kondo T. Relation of oxidative stress and glutathione synthesis to 095 (Fas/APO-1) mediated apoptosis of adult T cell leukemia cells. J Immunol 1996; 156:4722–4728.
22. Johnson TM, Yu ZX, Ferrans VJ, Lowenstein RA, Finkel T. Reactive oxygen species are downstream mediators of p53-dependent apoptosis. Proc Natl Acad Sci USA 1996; 93:11848–11852.
23. Hampton MB, Orrenius S. Dual regulation of caspase activity by hydrogen peroxide: implications for apotosis. FEBS Lett 1997; 414:552–556.
24. Mohr S, Zech B, Lapetina EG, Brune B. Inhibition of caspase-3 by S-nitrosation and oxidation caused by nitric oxide. Biochem Biophys Res Commun 1997; 238: 387–391.
25. Halliwell B. Oxidative stress, nutrition and health. Experimental strategies for optimization of nutritional antioxidant intake in humans. Free Rad Res 1996; 25:57–74.
26. Wiseman H, Halliwell B. Carcinogenic antioxidants: diethylstilboestrol, hexoestrol and 17α-ethynyl-oestradiol. FEBS Lett 1993; 322:159–163.
27. Totter JR. Spontaneous cancer and its possible relationship to oxygen metabolism. Proc Natl Acad Sci USA 1980; 77:1763–1767.
28. Ames BN, Shigenaga MK, Hagen TM. Oxidants, antioxidants and the degenerative diseases of aging. Proc Natl Acad Sci USA 1993; 90:7915–7922.
29. von Sonntag C. The Chemical Basis of Radiation Biology. London: Taylor and Francis, 1987.

30. Steenken S. Purine bases, nucleosides and nucleotides: aqueous solution redox chemistry and transformation reactions of their radical cations and e^- and $OH^\bullet$ adducts. Chem Rev 1989; 89:503–520.
31. Dizdaroglu M. Chemistry of free radical damage to DNA and nucleoproteins. In: Halliwell B, Aruoma OI, eds. DNA and Free Radicals. Chichester: Ellis Horwood UK, 1993:19–39.
32. Epe B. DNA damage induced by photosensitization. In: Halliwell B, Aruoma OI, eds. DNA and Free Radicals. Chichester: Ellis Horwood UK, 1993:41–65.
33. Cadet J, Ravanat JL, Buchko GW, et al. Singlet oxygen DNA damage: chromatographic and mass spectrometric analysis of damage products. Methods Enzymol 1994; 234:79–88.
34. Spencer JPE, Wong J, Jenner A, Aruoma OI, Cross CE, Halliwell B. Base modification and strand breakage in isolated calf thymus DNA and in DNA from human skin epidermal keratinocytes exposed to peroxynitrite or 3-morpholinosydnonimine. Chem Res Tox 1996; 9:1152–1158.
35. Whiteman M, Jenner A, Halliwell B. Hypochlorous acid-induced base modification in isolated calf thymus DNA. Chem Res Tox 1997; 10:1240–1246.
36. de Rojas-Walker T, Tamir S, Ji H, Wishnock JS, Tannenbaum SR. Nitric oxide induces oxidative damage in addition to deamination in macrophage DNA. Chem Res Toxicol 1995; 8:473–477.
37. Yermilov V, Rubio J, Oshima H. Formation of 8-nitroguanine in DNA treated with peroxynitrite in vitro and its rapid removal by depurination. FEBS Lett 1995; 376:207–210.
38. Floyd RA, Watson JJ, Wong PK, et al. Hydroxy-free radical adduct of deoxyguanosine: sensitive detection and mechanisms of formation. Free Rad Res Commun 1986; 1:163–172.
39. Stillwell WG, Xu HX, Adkins JA, et al. Analysis of methylated and oxidized purines in urine by capillary gas chromatography-mass spectrometry. Chem Res Toxicol 1989; 2:94–99.
40. Halliwell B. Oxygen and nitrogen are pro-carcinogens. Damage to DNA by reactive oxygen, chlorine and nitrogen species: measurement, mechanism and the effects of nutrition. Mutat Res 1999; 443:37–52.
41. Ames BN. Endogenous oxidative DNA damage, aging, and cancer. Free Rad Res Commun 1989; 7:121–128.
42. Loft S, Vistisen K, Ewertz M, et al. Oxidative DNA-damage estimated by 8-hydroxydeoxyguanosine excretion in man: influence of smoking, gender and body mass index. Carcinogenesis 1992; 13:2241–2247.
43. Loft S, Fischer-Nielsen A, Jeding IB, et al. 8-Hydroxydeoxyguanosine as a urinary marker of oxidative DNA damage. J Toxicol Environ Health 1993; 40:391–404.
44. Teixeira AJR, Gommers-Ampt JH, van de Werken G, et al. Method for the analysis of oxidized nucleosides by gas chromatography/mass spectrometry. Anal Biochem 1993; 214:474–483.
45. Sakumi K, Furuichi M, Tsuzuki T, et al. Cloning and expression of cDNA for

a human enzyme that hydrolyzes 8-oxo-dGTP, a mutagenic substrate for DNA synthesis J Biol Chem 1993; 268:23524–23530.

46. Dandona P, Thusu K, Cook S, Snyder B, Makowski J, Armstrong D, Nicotera T. Oxidative damage to DNA in diabetes mellitus. Lancet 1996; 347:444–445.
47. Leinonen J, Lehtimäki T, Toyokuni S, Okada K, Tanaka T, Hiai H, Ochi H, Laippala P, Rantalaiho V, Wirta O, Pasternack A, Alho H. New biomarker evidence of oxidative DNA damage in patients with non-insulin-dependent diabetes mellitus. FEBS Lett 1997; 417:150–152.
48. Rehman A, Nourooz-Zadeh J, Möller W et al. Increased oxidative damage to all DNA bases in patients with type II diabetes mellitus. FEBS Lett 1999; 448: 120–122.
49. Steinberg D, Parthasarathy S, Carew TE, et al. Beyond cholesterol. Modifications of low-density lipoprotein that increase its atherogenicity. N Engl J Med 1989; 320:915–924.
50. Heinecke JW. Mechanisms of oxidative damage of low density lipoprotein in atherosclerosis. Curr Opin Lipidol 1997; 8:268–274.
51. Esterbauer H, Gebicki J, Puhl H, Jurgens G. The role of lipid peroxidation and antioxidants in oxidative modification of LDL. Free Rad Biol Med 1992; 13: 341–390.
52. Pieper GM, Siebeneich W. Diabetes-induced endothelial dysfunction is prevented by long-term treatment with the modified iron chelator, hydroxyethyl starch conjugated-deferoxamine. J Cardiovasc Pharm 1997; 30:734–738.
53. Halliwell B, Chirico S. Lipid peroxidation: its mechanism, measurement and significance. Am J Clin Nutr 1993; 57:715S–725S.
54. Chirico S, Smith C, Marchant C, et al. Lipid peroxidation in hyperlipidaemic patients. A study of plasma using an HPLC-based thiobarbituric acid test. Free Rad Res Commun 1993; 19:51–57.
55. Akasaka K, Ohata A, Ohrui H, Meguro H. Automatic determination of hydroperoxides of phosphatidylcholine and phosphatidylethanolamine in human plasma. J Chromatogr 1995; B665:37–43.
56. Frei B, Yamamoto Y, Niclas D, Ames BN. Evaluation of an isoluminol chemiluminescence assay for the detection of hydroperoxides in human blood plasma. Anal Biochem 1988; 175:120–130.
57. Holley AE, Slater TF. Measurement of lipid hydroperoxides in normal human blood plasma using HPLC-chemiluminescence linked to a diode array detector for measuring conjugated dienes. Free Rad Res Commun 1991; 15:51–63.
58. Wilson R, Smith R, Wilson P, Shepherd MJ, Riemersma RA. Quantitative gas chromatography-mass spectrometry isomer-specific measurement of hydroxy fatty acids in biological samples and food as a marker of lipid peroxidation. Anal Biochem 1997; 248:76–85.
59. Yasuda M, Narita S. Simultaneous determination of phospholipid hydroperoxides and cholesteryl ester hydroperoxides in human plasma by high-performance liquid chromatography with chemiluminescence detection. J Chromatogr 1997; 693:211–217.

60. Morrow JD, Roberts LJ II. Mass spectrometry of prostanoids: F_2-isoprostanes produced by non-cyclooxygenase free radical-catalyzed mechanism. Methods Enzymol 1994; 233:163–174.
61. Pratico D, Lawson JA, Fitzgerald GA. Cyclooxygenase-dependent formation of the isoprostane, 8-epiprostaglandin $F_2\alpha$. J Biol Chem 1995; 270:9800–9808.
62. Wang Z, Ciabattoni G, Creminon C, et al. Immunological characterization of urinary 8-epi-prostaglandin $F_{2\alpha}$ excretion in man. J Pharmacol Exp Ther 1995; 275:94–100.
63. Nourooz-Zadeh J, Gopaul NK, Barrow S, et al. Analysis of F_2-isoprostanes as indicators of non-enzymatic lipid peroxidation in vivo by gas chromatography-mass spectrometry: development of a solid-phase extraction procedure. J Chromatogr 1995; B667:199–208.
64. Morrow JD, Frei B, Longmire AW, et al. Increase in circulating products of lipid peroxidation (F_2-isoprostanes) in smokers. N Engl J Med 1995; 332:1198–1203.
65. Gopaul NK, Nourooz-Zadeh J, Mallet AI, Anggard EE. Formation of F_2-isoprostanes during aortic endothelial cell-mediated oxidation of low density lipoprotein. FEBS Lett 1994; 348:297–300.
66. Nourooz-Zadeh J, Liu EHC, Änggård EE, Halliwell B. F_4-isoprostanes: a novel class of prostanoids formed during peroxidation of docosahexaenoic acid (DHA). Biochem Biophys Res Commun 1998; 242:338–344.
67. Griesmacher A, KinderHauser M, Andert S, et al. Enhanced serum levels of TBARS in diabetes mellitus. Am J Med 1995; 98:469–475.
68. Sundaram RK, Bhaskar A, Vijayalingam S, Viswanatthan M, Mohan R, Shanmugasundaram KR. Antioxidant status and lipid peroxidation in type II diabetes with and without complications. Clin Sci 1996; 90:255–260.
69. Velazques E, Winocour PH, Kesteven P, Alberti KGMM, Laker MF. Relation of lipid peroxides to macrovascular disease in type 2 diabetes. Diabet Med 1991; 8:752–758.
70. MacRury SM, Gordon D, Wilson R, et al. A comparison of different methods of assessing free radical activity in type 2 diabetes and peripheral vascular disease. Diabet Med 1993; 10:331–335.
71. Gopaul NK, Anggard EE, Mallet AI, Betteridge DJ, Wolff SP, Nourooz-Zadeh J. Plasma 8-epi-$PGF_{2\alpha}$ levels are elevated in individuals with non-insulin dependent diabetes mellitus. FEBS Lett 1995; 368:225–229.
72. Burk RF, Ludden TM. Exhaled alkanes as indices of in vivo lipid peroxidation. Biochem Pharmacol 1989; 38:1029–1032.
73. McGirr LG, Hadley M, Draper HH. Identification of N^{α}-acetyl-ε-(2-propenal) lysine as a urinary metabolite of malondialdehyde. J Biol Chem 1985; 260: 15427–15431.
74. Dhanakoti SN, Draper HH. Response of urinary malondialdehyde to factors that stimulate lipid peroxidation in vivo. Lipids 1987; 22:643–646.
75. Brown ED, Morris VC, Rhodes DG, et al. Urinary excretion of malondialdehyde in subjects fed meat cooked at high or low temperatures. Lipids 1995; 30:1053–1056.

76. Gutteridge JMC, Tickner TR. The characterisation of thiobarbituric acid reactivity in human plasma and urine. Anal Biochem 1978; 91:250–257.
77. Kosugi H, Kojima T, Kikugawa K. Characteristics of the thiobarbituric acid reactivity of human urine as a possible consequence of lipid peroxidation. Lipids 1993; 28:337–343.
78. Kneepkens CMF, Lepage G, Roy CC. The potential of the hydrocarbon breath test as a measure of lipid peroxidation. Free Rad Biol Med 1994; 17:127–160.
79. Springfield JR, Levitt MD. Pitfalls in the use of breath pentane measurements to assess lipid peroxidation. J Lipid Res 1994; 35:1497–1504.
80. Wade CR, van Rij AM. In vivo lipid peroxidation in Man as measured by the respiratory excretion of ethane, pentane and other low-molecular-weight hydrocarbons. Anal Biochem 1985; 150:1–7.
81. Kohlmüller D, Kochen W. Is *n*-pentane really an index of lipid peroxidation in humans and animals? A methodological reevaluation. Anal Biochem 1993; 210: 268–276.
82. Phillips M, Greenberg J, Sabas M. Alveolar gradient of pentane in normal human breath. Free Rad Res 1994; 20:333–337.
83. Aruoma OI, Halliwell B, Butler J, Hoey BM. Apparent inactivation of α_1-antiproteinase by sulphur-containing radicals derived from penicillamine. Biochem Pharmacol 1989; 38:4353–4357.
84. Beckman JS, Chen J, Ischiropoulos H, Crow JP. Oxidative chemistry of peroxynitrite. Methods Enzymol 1994; 233:229–240.
85. Halliwell B. What nitrates tyrosine? Is nitrotyrosine specific as a biomarker of peroxynitrite formation in vivo? FEBS Lett 1997; 411:157–160.
86. Davies MJ, Dean RT. Radical-Mediated Protein Oxidation. From Chemistry to Medicine. Oxford, England: Oxford University Press, 1997.
87. Wells-Knecht MC, Huggins TG, Dyer DG, et al. Oxidized amino acids in lens proteins with age. Measurement of *o*-tyrosine and dityrosine in the aging human lens. J Biol Chem. 1993; 268:12348–12352.
88. Lubec G, Weninger M, Anderson SR. Racemization and oxidation studies of hair protein in the *Homo tirolensis*. FASEB J 1994; 8:1166–1169.
89. Levine RL, Garland D, Oliver CN, Amici A, Climent I, Lenz AG, Ahn BW, Shaltiel S, Stadtman ER. Determination of carbonyl content in oxidatively modified protein. Methods Enzymol 1990; 186:464–487.
90. Amici A, Levine RL, Tsai L, Stadtman ER. Conversion of amino acid residues in proteins and amino acid homopolymers to carbonyl derivatives by metal-catalyzed oxidation reactions. J Biol Chem 1989; 264:3341–3346.
91. Lyras L, Shaw PJ, Evans PJ, Halliwell B. Oxidative damage and motor neurone disease. Difficulties in the measurement of protein carbonyls in human brain tissue. Free Rad Res 1996; 24:397–406.
92. Mayhan WG. Superoxide dismutase partially restores impaired dilatation of the basilar artery during diabetes mellitus. Brain Res 1997; 760:204–209.
93. Cosentino F, Hishikawa K, Katusic ZS, Lüscher TF. High glucose increases ni-

tric oxide synthase expression and superoxide anion generation in human aortic endothelial cells. Circulation 1997; 96:25–28.
94. Horie K, Miyata T, Maeda K, Miyata S, Sugiyama S, Sakai H, van Ypsersele de Strihou C, Monnier VM, Witztum JL, Kurokawa K. Immunohistochemical colocalization of glycoxidation products and lipid peroxidation products in diabetic renal glomerular lesions. Implications for glycoxidative stress in the pathogenesis of diabetic nephropathy. J Clin Invest 1997; 100:2995–3004.
95. Cominacini L, Young MMR, Capriati A, Garbin U, Fratta Pasini A, Campagnola M, Davoli, A, Rigoni A, Contessi GB, Lo Cascio V. Troglitazone increases the resistance of low density lipoprotein to oxidation in healthy volunteers. Diabetologia 1997; 40:1211–1218.
96. Viana M, Herrera E, Bonet B. Teratogenic effects of diabetes mellitus in the rat. Prevention by vitamin E. Diabetologia 1996; 39:1041–1046.
97. Hagay ZJ, Weiss Y, Zusman I, Peled-Kamar M, Reece EA, Eriksson UJ, Groner Y. Prevention of diabetes-associated embryopathy by overexpression of the free radical scavenger copper zinc superoxide dismutase in transgenic mouse embryos. Am J Obstet Gynecol 1995; 173:1036–1041.

4

Plasma Lipid Hydroperoxide and Vitamin E Profiles in Patients with Diabetes Mellitus

Jaffar Nourooz-Zadeh
University College London, London, England

Patients with non-insulin-dependent diabetes mellitus (NIDDM) are at increased risk of developing vascular and other complications. This excess risk is only partially explained by the traditional risk factors, including smoking, hypertension, and dyslipidemia (1–3). Therefore, oxidative stress has been proposed as a possible explanation for the accelerated complications in NIDDM (4–7). A major hypothesis is that low-density lipoprotein (LDL) modification by oxidation or glycosylation contributes to tissue damage through cytotoxic reactions with endothelial cells or through further reactions to generate ''modified'' LDL that is selectively accumulated by ''scavenger'' receptors (8).

Despite the biochemical importance of oxidative stress, its measurement in vivo has been difficult (9). Common approaches to assess oxidative stress in biological fluids are measurement of lipid peroxidation products, oxidatively modified DNA, or protein damage and measurement of the depletion of antioxidants.

Enhanced lipid peroxidation in diabetics has been reported using thiobarbituric acid reactive substances (TBARS) as an assay (10–14). The simple TBARS assay in fact measures many substances in addition to products of lipid peroxidation and is affected by the lipid content of the sample (15). Therefore,

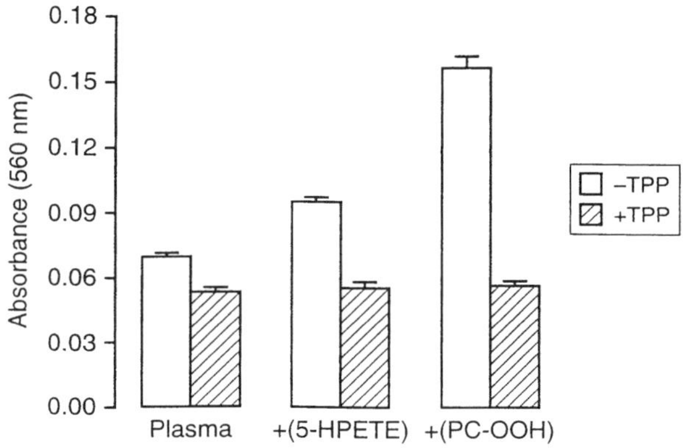

Figure 1 Detection of authentic ROOHs in plasma. PC-OOH, phospholipid hydroperoxides; 5-HPETE, 5-hydroperoxyeicotetraenoic acid.

it is unclear to what extent plasma lipoprotein peroxidation assessed by this method accounts for biological changes associated with oxidative stress.

We have used the ferrous oxidation with xylenol orange (FOX) assay coupled with triphenylphosphine (TPP) to determine plasma lipid hydroperoxide (ROOH) levels in health and disease (16,17). TPP is used to reduce ROOHs. This maneuver is necessary to generate a proper control for each individual plasma sample because plasma contains interfering components, mainly ferric ions that are detected by xylenol orange (Fig. 1). Other advantages of the FOX2 assay over existing techniques are kinetics of the reaction are independent of the chemical structure of the ROOHs and no extraction step is normally needed because the use of the 90% methanol–25 mM H_2SO_4 denatures proteins sufficiently allow access of the ferrous ions to available ROOHs. The coefficient of variation for individual plasma samples using this method is typically less than 5%, whereas that for the interassay coefficient of variation is <10% (16–19).

I. DIURNAL VARIATION OF PLASMA ROOHs

No information is available on the effect of diurnal variation on plasma lipid peroxidation products. Using the FOX assay, we examined this issue in two subjects (one woman, one man, aged 30 and 36, respectively) under fasting

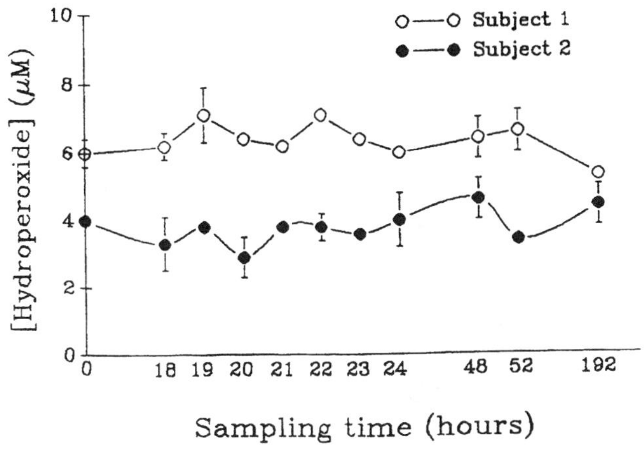

Figure 2 Diurnal change in plasma ROOHs. (From Ref. 18.)

and nonfasting conditions (17). As shown in Figure 2, little fluctuation around the mean ROOH value was associated with either the fasted or fed state. These data suggest that dietary input of ROOHs appears to be small by comparison with metabolic production of ROOH.

II. PLASMA ROOH LEVELS IN HEALTHY AND DIABETIC SUBJECTS

Mean levels of ROOH of 9.04 ± 4.3 and 9.4 ± 3.3 μmol/L were detected in freshly prepared plasma from type II diabetics from two different studies (n = 22 and 87, respectively) (17,18). The corresponding levels for healthy volunteers from three different studies were 3.02 ± 1.85, 3.76 ± 2.48, and 4.1 ± 2.2 μmol/L (n = 23, 21, and 41, respectively) (16–18). Data spread for plasma ROOHs and ratio of ROOHs/cholesterol standardized α-tocopherol in NIDDM and control subjects are shown in Figure 3. Clinical characteristics of NIDDM and control subjects are summarized in Table 1. Similar plasma ROOH concentrations have also been reported by other investigators using the FOX2 assay (20–22). These data together provide the evidence for the reliability of the FOX2 assay for the measurement of plasma ROOHs.

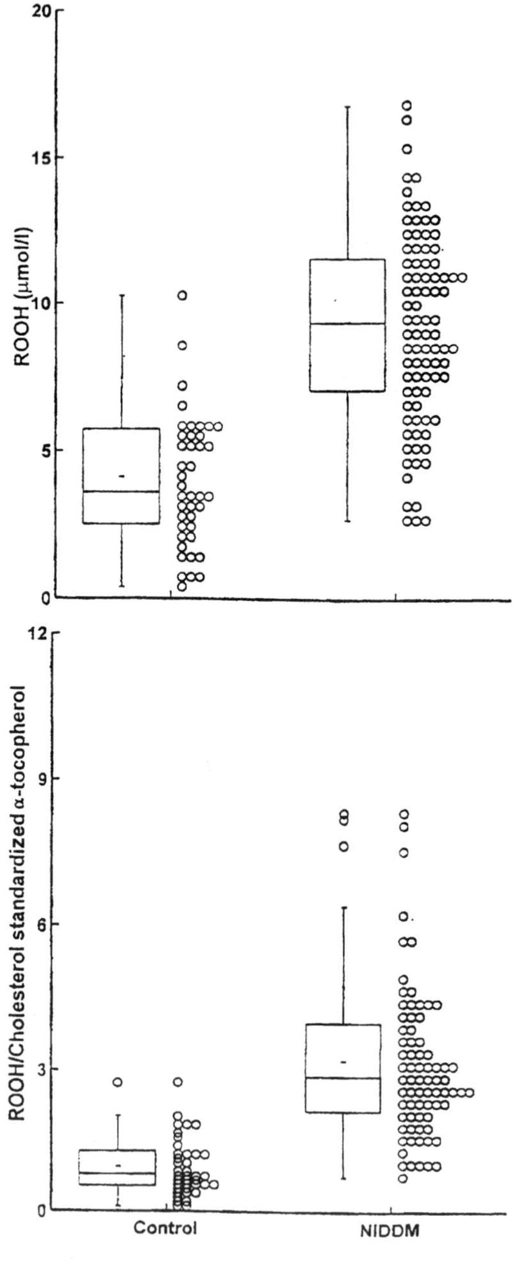

Figure 3 Data spread for ROOHs (top) and ROOHs/cholesterol-standardized α-tocopherol (bottom) in control and type II diabetic subjects.

Table 1 Clinical Characteristics of Healthy and NIDDM Individuals

Variables	Healthy	NIDDM	p
Numbers	41	87	—
Sex (F/M)	24/17	40/47	—
Age (yr)	38.2 ± 12.3	58.4 ± 14.7	<0.0005
	(21–69)*	(17–86)	
Diabetes duration (yr)	—	12.0 ± 8.3	—
		(0.0–44)	
Total cholesterol (mmol/L)	5.0 ± 1.1	6.0 ± 1.3	<0.002
	(1.4–6.9)	(3.3–9.9)	
Triglycerides (mmol/L)	0.9 ± 0.5	2.8 ± 1.8	<0.0005
	(0.3–2.5)	(0.6–3.5)	
Fasting glucose (mmol/L)	4.9 ± 0.4	12.1 ± 5.1	<0.0005
	(4.2–5.8)	(1.9–28.9)	
HbA1c (%)	—	11.0 ± 2.4	—
	(5–8)**	(5.9–17.8)	
ROOH (μM)	4.1 ± 2.2	9.4 ± 3.3	<0.0005
	(0.4–10.3)	(2.7–16.8)	
α-Tocopherol (μmol/L)	23.8 ± 8.3	19.6 ± 7.5	<0.05
	(10.6–47.0)	(8.6–44.3)	
α-Tocopherol/cholesterol (μmol/L)/(mmol/L)	5.1 ± 2.3	3.3 ± 1.0	<0.0005
	(1.9–13.0)	(1.5–6.2)	
ROOH/α-tocopherol/cholesterol	0.9 ± 0.6	3.2 ± 1.6	<0.0005
	(0.1–2.7)	(0.7–8.3)	

*Data in brackets are ranges.
**Data in parentheses are normal ranges.
Source: Ref. 18.

III. PLASMA ROOH IN DIABETICS WITH AND WITHOUT COMPLICATIONS

The association between diabetic complications and plasma lipid peroxidation as measured by nonspecific techniques (e.g., thiobarbituric acid- or ultraviolet-absorbing diene conjugates) has been examined by a number of investigators but has yielded contradictory results (10–12). We have shown that the elevated level of plasma ROOHs in diabetic subjects was not influenced by diabetic complications (Table 2). These data suggest that oxidative stress is an early stage in the disease pathology and not simply a consequence of the complications.

Table 2 Clinical Characterization for NIDDM Subjects With and Without Complications

Variables	No complications	Complications	*p*
Numbers	38	49	—
Age (yr)	53.3 ± 13.7 (17–82)*	62.3 ± 14.1 (31–86)	<0.005
Total cholesterol (mmol/L)	5.6 ± 1.2 (3.3–9.9)	6.4 ± 1.1 (4.2–9.9)	<0.05
Triglycerides (mmol/L)	2.5 ± 1.5 (0.7–6.2)	3.1 ± 1.9 (0.5–9.5)	NS
Fasting glucose (mmol/L)	11.4 ± 5.4 (1.9–28.9)	12.7 ± 5.1 (2.3–28.5)	NS
HbA1c (%)	10.9 ± 2.5 (5.9–16.8)	11.1 ± 2.3 (6.9–17.8)	NS
ROOH (μmol/L)	9.5 ± 3.3 (2.7–15.5)	9.4 ± 3.4 (2.7–16.8)	NS
α-Tocopherol (μmol/L)	18.6 ± 5.6 (9.2–30.9)	20.4 ± 8.7 (8.6–44.3)	NS
α-Tocopherol/cholesterol (μmol/L)/(mmol/L)	3.4 ± 0.9 (1.9–5.0)	3.2 ± 1.0 (1.5–6.2)	NS
ROOH/α-tocopherol/cholesterol	3.0 ± 1.4 (0.6–6.1)	3.3 ± 1.6 (0.9–8.3)	NS

*Data in brackets are ranges.
NS, not significant.
Source: Ref. 18.

IV. PLASMA VITAMIN E STATUS IN HEALTHY AND DIABETIC SUBJECTS

Data are conflicting on the α-tocopherol status in diabetic subjects. Some studies report no changes, others a decrease, and still others an increase (23–25). One problem with the previous studies was a failure to standardize α-tocopherol for lipid concentration, which would produce misleading results in hyperlipidemic patients. We have found that absolute plasma α-tocopherol levels in diabetic subjects were slightly, but significantly, lower than those of the control subjects (Table 1). Plasma α-tocopherol levels between the two groups differed markedly when α-tocopherol levels were expressed per unit of cholesterol. No difference was found in absolute plasma or cholesterol-standardized α-tocopherol in the diabetic patients with and without complications (Table 2). These findings have recently been confirmed by Borcea et al. (22). Further studies are needed to address the question whether the low plasma α-tocopherol in the diabetic patients is related to increased oxidative stress or chronic low dietary intake of vitamin E.

V. RELATIONSHIP BETWEEN ROOH AND GLYCEMIC CONTROL

Two independent studies from this laboratory have shown no correlation between plasma ROOHs and HbA1c (17,18). On the other hand, there was a scatter association between ROOH and fasting blood glucose ($r = 0.2$, $p < 0.05$) in the diabetic subjects but not in the control group (17,18). ROOH/cholesterol-standardized α-tocopherol ratio also showed a weak association with fasting blood glucose in the diabetic subjects but not in the control group ($r = 0.23$, $p < 0.05$) (18).

VI. INFLUENCE OF INSULIN THERAPY ON PLASMA ROOHs

Little information is available on the effect of glycemic control on plasma markers of oxidative stress. Berg et al. (26) compared the effect of continuous intensified insulin treatment (CIIT) and conventional insulin treatment (CIT) on plasma lipid peroxides as measured by the FOX assay. Plasma ROOHs in patients receiving CIIT fell by 31% as compared with baseline over a period of 24 months. HbA1c fell by 15% during the same period (Fig. 4). By contrast, no difference was seen in patients receiving CIT over the same period. Faure et al. (27) also examined the effect of CIIT on plasma lipid peroxides using the TBA assay. They too reported a marked reduction in TBARs after CIIT as compared with the baseline level (2.42 ± 0.25 vs. 3.03 ± 0.27 μmol/L; $n = 16$) over a period of 7 years (27). These observations provide further support for the hypothesis of a beneficial effect of insulin therapy on lipid peroxidation brought about by decreasing circulating HbA1c levels

VII. EFFECT OF ANTIOXIDANT TREATMENT ON PLASMA ROOHs

To the best of our knowledge, there is one study addressing the effect of antioxidant therapy on plasma markers of oxidative stress in diabetic patients.

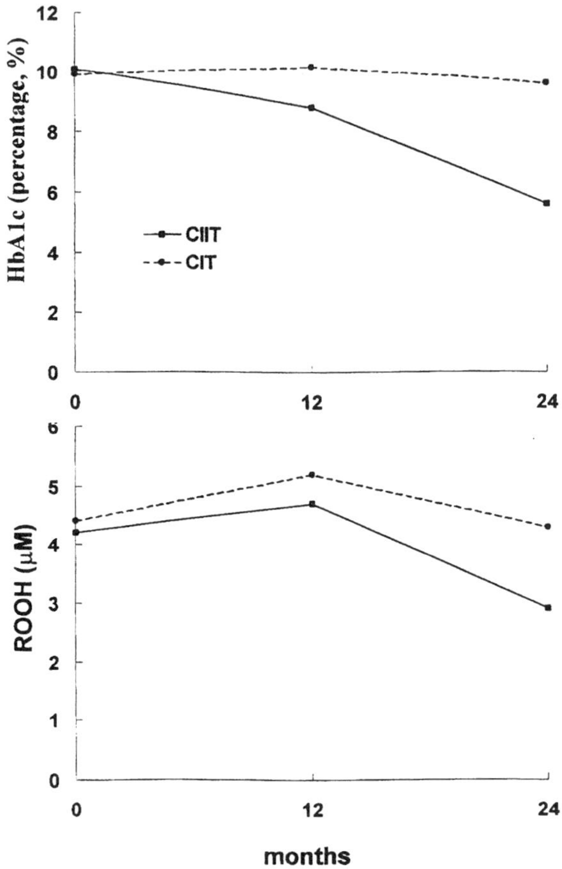

Figure 4 Change in plasma ROOHs and HbA1c during continuous intensified insulin therapy (CIIT) and conventional insulin therapy (CIT).

Borcea et al. (22) studied the effect of the antioxidant α-lipoic acid on plasma ROOHs in diabetic patients ($n = 33$) receiving α-lipoic acid for 12 weeks (600 mg/day). Diabetics treated with α-lipoic acid had markedly lower levels of plasma ROOHs than the control group. A trend toward higher α-tocopherol concentration was seen in the α-lipoic acid-treated subjects as compared with control subjects. α-Lipoic acid exists naturally in physiological systems as a cofactor for enzymatically catalyzed acyl transfer reactions (28). α-Lipoic acid and its intracellularly reduced form, dehydrolipoate, have been shown to scavenge a variety of reactive species such as HO$^{\bullet}$, ROO$^{\bullet}$, HOCl, and peroxynitrite; to regenerate both α-tocopherol and ascorbate; and to raise intracellular glutathione levels. Thus, these data provide the first direct evidence for the hypothesis that treatment with the antioxidant α-lipoic acid reduces accumulation of ROOHs in the circulation.

VIII. CONCLUSION

Diabetes mellitus has been proposed to be associated with a high risk of atherosclerosis and kidney and nerve damage. Preliminary work from this laboratory has shown that plasma from individuals with diabetes mellitus contains elevated levels of ROOHs. The diabetic subjects also had lower levels of plasma α-tocopherol as compared with control subjects, which was unrelated to dyslipidemia. Another important point from our data is that ROOH levels were similar in diabetics with and without complications, suggesting that oxidative stress occurs at an early stage in the disease pathology. It predates the complications, not simply a consequence of the complications. In addition, we have shown that insulin therapy and antioxidant therapy have a beneficial effect on oxidative stress.

ACKNOWLEDGMENT

Supported by the British Heart Foundation.

REFERENCES

1. Pyorala K, Laakso M, Uusitupa M. Diabetes and atherosclerosis: an epidemiological view. Diabetes 1987; 3:463–524.
2. Kanell WB, Hjorland M, Castelli WP. Role of diabetes in cardiac disease: conclusion from population studies. Am J Cardiol 1974; 34:29–34.
3. Uusittupa M, Niskanen LK, Siitonen O, Voutilainen E, Pyorala K. Five-years incidence of atherosclerotic vascular disease in relation to general risk factors, insulin level, and abnormalities in lipoprotein composition in NIDDM and non-diabetic subjects. Circulation 1990; 82:27–36.
4. Oberley LW. Free radicals and diabetes. Free Rad Biol Med 1988; 5:113–124.
5. Baynes JW. Perspectives in diabetes: role of oxidative stress in development of complications in diabetes. Diabetes 1991; 40:405–412.

6. Wolff SP. Diabetes and free radicals. Br Med Bull 1993; 49:642–652.
7. Giugliano D, Ceriello A, Paolisso G. Diabetes mellitus, hypertension, and cardiovascular disease: which role for oxidative stress? Metabolism 1995; 44:363–368.
8. Steinberg D, Parthasarathy S, Carew TE, Khoo JC, Witztum JL. Beyond cholesterol: modification of LDL that increase atherogenicity. N Engl J Med 1989; 320:915–924.
9. Halliwell B. Oxidative stress, nutrition and health: experimental strategies for optimization of nutritional antioxidants intakes in humans. Free Rad Res Comm 1996; 25:57–74.
10. Velazques E, Winocour PH, Kesteven P, Alberti KGMM, Laker MF. Relation of lipid peroxides to macrovascular disease in type 2 diabetes. Diabetic Med 1991; 8:752–758.
11. MacRury SM, Gordon D, Wilson R, Bradley H, Gemmell CG, Paterson JR, Rumley AG, MacCuish AC. A comparison of different methods of assessing free radical activity in type 2 diabetes and peripheral vascular disease. Diabetic Med 1993; 10:331–335.
12. Griesmacher A, Kinder-Hauser M, Andert S, Schreiner W, Toma C, Knoebl P, Pietschmann P, Prager R. Enhanced serum levels of TBARS in diabetes mellitus. Am J Med 1995; 98:469–475.
13. Niskanen LK, Salonen JT, Nyssonen K, Uusitupa MIJ. Plasma lipid peroxidation and hyperglycaemia: a connection through hyperinsulinaemia. Diabetic Med 1995; 12:802–808.
14. Sundaram RK, Bhaskar A, Vijayalingam S, Viswanatthan M, Mohan R, Shanmugasundaram KR. Antioxidant status and lipid peroxidation in type II diabetes with and without complications. Clin Sci 1996; 90:255–260.
15. Chirico S, Smith C, Marchant C, Mitchinson MJ, Halliwell B. Lipid peroxidation in hyperlipidaemic patients. A study of plasma using an HPLC-based thiobarbituric acid test. Free Rad Res Commun 1993; 19:51–57.
16. Nourooz-Zadeh J, Tajaddini-Sarmadi J, Wolff SP. Measurement of plasma hydroperoxide concentrations by the ferrous-oxidation in xylenol (FOX) assay in conjunction with triphenylphosphine. Anal Biochem 1994; 220:403–409.
17. Nourooz-Zadeh J, Tajaddini-Sarmadi J, McCarthy S, Betteridge DJ, Wolff SP. Elevated levels of authentic plasma hydroperoxides in NIDDM. Diabetes 1995; 44:1054–1058.
18. Nourooz-Zadeh J, Rahimi A, Tajaddini-Sarmadi J, Tritschler H, Rosen P, Halliwell B, Betteridge DJ. Relationship between plasma measures of oxidative stress and metabolic control in NIDDM. Diabetologia 1997; 40:647–653.
19. Södergren E, Nourooz-Zadeh J, Berglund L, Vessby B. Re-evaluation of the ferrous oxidation in xylenol orange assay for the measurement of lipid hydroperoxides. J Biochem Biophys Methods 1998; 37:137–146.
20. Santini SA, Marra G, Giardina B, Cotroneo P, Mordente A, Martorana GE, Manto A, Ghirlanda G. Detective plasma antioxidant defenses and enhanced susceptibility to lipid peroxidation in uncomplicated IDDM. Diabetes 1997; 46: 1853–1858.

21. Nuttall SL, Martin U, Sinclair AJ, Kendall. Glutathione: in sickness and in health. Lancet 1998; 351:645–646.
22. Borcea V, Nourooz-Zadeh J, Wolff SP, Zumbach M, Hofmann M, Urich H, Wahl P, Ziegler R, Tritschler HJ, Nawroth PP. Oxidative stress and antioxidant depletion in patients with diabetes mellitus. Diabetes Care (submitted).
23. Thompson KH, Godin DV. Micronutrients and antioxidants in the progression of diabetes. Nutr Res 1995; 15:1377–1410.
24. Tsai EC, Hirsch IB, Brunzell JD, Chait A. Reduced plasma peroxyl radical trapping capacity and increased susceptibility of LDL to oxidation in poorly controlled IDDM. Diabetes 1994; 43:1010–1014.
25. Asayama K, Uchida N, Nakane T, Hayashibe H, Dobashi K, Amemiya S, Kato K, Nakazawa S. Antioxidants in the serum of children with IDDM. Free Rad Biol Med 1993; 15:597–602.
26. Berg TJ, Nourooz-Zadeh J, Wolff SP, Tritschler HJ, Bangstad HJ, Hanssen KE. Hydroperoxides in plasma are reduced by intensified insulin treatment: a randomised, controlled study of IDDM patients with microalbuminuria. Diabetes Care (in press).
27. Faure P, Corticelli P, Richard MJ, Arnaud J, Coudray C, Halimi S, Favier A, Roussel AM. Lipid peroxidation and trace element status in diabetic ketonic patients: Influence of insulin therapy. Clin Chem 1993; 39:789–793.
28. Packer L, Witt EH, Tritschler HJ. Alpha-lipoic acid as a biological antioxidant. Free Rad Biol Med 1995; 19:227–250.

5
Concentrations of Antioxidative Vitamins in Plasma and Low-Density Lipoprotein of Diabetic Patients

Wolfgang Leonhardt
Technical University, Dresden, Germany

Several recent studies indicate that oxidative stress is increased in diabetic patients. Oxidative stress is a major component in the development of late complications in diabetic patients (1–4). It is mainly based on hyperglycemia. During the cellular metabolization of glucose, superoxide anions can be formed that shift the pro/antioxidative balance in blood (5,6). Intracellular activation of the polyol pathway produces an imbalance in the ratio of NADH/ NAD^+. Elevated blood glucose concentrations also cause increased glycation of lipoproteins. Because of these factors, reactive oxygen species and lipoperoxides are formed in the blood of diabetic patients (7–12) and their lipoproteins are more prone to in vitro oxidation (13,14). Glucose can act prooxidatively on low-density lipoprotein (LDL) in vitro (1,6,15,16). Impaired protection of lipid membranes against damage by free radicals is important in insulin-dependent diabetes mellitus (IDDM) because islet cell destruction by leukocytes may be mediated through the generation of toxic oxygen radicals (17).

There are many defenses to protect the organism from free radical processes (18). Antioxidant enzymes such as superoxide dismutase, catalase, and glutathione peroxidase are preventive antioxidants because they eliminate species involved in the initiation of free radical chain reactions. Some small molecule antioxidants, such as ascorbate, the tocopherols, ubiquinol, urate, and glutathione, are able to repair oxidizing radicals directly and therefore are chain-breaking antioxidants.

I. VITAMIN E IN DIABETES

Vitamin E (RRR-α-tocopherol) is the most important lipid-soluble antioxidant, which protects lipoproteins and cell membrane lipids from oxidative damage. This ability is coupled to other antioxidant systems (vitamin C, glutathione, lipoic acid) that can recycle the vitamin E radical (19). In the absence of such systems, vitamin E can behave as an oxidant (20). Dietary vitamin E is transported to the liver and secreted from the liver within very-low-density lipoproteins (VLDL). It is distributed among VLDL and LDL during the transfer and metabolism of the lipoprotein lipids (21). Thermodynamic partitioning also permits some transfer into high-density lipoproteins (22). An important part of vitamin E is constituent of cell membranes where it protects the lipid moiety against peroxidation (23).

About one-half of the total plasma vitamin E is a constituent of circulating LDL. Interindividual variations in plasma vitamin E are closely related to those in LDL (24,25). The concentration of vitamin E per LDL particle is rather low (i.e., in the order of 5–9 molecules compared with 2200 molecules of cholesterol and 170 molecules of triglycerides) (26). Nevertheless, the level of vitamin E in LDL is an independent factor that influences susceptibility of LDL to oxidation. The lagtime of in vitro LDL oxidation was found to be related to the level of vitamin E in LDL when diabetic patients were supplemented with vitamin E (27,28). For persons with usual nutritional habits, the corresponding relationship was observed in two studies (29,30) but not in others (3,31,32).

There are several publications on vitamin E concentrations in the plasma of diabetic patients. The assumption that the oxidative stress in diabetes is due to deficient vitamin E in plasma could not be confirmed. In most studies, no statistically significant differences in the concentrations between diabetic and control persons were observed. Two studies exhibited even significantly higher levels in diabetes (Table 1). The weighted mean values (control subjects 26.4 ± 1.9 μmol/L, IDDM 24.4 ± 1.6 μmol/L, NIDDM 22.4 ± 2.0 μmol/L) are only marginally different for the plasma of control persons, IDDM, and non-IDDM (NIDDM).

Published data on vitamin E concentrations in LDL (Table 2) show very similar mean values for diabetic persons and control subjects (control subjects 7.5 mol/mol, IDDM 7.0 mol/mol, NIDDM 6.8 mol/mol). One study demon-

Table 1 Plasma (Serum) Vitamin E Concentrations in Diabetes

Group	Vitamin E (μmol/L)	*n*	Sign.	Ref.
Control subjects	21.4 ± 0.6	29		
IDDM	23.7 ± 0.8	27	*	33
Control subjects	24.9 ± 1.4	20		
IDDM	24.6 ± 1.6	15		3
Control subjects	26.5	62		
IDDM	22.7	77		34
NIDDM	21.4	81		
Control subjects	24.8 ± 2.3	180		
NIDDM	21.1 ± 1.5	164	*	35
Control subjects	23.9 ± 1.4	20		
IDDM	28.3 ± 1.5	20		36
Control subjects	17.0 ± 2.1	12		
NIDDM	16.2 ± 2.9	9		37
Control subjects (vs. NIDDM)	20.1 ± 2.7	15		
Control subjects (vs. IDDM)	18.0 ± 1.9	10		30
NIDDM	22.6 ± 6.5	53		
IDDM	21.0 ± 4.1	10		
Control subjects	27.8 ± 2.4	47		
NIDDM	25.8 ± 2.1	59		38
Control subjects	20.6 ± 0.7	40		
NIDDM	24.2 ± 1.0	40	*	39
Control subjects	27.9 (16.3–39.5)	28		
NIDDM	27.5 (8.7–46.3)	21		40
Control subjects (M/F)	28.6/27.9*	210/240		
IDDM (M/F)	23.6/26.2	60/63	*	41
Control subjects	23.8 ± 1.3	41		
NIDDM	19.5 ± 0.8	87		42
Control subjects (vs. NIDDM)	33.3 ± 3.3	20		
Control subjects (vs. IDDM)	27.5 ± 1.4	24		43
NIDDM	32.0 ± 1.8	24		
IDDM	25.2 ± 1.4	28		

*Median.

Table 2 LDL Vitamin E Concentrations in Diabetes

Group	Vitamin E (mol/mol)	*n*	Sign.	Ref.
Control subjects (vs. NIDDM)	7.5 ± 1.0	20		31
Control subjects (vs. IDDM)	7.1 ± 1.3	20		
NIDDM	8.5 ± 3.5	20		
IDDM	7.7 ± 2.1	20		
Control subjects (vs. NIDDM)	8.1 (1.20)*	15		30
Control subjects (vs. IDDM)	7.4 (1.33)	10		
NIDDM	6.1 (1.33)	53	*	
IDDM	5.7 (1.32)	10		

*Geometric mean and geometric standard deviation (in parentheses).

strated significantly lowered levels in NIDDM; vitamin E in LDL was inversely related to HbA1c and positively related to the lagtime of ex vivo oxidation of LDL. This means that vitamin E in LDL is a better marker of antioxidant deficiency in diabetes than vitamin E in plasma (30).

II. PROBLEM WITH LIPID STANDARDIZATION OF VITAMIN E

There are close correlations between the concentrations of vitamin E and lipids (triglycerides, cholesterol, and phospholipids) in plasma. They are due to the lipophilic properties of vitamin E, and moreover they reflect that the antioxidative capacity of lipids is regulated in progression with the lipid mass.

Epidemiological studies revealed that the mathematical relationship between vitamin E and lipid concentrations (44) has the feature that it does not pass the origin. Rather it has a large ordinate section. This means that low lipid concentrations are associated with relatively more vitamin E and high lipid concentrations with relatively less vitamin E. Lipid standardization has the purpose to make vitamin E concentrations comparable irrespective of the corresponding lipid concentrations. The ratio of vitamin E to lipid concentration does not fulfill this condition. It can be shown that this ratio is inversely related to the lipid concentrations. Therefore, the widely used division of vitamin E by cholesterol (3,37,39,41,42,45) or cholesterol plus triglyceride (34, 40,45) concentrations is inadequate. By this procedure, most persons with above-normal lipid concentrations appear vitamin deficient. An alternative is a correction formula derived from the multiple regression of vitamin E on cholesterol and triglyceride concentrations. The constants in this formula should be derived from the population under study. For this purpose, 15–20 complete data sets may be sufficient (44). Recently, the formula was published with constants as follows (vitamin E in μmol/L) (46):

$$\begin{aligned}\text{Standardized vitamin E} = {} & \text{measured vitamin E} \\ & -2.9\ (\text{cholesterol } -5.2) \\ & -1.5\ (\text{triglycerides } -1.3)\end{aligned}$$

The multiple regression on cholesterol and triglyceride concentrations was used for vitamin E standardization by several authors (44,46–48). No statistically significant difference of standardized values between diabetic patients and control persons was observed.

III. VITAMIN A IN DIABETES

Vitamin A (*trans*-retinol) is required for normal growth, vision, and resistance to radical-mediated processes during infections. The fat-soluble vitamin is taken up with animal food and partly formed from other carotenoids. After absorption, vitamin A is transported in chylomicrons from the gut via the lymph duct and blood to the liver. Although the liver secretes a specific retinol-binding protein (38,49) into the bloodstream, plasma vitamin A correlates with plasma lipids almost as strongly as vitamin E does (50).

The level of vitamin A in diabetes has found much attention in recent literature. Vitamin A deficiency may cause blindness. Poorly controlled diabetes mellitus is attributed to a decreased availability of retinol carrier protein and subsequently to depressed vitamin A levels in blood. The impaired vitamin A status may not be improved by vitamin A supplementation but by insulin administration (51). In persons with well-controlled NIDDM without insulin deficiency, the metabolism of vitamin A appears not to be impaired. Interestingly, persons with impaired glucose tolerance show increased (2.5 μmol/L) vitamin A versus persons with normal glucose tolerance (2.1 μmol/L) (46). Most studies demonstrated lowered levels in IDDM, the difference being significant in six studies. Significantly lowered levels in NIDDM were found in two studies (Table 3). The weighed mean values are similar for control subjects and NIDDM and lower for IDDM (control subjects 1.95 ± 0.23 μmol/L, IDDM 1.52 ± 0.46 μmol/L, NIDDM 2.29 ± 0.23 μmol/L).

Table 3 Plasma (Serum) Vitamin A (Retinol) Concentrations in Diabetes

Group	Vitamin A (μmol/L)	*n*	Sign.	Ref.
Control subjects	2.32 ± 0.36			52
IDDM	1.68 ± 0.83		*	
Control subjects	1.86 ± 0.35			53
IDDM	1.63 ± 0.33		*	
Control subjects	1.82 ± 0.45			
IDDM	1.45 ± 0.36		*	54
Control subjects	1.95 ± 0.11	20		
IDDM	1.55 ± 0.07	15	*	3
Control subjects	1.89 ± 0.56	20		
IDDM	1.71 ± 0.99	20		36
Control subjects	2.14 ± 0.10	47		
NIDDM	2.23 ± 0.10	59		38
Control subjects	2.3 ± 0.18	180		
NIDDM	2.2 ± 0.11	164	*	35
Control subjects	1.7 ± 0.1	47		
NIDDM	1.5 ± 0.1	46	*	39
Control subjects	2.7 (0.8–4.4)	28		40
NIDDM	2.6 (1.6–3.6)	21		
Control subjects (M/F)	1.86/1.54*	210/240		
IDDM (M/F)	1.46/1.28	60/63	*	41
Control subjects (vs. NIDDM)	2.23 ± 0.18	20		
Control subjects (vs. IDDM)	1.94 ± 0.10	24		43
NIDDM	2.23 ± 0.14	24		
IDDM	1.30 ± 0.05	28	*	
Control subjects	2.9 ± 0.6	35		
IDDM	3.3 ± 1.0	10		51
NIDDM	3.2 ± 0.9	53		

*Median.

IV. VITAMIN C IN DIABETES

Vitamin C (ascorbic acid) is a powerful antioxidant and a cofactor in collagen biosynthesis, which affects platelet activation, prostaglandin biosynthesis, and the polyol pathway. Vitamin C acts as an antioxidant both in vitro and in vivo and protects plasma lipids and lipid membranes. It has the power to spare and to increase plasma-reduced glutathione (56). The antioxidative ability of vitamin E can be continuously restored through its recycling by other antioxidants, mainly vitamin C (18,19).

Table 4 Plasma Vitamin C Concentrations in Diabetes

Group	Vitamin C (μmol/L)	*n*	Sign.	Ref.
Control subjects	82.9 ± 30.9	22		
NIDDM	55.6 ± 20.0	21		
NIDDM + Complic.	42.1 ± 19.3	20		57
Control subjects	60.0 ± 5.5	180		
NIDDM	48.8 ± 2.3	164	*	
NIDDM + Complic.	29.9 − 41.2	163	*	35
Normal persons	61.3 ± 9.7	20		
Borderline FBG	47.7 ± 7.4	10	*	
NIDDM	28.4 ± 5.7	30	*	58
Control subjects	71.6 (37.5–105.6)	28		
NIDDM	57.9 (51.7–64.2)	21		40
ND, PVD	47.1 (7.4–86.9)	21	*	
NIDDM, PVD	48.3 (15.3–80.1)	11	*	
Control subjects A = 28 yr	87.5 ± 4.9	24		
IDDM	63.6 ± 6.0	28	*	43
Control A = 63 yr	58.5 ± 5.3	20		
NIDDM	38.6 ± 5.7	24	*	

Complic., diabetic complications; FBG, fasting blood glucose; PVD, peripheral vascular disease.

Abnormalities of vitamin C metabolism have been reported in experimentally induced diabetes and in diabetic patients. Hyperglycemia may be directly responsible for a vitamin C deficit. Exposure to glucose may inactivate antioxidant enzymes and impair the intracellular regeneration of vitamin C by removing reducing equivalents in the form of NADPH for the polyol pathway (59).

Nearly all studies demonstrated significantly diminished levels of vitamin C in the plasma of NIDDM. The reduction was also observed in IDDM and in borderline fasting blood glucose, and it was more pronounced when diabetic complications occurred in addition (Table 4). The weighed mean values are very different for control subjects and NIDDM (control subjects 65.0 ± 7.8 μmol/L, NIDDM 46.8 ± 4.6 μmol/L).

V. CONCLUSION

The epidemiological data of this chapter refer to diabetic patients and control persons who are not supplemented with antioxidant vitamins and who do not take antioxidative medications. There are many reports showing that increased dietary intake or supplementation with vitamins E, A, and C can largely increase the plasma levels of the antioxidant vitamins, with positive consequences concerning metabolic control and late complications of diabetes.

REFERENCES

1. Hunt JV, Smith CC, Wolff SP. Autoxidative glycosylation and possible involvement of peroxides and free radicals in LDL modification by glucose. Diabetes 1990; 39:1420–1424.
2. Ceriello A, Giugliano D, Quatraro A, Donzella C, Dipalo G, Lefebvre PJ. Vitamin E reduction of protein glycosylation in diabetes: new prospect for prevention of diabetic complications? Diabetes Care 1991; 14:68–72.
3. Tsai EC, Hirsch IB, Brunzell JD, Chait A. Reduced plasma peroxyl radical trapping capacity and increased susceptibility of LDL to oxidation in poorly controlled IDDM. Diabetes 1994; 43:1010–1014.
4. Giugliano D, Ceriello A, Paolisso G. Diabetes mellitus, hypertension, and cardiovascular disease: which role for oxidative stress? Metabolism 1995; 44:363–368.
5. Thornalley P. Monosaccharide auto-oxidation in health and disease. Environ Health Perspect 1985; 64:297–307.
6. Rifici VA, Schneider SH, Khachadurian AK. Stimulation of low density lipoprotein oxidation by insulin and insulin like growth factor I. Atherosclerosis 1994; 107:99–108.
7. Altomare F, Vendemiale G, et al. Increased lipid peroxidation in type 2 poorly controlled diabetic patients. Diabetes Metab 1992; 18:264–271.
8. Chittar HS, Nihalani KD, Varthakavi PK, Udipi SA. Lipid peroxide levels in diabetics with micro- and macroangiopathies. J Nutr Biochem 1994; 5:442–445.
9. Evans RW, Orchard TJ. Oxidized lipids in insulin-dependent diabetes mellitus: a sex-diabetes interaction? Metabolism 1994; 43:1196–1200.
10. Gallou G, Ruelland A, Campion L, Maugendre D, Lemoullec N, Legras B, Allannic H, Cloarec L. Increase in thiobarbituric acid-reactive substances and vascular complications in type 2 diabetes mellitus. Diabetes Metab 1994;20:258–264.
11. Haffner SM, Agil A, Mykkanen L, Stern MP, Jialal I. Plasma oxidizability in subjects with normal glucose tolerance, impaired glucose tolerance, and NIDDM. Diabetes Care 1995; 18:646–653.
13. Babiy AV, Gebicki JM, Sullivan DR, Willey K. Increased oxidizability of plasma lipoproteins in diabetic patients can be decreased by probucol therapy and is not due to glycation. Biochem Pharmacol 1992; 43:995–1000.
14. Cestaro B, Gandini R, Viani P, Maraffi F, Cervato G, Montalto C, Gatti P, Megali R. Fluorescence-determined kinetics of plasma high oxidizability in diabetic patients. Biochem Mol Biol Int 1994; 32:983–994.
15. Hicks M, Delbridge L, Yue DK, Reeve TS. Catalysis of lipid peroxidation by

glucose and glycosylated collagen. Biochem Biophys Res Commun 1988; 151: 649–655.
16. Kawamura M, Heinecke JW, Chait A. Pathophysiological concentrations of glucose promote oxidative modification of low density lipoprotein by a superoxide-dependent pathway. J Clin Invest 1994; 94:771–778.
17. Oberley LW. Free radicals and diabetes. Free Rad Biol Med 1988; 5:113–124.
18. Frei B, Stocker R, Ames BN. Antioxidant defenses and lipid peroxidation in human blood plasma. Proc Natl Acad Sci USA 1988; 85:9748–9752.
19. Kagan VE, Serbinova EA, Forte T, Scita G, Packer L. Recycling of vitamin E in human low density lipoproteins. J Lipid Res 1992;33:385–397.
20. Stocker R, Bowry VW, Frei B. Ubiquinol-10 protects human low density lipoprotein more efficiently against lipid peroxidation than does alpha-tocopherol. Proc Natl Acad Sci USA 1991; 88:1646–1650.
21. Kostner GM, Oettl K, Jauhiainen M, Ehnholm C, Esterbauer H, Dieplinger H. Human plasma phospholipid transfer protein accelerates exchange/transfer of α-tocopherol between lipoproteins and cells. Biochem J 1995; 305:659–667.
22. Behrens WA, Thompson JN, Madere R. Distribution of α-tocopherol in human plasma lipoproteins. Am J Clin Nutr 1982; 35:691–696.
23. Buettner GR. The pecking order of free radicals and antioxidants: lipid peroxidation, alpha-tocopherol, and ascorbate. Arch Biochem Biophys 1993; 300:535–543.
24. Davies T, Kelleher J, Losowsky MS. Interrelation of serum lipoprotein and tocopherol levels. Clin Chim Acta 1969; 24:431–436.
25. Rubba P, Mancini M, Fidanza F, Leccia G, Riemersma RA, Gey KF. Plasma vitamin E, apolipoprotein B, and HDL-cholesterol in middle-aged men from southern Italy. Atherosclerosis 1989;77:25–29.
26. Esterbauer H, Gebicky J, Puhl H, Jürgens G. The role of lipid peroxidation and antioxidants in oxidative modification of LDL. Free Rad Biol Med 1992; 13: 341–390.
27. Reaven PD, Herold DA, Barnett J, Edelman S. Effects of vitamin E on susceptibility of low-density lipoprotein and low-density lipoprotoin subfractions to oxidation and on protein glycation in NIDDM. Diabetes Care 1995; 18:807–816.
28. Fuller CJ, Chandalia M, Garg A, Grundy SM, Jialal I. RRR-alpha-tocopheryl acetate supplementation at pharmacologic doses decreases low density lipoprotein oxidative susceptibility but not protein glycation in patients with diabetes mellitus. Am J Clin Nutr 1996; 63:753–759.
29. Frei B, Gaziano JM. Content of antioxidants, preformed lipid hydroperoxides, and cholesterol as predictors of the susceptibility of human LDL to metal ion-dependent and ion-independent oxidation. J Lipid Res 1993; 34:2135–2145.
30. Leonhardt W, Hanefeld M, Muller G, Hora C, Meissner D, Lattke P, Paetzold A, Jaross W, Schroeder HE. Impact of concentrations of glycated hemoglobin, alpha-tocopherol, copper, and manganese on oxidation of low density lipoproteins in patients with type I diabetes, type II diabetes and control subjects. Clin Chim Acta 1996; 254:173–186.
31. Beaudeux JL, Guillausseau PJ, Peynet J, Flourie F, Assayag M, Tielmans D, Warnet A, Rousselet F. Enhanced susceptibility of low density lipoprotein to in

vitro oxidation in type 1 and type 2 diabetic patients. Clin Chim Acta 1995; 239: 131–141.

32. Dimitriadis E, Griffin M, Owens D, Johnson A, Collins P, Tomkin GH. Oxidation of low density lipoprotein in NIDDM: its relationship to fatty acid composition. Diabetologia 1995; 38:1300–1306.
33. Asayama K, Uchida N, Nakane T, Hayashibe H, Dobashi K, Amemiya S, Kato K, Nakazawa S. Antioxidants in the serum of children with insulin-dependent diabetes mellitus. Free Rad Biol Med 1993; 15:597–602.
34. Griesmacher A, Kindhauser M, Andert SE, Schreiner W, Toma C, Knoebl P, Pietschmann P, Prager R, Schnack C, Schernthaner G, Mueller MM. Enhanced serum levels of thiobarbituric-acid-reactive substances in diabetes mellitus. Am J Med 1995; 98:469–475.
35. Sundaram RK, Bhaskar A, Vijayalingam S, Viswanthan M, Mohan R, Shanmugasundaram KR. Antioxidant status and lipid peroxidation in type II diabetes mellitus with and without complications. Clin Sci 1996; 90:255–260.
36. Osterode W, Holler C, Ulberth F. Nutritional antioxidants, red cell membrane fluidity, and blood viscosity in type 1 (insulin dependent) diabetes mellitus. Diabetic Med 1996; 13:1044–1050.
37. Galvan AQ, Muscelli E, Catalano C, Natali A, Sanna G, Masoni A, Bernardini B, Barsacchi R, Ferrannini E. Insulin decreases circulating vitamin E levels in humans. Metabolism 1996; 45:998–1003.
38. Basualdo CG, Wein EE, Basu TK. Vitamin A (retinol) status of first nation adults with non-insulin-dependent diabetes mellitus. J Am Coll Nutr 1997; 16:39–45.
39. Ceriello A, Bortolotti N, Falleti E, Taboga C, Tonutti L, Crescentini A, Motz E, Lizzio S, Russo A, Bartoli E. Total radical-trapping antioxidant parameter in NIDDM patients. Diabetes Care 1997; 20:194–197.
40. Dyer RG, Stewart MW, Mitcheson J, George K, Alberti MM, Laker MF. 7-Ketocholesterol, a specific indicator of lipoprotein oxidation, and malondialdehyde in non-insulin dependent diabetes and peripheral vascular disease. Clin Chim Acta 1997; 260:1–13.
41. Olmedilla B, Granado F, Gilmartinez E, Blanco I, Rojashidalgo E. Reference values for retinol, tocopherol, and main carotenoids in serum of control and insulin dependent diabetic Spanish subjects. Clin Chem 1997; 43:1066–1071.
42. Nourooz-Zadeh J, Rahimi A, Tajaddinisarmadi J, Tritschler H, Rosen P, Halliwell B, Betteridge DJ. Relationships between plasma measures of oxidative stress and metabolic control in NIDDM. Diabetologia 1997; 40:647–653.
43. Maxwell SRJ, Thomason H, Sandler D, Leguen C, Baxter MA, Thorpe GHG, Jones AF, Barnett AH. Antioxidant status in patients with uncomplicated insulin-dependent and non-insulin-dependent diabetes mellitus. Eur J Clin Invest 1997; 27:484–490.
44. Jordan P, Brubacher D, Moser U, Stähelin HB, Gey KF. Vitamin E and vitamin A concentrations in plasma adjusted for cholesterol and triglycerides by multiple regression. Clin Chem 1995; 41:924–927.
45. Thurnham DI, Davies JA, Crump BJ, Situnayake RD, Davis M. The use of differ-

ent lipids to express serum tocopherol: lipid ratios for the measurement of vitamin E status. Ann Clin Biochem 1986; 23:514–520.
46. Tavridou A, Unwin NG, Laker MF, White M, Alberti KGMM. Serum concentrations of vitamins A and E in impaired glucose tolerance. Clin Chim Acta 1997; 266:129–140.
47. Salonen JT, Nyyssönen K, Tuomainen T-P, Mäenpää TH, Korpela H, Kaplan GA, Lynch J, Helmrich SP, Salonen R. Increased risk of non-insulin-dependent diabetes mellitus at low plasma vitamin E concentrations: a 4-year follow-up study in men. Br Med J 1995; 311:1124–1127.
48. Nyyssönen K, Porkkalasarataho E, Kaikkonen J, Salonen JT. Ascorbate and urate are the strongest determinants of plasma antioxidative capacity and serum lipid resistance to oxidation in Finnish men. Atherosclerosis 1997; 130:223–233.
49. Krill D, Oleary L, Koehler AN, Kramer MK, Warty V, Wagner MA, Dorman JS. Association of retinol-binding protein in multiple-case families with insulin-dependent diabetes. Hum Biol 1997; 69:89–96.
50. Gey KF, Puska P, Jordan P, Moser UK. Inverse correlation between plasma vitamin E and mortality from ischemic heart disease in cross-cultural epidemiology. Am J Clin Nutr 1991; 53:326S–334S.
51. Basu TK, Basualdo C. Vitamin A homeostasis and diabetes mellitus. Nutrition 1997; 13:804–806.
52. Wako Y, Suzuki K, Goto Y, Kimura S. Vitamin A transport in plasma of diabetic patients. Tohoku J Exp Med 1986; 49:133.
53. Basu TK, Tze WJ, Leichter J. Serum vitamin A and retinol-binding protein in patients with insulin-dependent diabetes mellitus. Am J Clin Nutr 1989; 50:329.
54. Martinoli L, De Felice M, Seghieri G, et al. Plasma retinol and alpha-tocopherol concentrations in insulin-dependent diabetes mellitus: the relationship to microvascular complications. Int J Vitam Nutr Res 1993; 63:87.
55. Leonhardt W, Hanefeld M, Lattke P, Jaroß W. Vitamin E-Mangel und Oxidierbarkeit der Low-Density-Lipoproteine bei Typ-I-und Typ-II-Diabetes: Einfluß der Qualität der Stoffwechselkontrolle. Diabetes 1997; 6(suppl 2):24–28.
56. Paolisso G, D'Amore A, Balbi V, Volpe C, Galzerano D, Giugliano D, Sgambato S, Varricchio M, D'Onofrio F. Plasma vitamin C affects glucose homeostasis in healthy subjects and in non-insulin-dependent diabetics. Am J Physiol 1994; 266: E261–E268.
57. Sinclair AJ, Girling AJ, Gray L, Le Guen C, Lunec J, Barnett AH. Disturbed handling of ascorbic acid in diabetic patients with and without microangiopathy during high-dose ascorbate supplementation. Diabetologia 1997; 34:171–175.
58. Srinivasan KN, Pugalendi KV, Sambandam G, Rao MR, Menon PV. Diabetes mellitus, lipid peroxidation, and antioxidant status in rural patients. Clin Chim Acta 1997; 259:183–186.
59. Maxwell SRJ, Thomason H, Sandler D, Leguen C, Baxter AM, Thorpe GHG, Jones AF, Barnett AH. Poor glycaemic control is associated with reduced serum free radical scavenging (antioxidant) activity in non-insulin-dependent diabetes mellitus. Ann Clin Biochem 1997; 34:638–644.

6
Oxidative Stress in Diabetes

John W. Baynes and Suzanne R. Thorpe
University of South Carolina, Columbia, South Carolina

I. DEFINING OXIDATIVE STRESS

The first step in addressing the role of oxidative stress (OxS) in diabetic complications is to define OxS. It is often defined as a shift in the pro-oxidant–antioxidant balance in the pro-oxidant direction. This definition of OxS is more descriptive than quantitative and chemical in nature. Philosophically, it implies a null point, a balance point at which there is no OxS—OxS occurs only when the balance is shifted toward the pro-oxidant direction. There is a conceptual flaw in this definition because it fails to recognize that OxS is a constant feature of biological systems. Peroxides, superoxide, hydroxyl radicals, and other reactive oxygen species (ROS), the mediators of OxS, are being formed continuously in the body and always exist at some steady-state concentration. The resulting oxidative damage to protein, DNA, and other biomolecules is a ubiquitous and universal consequence of life under aerobic conditions.

OxS might be better defined as "a measure of the prevailing level of ROS in a biological system." This definition acknowledges the continuous presence of ROS in biological systems, at some level determined by the relative rates of their formation and consumption. It accepts OxS as a normal feature of cellular metabolism rather than a disturbance in an equilibrium—OxS waxes and wanes but never disappears from the biological scene. Like metabolites, levels of ROS may differ at different stages in the feeding–fasting and diurnal cycles, among different subcellular compartments, among different cell types, in a cell at different stages in its growth and development, and even among cells of the same type but in different regions of a tissue. ROS are mediators of hormone action and growth factor and cytokine activity, and variations in ROS concentrations and OxS in intracellular and extracellular environments appear to be a central feature of regulatory biology (1).

From a quantitative viewpoint, OxS may be considered the sum of the products of the concentration and reactivity of numerous ROS in the cell. Should cells in which redox coenzyme systems are off-balance or in which reduced glutathione (GSH) is depleted also be considered oxidatively stressed? This is not a trivial question because alterations in ascorbate or GSH homeostasis are often cited as evidence of OxS. However, even a poor defense may be adequate in the absence of an oxidative challenge. Persons with glucose 6-phosphate dehydrogenase deficiency, for example, are asymptomatic until they are challenged by drugs or infection, leading to hemolytic anemia. Thus, a shift in the set point or concentration of redox coenzymes in a cell may predispose to oxidative stress, but the perturbation per se does not necessarily indicate that the cell is oxidatively stressed.

At this time it is not possible to quantify OxS, but this may eventually be achievable. The total radical antioxidant potential (TRAP) of plasma can now be estimated, for example, as the sum of a variety of antioxidant concentrations in plasma, including ascorbate, tocopherols, uric acid, and protein (2). Plasma TRAP is commonly expressed relative to that of a concentration of an antioxidant standard, such as Trolox (3). It may eventually be possible to develop a standard, such as ''H_2O_2 equivalents'' for assessing OxS in cells and tissues or actually to measure the concentration of specific oxyradicals by electron paramagnetic resonance spectroscopy (4).

Because of the many components and factors affecting OxS (Fig. 1), it is difficult, if not impossible, to assess the overall status of OxS in a biological system by measurement of the status of an individual or even several enzymes or antioxidant systems. Indeed, the interpretation of these data is often gratuitous. A low level of antioxidant enzyme is often interpreted as evidence of OxS, but high levels of superoxide dismutase are associated with OxS in the lungs in response to hyperbaric oxygen. Similarly, high plasma levels of uric acid are associated with inflammation in gout, whereas high levels of ascorbic may be pro-oxidant in the presence of free or heme iron.

In the absence of unambiguous assays or standards for measuring OxS, measurement of the consequences of OxS has been used as a surrogate. One approach for assessing the status of OxS is to measure the rate of excretion of products of oxidation of DNA, such as thymi(di)ne glycol or 8-oxodeoxyguan(os)ine (5,6). Another is to measure the level of activation or expression of protein kinases, activator protein-1 or nuclear factor kappa B, growth factors (transforming growth factor-β, insulin-like growth factor-1, and vascular en-

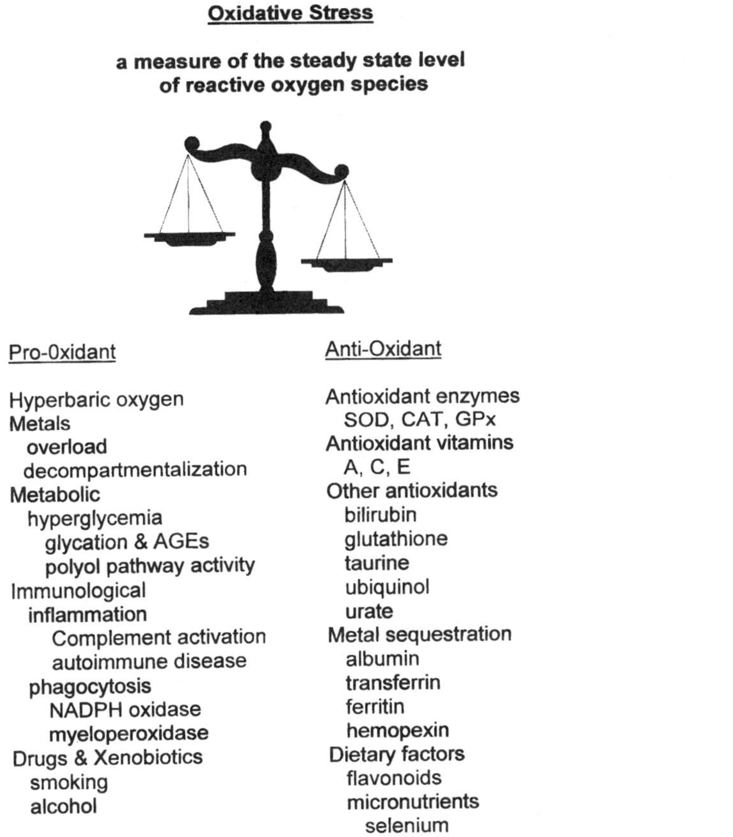

Figure 1 Some factors determining the status of OxS in biological systems.

dothelial growth factor) or heme oxygenase, all of which are involved in the response to oxidative stress (1,7) but also respond to other stresses such as reductive, thermal (heat/cold), and osmotic shock. A third approach, the focus of our research and of this article, is the measurement of the extent of oxidative damage to long-lived proteins, such as collagen, which integrates the time-averaged ambient level of OxS.

II. NATURE OF OXIDATIVE DAMAGE

Oxidative damage to protein may be divided chemically into primary and secondary damage (Table 1). Primary damage results from direct reaction of pro-

Table 1 Biomarkers of Oxidative Stress

Precursors: Reactive Oxygen Species			
H_2O_2, $O_2^{-\bullet}$, $OOH^\bullet$, $OH^\bullet$, HOCl, ONOOH, metal:oxo complexes			
Primary Products of Oxidation of Protein			
Class	Example		
Aromatic	*o*-Tyrosine, dityrosine, chlorotyrosine nitrotyrosine, ditytrosine, dihydroxyphenylalanine		
Sulfhydryl	Protein disulfides, methionine sulfoxide		
Amino acid hydroperoxides	Valine, leucine, isoleucine		
Protein carbonyls	Oxohistidine, adipic semialdehyde		
Secondary Products of Oxidation of Protein			
	Lipid	Carbohydrate	Mixed
Precursor	MDA-Lys	Pentosidine	CML, CEL
Products	HNE-(Lys, His, Cys)	Crosslines	GOLD, MOLD
	Pyrroles	Vesperlysines	Argpyrimidine

teins with ROS. Products of these reactions include stable compounds, isolable by acid hydrolysis of proteins, such as *o*-tyrosine and methionine sulfoxide (MetSO). Some products, such as nitrotyrosine and chlorotyrosine, provide insight into the source of the damage, peroxynitrite and HOCl, respectively. Other products, such as protein carbonyls, may be derived from several sources, are unstable to acid hydrolysis, and may be transient but important intermediates in the cell, e.g., in marking proteins for turnover (8).

Secondary oxidative damage results from reaction of proteins with products of oxidation of small molecules, including lipids, carbohydrates, and amino acids. The intermediates in this process are reactive carbonyl and dicarbonyl compounds, such as malondialdehyde, α, β-unsaturated and hydroxyaldehydes, glyoxal, and methylglyoxal (MGO), which react with nucleophilic groups on protein to form lipoxidation (9) and glycoxidation (10,11) products (Table 1). Lipoxidation products require oxidation (peroxidation) for their formation from lipids, whereas glycoxidation products are a subclass of advanced glycation end products (AGEs), requiring autoxidation chemistry (oxidation by molecular oxygen) for their formation from reducing sugars or ascorbate. Some AGEs (e.g., pyrraline and imidazolones formed by reaction of 3-deoxyglucosone [3DG] with lysine and arginine residues in protein) do not require oxidation for their formation from reducing sugars. These AGEs are useful indicators of nonoxidative chemical modification of proteins.

Some secondary oxidation products, such as carboxymethyllysine (CML), carboxyethyllysine (CEL), pentosidine (12,13), and vesperlysines (14), are stable to acid hydrolysis, whereas others, such as crosslines (15) and the malondialdehyde and 4-hydroxynonenal adducts to lysine (MDA-lysine, HNE-lysine) (16), are labile. Some are characteristic of lipid peroxidation, such as MDA-Lys and HNE adducts to Lys, His, and Cys, whereas pentosidine, vesperlysines and crosslines are derived exclusively from carbohydrates. CML and CEL are more general markers that may be formed after oxidation of carbohydrates, lipids, or amino acids (17,18). Some of these compounds, such as CML, CEL, and the imidazolium salts, glyoxal- and methylglyoxal-lysine dimer (GOLD, MOLD) (19), are end products, whereas others, such as MDA and HNE adducts to lysine, may progress to form crosslinks and pyrrole adducts in protein.

Both primary and secondary oxidation products are measured as indicators of OxS. In the several cases in which stable end products are formed, such as *o*-tyrosine, MetSO, CML, CEL, pentosidine, GOLD, and MOLD, the products accumulate with age in long-lived proteins, such as collagens and crystallines (12,13,17,19,20). Because they are oxidation products, these compounds are biomarkers of oxidative damage to protein and should provide insight into levels of oxidative stress. Primary oxidation products are formed directly by reaction of ROS with protein, and their concentration in tissue proteins should provide a direct index of OxS. In contrast, secondary oxidation products should be second-order products of OxS (Fig. 2), that is, their levels in tissues are determined by both the prevailing level of OxS and the ambient concentration of oxidizable substrates.

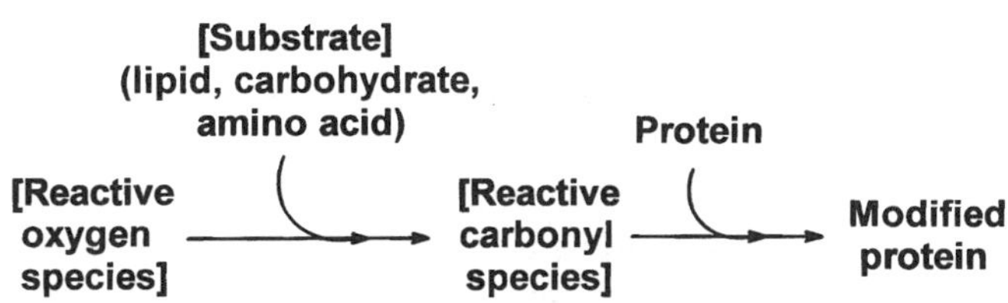

Figure 2 Reaction pathway illustrating the role of both prevailing oxidative stress (ROS concentration) and ambient substrate concentration in formation of secondary oxidation products. According to this scheme, the rate of production of reactive carbonyl species, intermediates in the formation of secondary oxidation products, is first order in ROS, first order in substrate, and second order overall. Increases in either ROS or substrate may increase the rate of formation of reactive carbonyl species and secondary oxidation products.

III. IS OxS INCREASED IN DIABETES?

OxS is a feature of all chronic diseases. Free Radicals in Biology and Medicine (21), one of the early monographs in this field, lists a full page of diseases in which OxS is implicated as a pathogenic agent. OxS is a sign of cellular stress, injury, and apoptosis. At sites of overt pathology, such as in the kidney in diabetes and in plaque formed in atherosclerosis, Alzheimer's disease, and dialysis-related amyloidosis, both primary and secondary biomarkers of OxS are detected together by immunohistochemical techniques (22–28). Although these observations indicate a broad spectrum of oxidative damage to tissue proteins in chronic disease, it is unlikely that OxS is a primary pathogenic mechanism in most chronic diseases. This is most obvious in autoimmune diseases where an errant immunological response underlies the development of pathology. Even in the case of disease induced by environmental agents, such as chronic pulmonary disease, OxS associated with phagocytosis and complement activation is probably the major source of tissue damage. The question about the role of OxS in diabetes is, therefore, not whether OxS in increased but whether OxS is a primary pathogenic mechanism in diabetes.

IV. WHAT DO CHEMICAL BIOMARKERS OF OxS TELL US ABOUT THE STATUS OF OxS IN DIABETES?

As summarized below and presented in greater detail elsewhere (11), there are several lines of evidence that OxS is not a primary pathogenic mechanism underlying diabetic complications.

1. Age-adjusted levels of the primary oxidation products, *o*-Tyr and MetSO, in skin collagen are not increased in diabetes (Fig. 3) (20).
2. Increases in secondary oxidation (lipoxidation and glycoxidation) products in plasma and tissue proteins and in urine can be explained by increases in substrate concentrations alone, without invoking an increase in oxidative stress (11,13).
3. Increases in lipoxidation and glycoxidation products in plasma are more closely associated with the presence of vascular (29,30) and renal (31) complications rather than diabetes itself, suggesting that OxS is apparent only when advanced tissue damage has occurred.
4. Increased levels of 3DG, a nonoxidative AGE precursor, are ob-

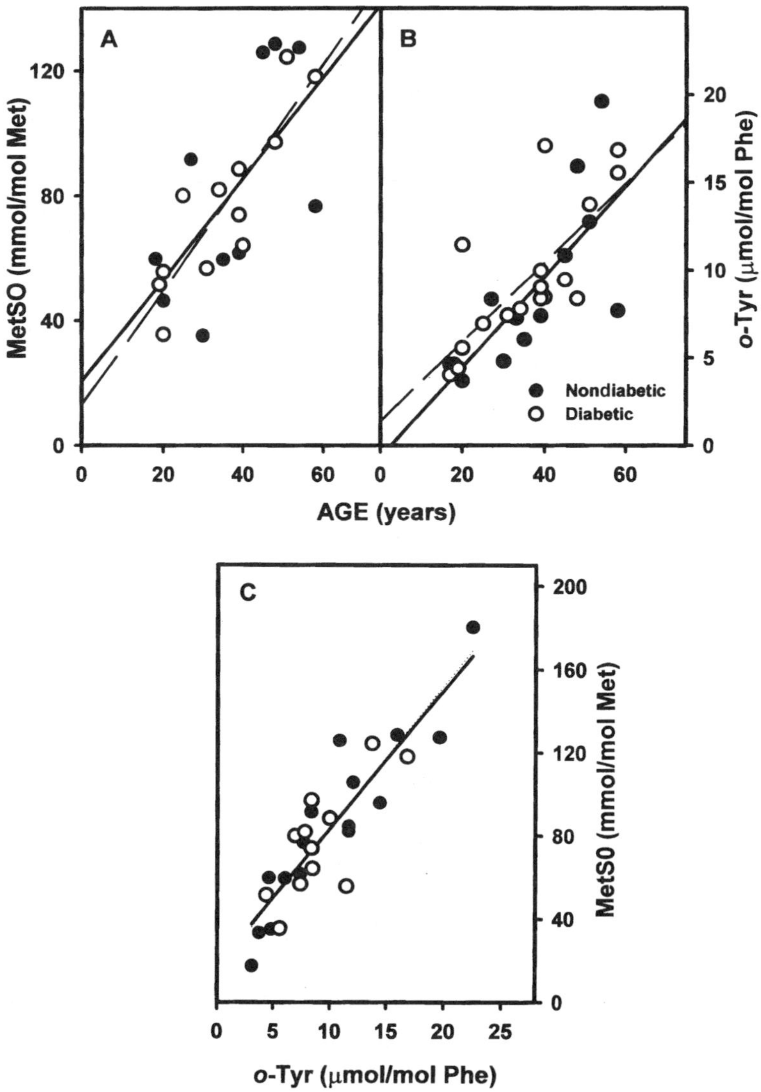

Figure 3 Age-dependent increase in (A) MetSO and (B) *o*-tyrosine in human skin collagen from diabetic and nondiabetic subjects. Despite significant differences in the absolute concentrations of these biomarkers, there is a strong correlation (C) between levels of these primary oxidation products in skin collagen. (From Ref. 20.)

served in diabetic serum (32,33), suggesting a more generalized increase in carbonyl stress (11) in diabetes.

V. CARBONYL STRESS IN DIABETES

The increase in lipoxidation and glycoxidation products in diabetes is the direct result of an increase in carbonyl precursors; however, not all of these intermediates are derived from oxidative reactions. 3DG, for example, is formed nonoxidatively from Amadori compounds (34) or fructose-3-phosphate (35) and is also increased in diabetes, along with increases in both pyrraline and 3DG-arginine imidazolone (36) adducts that are derived from 3DG by nonoxidative mechanisms. MGO adducts to protein, including CEL and MOLD, are also increased in diabetes (37,38). Like 3DG, MGO is formed by anaerobic mechanisms, either enzymatically as an intermediate in amino acid catabolism or by β-elimination reactions of triose phosphates (39,40). However, MGO may also be produced during the oxidative chemistry of both lipids and carbohydrates, so that its precise origin in vivo is unknown. In any case, the increase in 3DG, and possibly MGO, and their adducts to proteins suggests that limitations in the detoxification of reactive carbonyl compounds, produced by both oxidative and nonoxidative mechanisms, underlie the increased chemical modification of proteins in diabetes (Fig. 4).

There are three major routes for detoxification of reactive carbonyl compounds: NAD^+-dependent oxidation of aldehydes to carboxylic acids, NADPH-dependent reduction of aldehydes to alcohols, and rearrangement of ketoaldehydes to hydroxyacids. The first pathway is illustrated by the oxidation of HNE to hydroxynonenoic acid (41,42) or of 3DG to 2-keto-3-deoxygluconic acid (43), the second by reduction of 3DG to 3-deoxyfructose (44,45), and the third by the GSH-dependent glyoxalase pathway (40). Conjugation of reactive aldehydes to GSH thiohemiacetals by GSH S-transferases is also important in presenting substrates for oxidation by dehydrogenases (42,46), for metabolism of MGO in the glyoxalase pathway (38), or for export of the GSH conjugates from cells (42,47). There is widespread evidence that these pathways are compromised in diabetes as a result of shifts in redox coenzyme systems or that they are overwhelmed by an excess of carbonyl substrates. The shift in the redox potential of the $NAD^+ \parallel NADH$ couple during pseudohypoxia (48,49) may limit NAD^+-dependent oxidation reactions, contributing to the increase in diacylglycerol concentration and activation of protein kinase C. Shifts in the $NADP^+ \parallel NADPH$ system as a result of polyol pathway activity

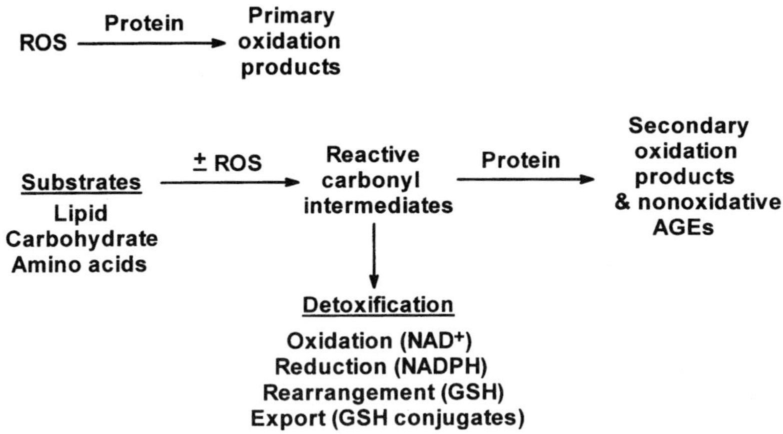

Figure 4 Reaction scheme illustrating the role of impaired detoxification pathways in increased formation of lipoxidation and glycoxidation products and nonoxidative AGEs in tissues in diabetes. The increase in substrate concentrations and impairment of detoxification systems, rather than increased oxidative stress, is considered the most significant factor contributing to the increased chemical modification of proteins in diabetes.

may limit the efficiency of NADPH-dependent reduction reactions (50), explaining the increase in both 3DG (30,31) and 3-deoxyfructose (51) in plasma of diabetic patients, and decreases in GSH (52). Similarly, the parallel increases in MGO, D-lactate and S-lactoylglutathione (40), in diabetic blood suggests an overload on the glyoxalase pathway in diabetes resulting from a combination of increased substrate flux, rate-limiting GSH production, and excessive GSH-conjugate efflux from tissues.

The combination of increased concentration of oxidizable substrates and decreased efficiency of detoxification pathways can cause an increase in the concentration of reactive carbonyl intermediates, even in the absence of an increase in OxS. The resultant increase in secondary oxidation products (lipoxidation and glycoxidation products) in tissues may appear, at first glance, to be the result of an increase in OxS. However, the increase in secondary oxidation products (lipoxidation and glycoxidation products) (13) without a corresponding increase in primary oxidation products (MetSO and *o*-tyrosine) (20) suggests that this is not the case in diabetes. At least in the early stages of the disease, before the appearance of overt complications, the increase in secondary oxidation products can be attributed to an increase in oxidizable substrates, coupled with insufficient detoxification activity, without invoking an increase in oxidative stress.

VI. IS THERE A RATIONALE FOR ANTIOXIDANT THERAPY IN DIABETES?

In principle, all chronic disease should respond to antioxidant therapy. In fact, however, antioxidant therapy has had limited impact on the progress of chronic diseases, such as chronic pulmonary disease, or autoimmune diseases, such as lupus erythematosus or rheumatoid arthritis. There is epidemiological evidence that antioxidants may limit atherogenesis, but alternative therapies, such as antihypertensive and lipid-lowering drugs, are substantially more effective than antioxidant therapy. Antioxidant therapy in autoimmune diseases is also symptomatic therapy, directed at limiting the damage rather than suppressing the pathogenic mechanism. Likewise, antioxidant therapy to address the fulminating OxS characteristic of advanced complications in diabetes may have limited effect in retarding the development of early diabetic complications. However, ''antioxidant'' therapy with agents such as *N*-acetylcysteine and lipoic (thioctic) acid, which yield an increase in cellular GSH, may provide protection against tissue damage by enhancing detoxification systems for reactive carbonyl compounds. GSH is a bifunctional coenzyme—it supports both antioxidant and other detoxification activities in the cell. It is oxidized (to GSSG) when it functions as a coenzyme for antioxidant reactions (e.g., in reduction of protein disulfides or in detoxification of hydrogen or organic peroxides) catalyzed by GSH peroxidase. However, GSH is regenerated intact when it participates in the glyoxalase pathway or as a substrate for GSH S-transferases. In these instances, it acts as a coenzyme, not as an antioxidant. The therapeutic benefits of *N*-acetylcysteine and lipoic acid therapy may therefore be attributable to their role in enhancing GSH-dependent detoxification rather than antioxidant pathways. At the same time, other antioxidants, such as ascorbate and vitamin E, may spare GSH for use in detoxification functions, providing some protective advantage to cells challenged by increase rates of reactive carbonyl formation in diabetes. The interplay between the antioxidant and carbonyl detoxification roles of GSH is critical for protecting the cell against both oxidative and carbonyl stress.

VII. SUMMARY AND CONCLUSION

In the foregoing discussion we have tried to define the nature of OxS and then, using that definition, to assess the status of OxS in diabetes. Based on analysis of various biomarkers of OxS in long-lived proteins, we conclude that OxS is not overtly or systemically increased in diabetes, except at later stages in the development of complications. Metabolic derangements in diabetes lead to an increase in concentration of oxidizable substrates and compromised detoxification pathways. The resulting increase in reactive carbonyls in tissues, known as carbonyl stress, leads directly to increased chemical modification of proteins in diabetes. Efforts directed at decreasing substrate concentration (maintenance of euglycemia and normolipidemia), bolstering detoxification pathways (GSH precursors or enhancers), and trapping reactive carbonyl species (AGE inhibitors, carbonyl traps) represent reasonable therapeutic approaches for limiting the chemical modification and crosslinking of proteins in diabetes and inhibiting the development of diabetic complications. Antioxidant vitamins and drugs may spare coenzymes for detoxification pathways during early stages of diabetes and may be useful as supportive therapy at later stages of the disease.

ACKNOWLEDGMENT

Supported by research grant DK-19971 from the National Institutes of Diabetes and Digestive and Kidney Diseases.

REFERENCES

1. Suzuki YJ, Forman HJ, Sevanian A. Oxidants as stimulators of signal transduction. Free Rad Biol Med 1997; 22:269–285.
2. Ghiselli A, Serafini M, Maiani G, Azzini E, Ferro-Luzzi A. A fluorescence-based method for measuring total plasma antioxidant capability. Free Rad Biol Med 1995; 18:29–36.
3. Tubaro F, Ghiselli A, Rapuzzi P, Maiorino M, Ursini F. Analysis of plasma antioxidant capacity by competition kinetics. Free Rad Biol Med 1998; 24:1228–1234.
4. Delmas-Beauvieux MC, Peuchant E, Thomas MJ, Dugourg L, Pinto AP, Clerc M, Gin H. The place of electron spin resonance methods in the detection of

oxidative stress in type 2 diabetes with poor glycemic control. Clin Biochem 1998; 31:221–228.
5. Beckman KB, Ames BN. Detection and quantification of oxidative adducts of mitochondrial DNA. Methods Enzymol 1996;264:442–453.
6. Cadet J, Berger M, Douki T, Ravanat JL. Oxidative damage to DNA: formation, measurement and biological significance. Rev Physiol Biochem Pharmacol 1997; 131:1–87.
7. Camhi SL, Lee P, Choi AM. The oxidative stress response. New Horizons 1995; 3:170–182.
8. Stadtman ER. Covalent modification reactions are marking steps in protein turnover. Biochemistry 1990; 29:6323–6331.
9. Requena JR, Fu MX, Ahmed MU, Jenkins AJ, Lyons TJ, Thorpe SR. Lipoxidation products as biomarkers of oxidative damage to proteins during lipid peroxidation reactions. Nephrol Dial Transplant 1996; 11(suppl 1):48–53.
10. Wells-Knecht KJ, Brinkmann E, Wells-Knecht MC, Ahmed MU, Zyzak DV, Thorpe SR, Baynes JW. New biomarkers of Maillard reaction damage to proteins. Nephrol Dial Transplant 1996; 11(suppl 5):41–47.
11. Baynes JW, Thorpe SR. The role of oxidative stress in diabetic complications: a new perspective on an old paradigm. Diabetes 1999; 48:1–9.
12. Ahmed MU, Brinkmann-Frye E, Degenhardt TP, Thorpe SR, Baynes JW. N^{ϵ}-(carboxyethyl)lysine, a product of chemical modification of protein by methylglyoxal, increases with age in human lens proteins. Biochem J 1997; 324:565–570.
13. Dyer DG, Dunn JA, Thorpe SR, Baillie KE, Lyons TJ, McCance DR, Baynes JW. Accumulation of Maillard reaction products in skin collagen in diabetes and aging. J Clin Invest 1993; 91:2463–2469.
14. Nakamura K, Nakazawa Y, Ienaga K. Acid-stable fluorescent advanced glycation end products: vesperlysines A, B, and C are formed as crosslinked products in the Maillard reaction between lysine or proteins with glucose. Biochem Biophys Res Commun 1997; 232:227–230.
15. Ienaga K, Nakamura K, Hochi T, Nakazawa Y, Fukunaga Y, Kakita H, Nakano K. Crosslines, fluorophores in AGE-related cross-linked proteins. Contrib Nephrol 1995; 112:42–51.
16. Requena JR, Fu M-X, Ahmed MU, Jenkins AJ, Lyons TJ, Baynes JW, Thorpe SR. Quantitation of malondialdehyde and 4-hydroxynonenal adducts to lysine residues in native and oxidized human low density lipoprotein. Biochem J 1997; 322:317–325.
17. Fu M-X, Requena JR, Jenkins AJ, Lyons TJ, Baynes JW, Thorpe SR. The advanced glycation end-product, N^{ϵ}-(carboxymethyl)lysine, is a product of both lipid peroxidation and glycoxidation reactions. J Biol Chem 1996; 271:9982–9986.
18. Hazen SL, Hsu FF, d'Avignon A, Heinecke JW. Human neutrophils employ myeloperoxidase to convert alpha-amino acids to a battery of reactive aldehydes: a pathway for aldehyde generation at sites of inflammation. Biochemistry 1998; 37:6864–6873.

19. Brinkmann Frye E, Degenhardt TP, Thorpe SR, Baynes JW. Role of the Maillard reaction in aging of tissue proteins: age-dependent increase in imidazolium cross-links in human lens protein. J Biol Chem 1998; 273:18714–18719.
20. Wells-Knecht MC, Lyons TJ, McCance DR, Thorpe SR, Baynes JW. Age-dependent accumulation of *ortho*-tyrosine and methionine sulfoxide in human skin collagen is not increased in diabetes: evidence against a generalized increase in oxidative stress in diabetes. J Clin Invest 1997; 100:839–846.
21. Halliwell B, Gutteridge JMC. Free Radicals in Biology and Medicine. 2d ed. Oxford: Clarendon Press, 1989.
22. Niwa T, Katsuzaki T, Miyazaki S, Miyazaki T, Ishizaki Y, Hayase F, Tatemichi N, Takei Y. Immunohistochemical detection of imidazolone, a novel advanced glycation end product, in kidneys and aortas of diabetic patients. J Clin Invest 1997; 99:1272–1280.
23. Horie K, Miyata T, Maeda K, Miyata S, Sugiyama S, Sakai H, van Ypersele C, Monnier VM, Witztum JL, Kurokawa K. Immunohistochemical colocalization of glycoxidation and lipid peroxidation products in diabetic renal disease: implication of glycoxidative stress in the pathogenesis of diabetic nephropathy. J Clin Invest 1997; 100:2995–3004.
24. Beckmann JS, Yao ZY, Anderson PG, Chen J, Accavitti MA, Tarpey MM, White CR. Extensive nitration of protein tyrosines in human atherosclerosis detected by immunohistochemistry. Biol Chem Hoppe-Seyler 1994; 375:81–86.
25. Hazen SL, Heinecke JW. 3-Chlorotyrosine, a specific marker of myeloperoxidase-catalyzed oxidation, is markedly elevated in low density lipoprotein isolated from human atherosclerotic plaque. J Clin Invest 1997; 99:2075–2081.
26. Haberland ME, Fong D, Cheng L. Malondialdehyde-altered protein occurs in atheroma of Watanabe heritable hyperlipidemic rabbits. Science 1988; 241:215–218.
27. Kume S, Takeya M, Mori T, Araki N, Suzuki H, Horiuchi S, Kodama T, Miyauchi Y, Takahashi K. Immunohistochemical and ultrastructural detection of advanced glycation end products in atherosclerotic lesions of human aorta with a novel specific monoclonal antibody. Am J Pathol 1995; 147:654–667.
28. Sayre LM, Zelasko DA, Harris PL, Perry G, Salomon RG, Smith MA. 4-Hydroxynonenal-derived advanced lipid peroxidation end products are increased in Alzheimer's disease. J Neurochem 1997; 68:2092–2097.
29. Stringer MD, Görög PG, Freeman A, Kakkar VV. Lipid peroxides and atherosclerosis. Br Med J 1989; 298:281–284.
30. Willems D, Dorchy H, Dufrasne D. Serum antioxidant status and oxidized LDL in well-controlled young type 1 diabetic patients and without subclinical complications. Atherosclerosis 1998; 137(suppl):S61–64.
31. Miyata T, Fu MX, Kurokawa K, van Ypersele C, Thorpe SR, Baynes JW. Autoxidation products of both carbohydrates and lipids are increased in uremic plasma: is the oxidative stress in uremia? Kidney Int 1998; 54:1290–1295.
32. Niwa T, Takeda H, Yoshizumi H, Tatematsu A, Ohara M, Timiyama S, Niimura

K. Presence of 3-deoxyglucosone, a potent protein crosslinking intermediate of the Maillard reaction. Biochem Biophys Res Commun 1993; 196:837–843.

33. Hamada Y, Nakamura J, Fujisawa H, Yago H, Nakashima E, Koh N, Hotta N. Effects of glycemic control on plasma 3-deoxyglucosone levels in NIDDM patients. Diabetes Care 1997; 20:1466–1469.
34. Hayashi T, Namiki M. Role of sugar fragmentation in the Maillard reaction. In: Fujimaki M, Namiki FM, Kato H, eds, Amino-carbonyl Reactions in Food and Biological Systems. Amsterdam: Elsevier, 1986:29–38.
35. Lal S, Szwergold BS, Taylor AH, Randall WC, Kappler F, Wells-Knecht KJ, Baynes JW, Brown TR. Metabolism of fructose 3-phosphate in the diabetic rat lens. Arch Biochem Biophys 1995; 318:191–199.
36. Niwa T, Katsuzaki T, Miyazaki S, Miyazaki T, Ishizaki Y, Hayase F, Tatemichi N, Takei Y. Immunohistochemical detection of imidazolone, a novel advanced glycation end product, in kidneys and aortas of diabetic patients. J Clin Invest 1997; 99:1272–1280.
37. Degenhardt TP, Thorpe SR, Baynes JW. Chemical modification of proteins by methylglyoxal. Cell Mol Biol 1998; 44:1139–1145.
38. Nagaraj RH, Shipanova IN, Faust FM. Protein crosslinking by the Maillard reaction. Isolation, characterization, and in vivo detection of a lysine-lysine crosslink derived from methylglyoxal. J Biol Chem 1996; 271:19339–19345.
39. Richard JP. Kinetic parameters for elimination reaction catalyzed by triosephosphate isomerase and an estimation of the reaction's physiological significance. Biochemistry 1991; 30:4581–4585.
40. Thornalley PJ. The glyoxalase system in health and disease. Mol Aspects Med 1993; 14:287–371.
41. Siems W, Grune T, Beierl B, Zollner H, Esterbauer H. The metabolism of 4-hydroxynonenal, a lipid peroxidation product, is dependent on tumor age in Ehrlich mouse ascites cells. In: Emerit I, Chance B, eds. Free Radicals and Aging. Basel: Birkhäuser, 1992:124–135.
42. Srivastava S, Chandra A, Wang LF, Seifert WE, DaGue BB, Ansari NH, Srivastava SK, Bhatnagar A. Metabolism of the lipid peroxidation product, 4-hydroxy-*trans*-2-nonenal, in isolated perfused rat heart. J Biol Chem 1998; 273:10893–10900.
43. Fujii E, Iwase H, Ishii-Karakasa I, Yajima Y, Hotta K. The presence of 2-keto-3-deoxygluconic acid and oxoaldehyde dehydrogenase activity in human erythrocytes. Biochem Biophys Res Commun 1995; 210:852–857.
44. Kato H, van Chuyen N, Shinoda T, Sekiya F, Hayase F. Metabolism of 3-deoxyglucosone, an intermediate compound in the Maillard reaction, administered orally or intravenously to rats. Biochim Biophys Acta 1990; 1035:71–76.
45. Kanazu T, Shinoda M, Nakayama T, Deyashiki Y, Hara A, Sawada H. Aldose reductase is a major protein associated with 3-deoxyglucosone reductase activity in rat, pig and human livers. Biochem J 1991; 279:903–906.
46. Srivastava S, Chandra A, Bhatnagar A, Srivastava S, Ansari NH. Lipid peroxidation product, 4-hydroxynonenal and its conjugate with GSH are excellent sub-

strates of bovine lens aldose reductase. Biochem Biophys Res Commun 1995; 217:741–746.

47. Ishikawa T, Esterbauer H, Sies H. Role of cardiac glutathione transferase and of the glutathione S-conjugate export system in biotransformation of 4-hydroxynonenal in the heart. J Biol Chem 1986; 261:1576–1581.
48. Williamson JR, Chang K, Frangos M, Hasan KS, Ido Y, Kawamura T, Nyengaard JR, Van den Enden M, Kilo C, Tilton RG. Hyperglycemic pseudohypoxia and diabetic complications. Diabetes 1993; 42:801–813.
49. Ido Y, Kilo C, Williamson JR. Cytosolic NADH/NAD^+, free radicals, and vascular dysfunction in early diabetes mellitus. Diabetologia 1997; 40:S115–S117.
50. Bravi MC, Pietrangeli P, Laurenti O, Basili S, Cassone-Faldetta M, Ferri C, De Mattia G. Polyol pathway activation and glutathione redox status in non-insulin-dependent diabetic patients. Metabolism 1997; 46:1194–1198.
51. Wells-Knecht KJ, Lyons TJ, McCance DR, Thorpe SR, Feather MS, Baynes JW. 3-Deoxyfructose concentrations are increased in human plasma and urine in diabetes. Diabetes 1994; 43:1152–1156.
52. Samiec PS, Drews-Botsch C, Flagg EW, Kurtz JC, Sternberg P Jr, Reed RL, Jones DP. Glutathione in human plasma: decline in association with aging, age-related macular degeneration, and diabetes. Free Rad Biol Med 1998; 24:699–704.

7

Antioxidative Defense in Diabetic Peripheral Nerve: Effects of DL-α-Lipoic Acid, Aldose Reductase Inhibitor, and Sorbitol Dehydrogenase Inhibitor

Irina G. Obrosova and Douglas A. Greene
University of Michigan Medical Center, Ann Arbor, Michigan

Hans-Jochen Lang
Hoechst Marion Roussel, Frankfurt, Germany

Diabetes-induced oxidative stress in target tissues for diabetic complications, including peripheral nerve, results from at least three mechanisms (Fig. 1), including glucose autooxidation, formation of advanced glycation end products, and increased aldose reductase (AR) activity (1). The contribution of oxidative stress to peripheral diabetic neuropathy has been well established (1–6). Diabetes-induced oxidative stress leads to decreased endoneurial blood flow with resulting endoneurial hypoxia (1–4,6,7). Increased formation of reactive oxygen species (ROS) impairs neurotrophic support (8) and causes redox imbalances (9), energy deficiency (9), and perhaps defects in ion-transport mechanisms, which theoretically can be both mediated by and be independent of the corresponding changes in nerve blood flow.

Although the role of oxidative stress in diabetes-induced nerve vascular dysfunction and nerve conduction deficits is no longer a subject for debate, there is still a number of questions that need to be addressed. It is still unclear

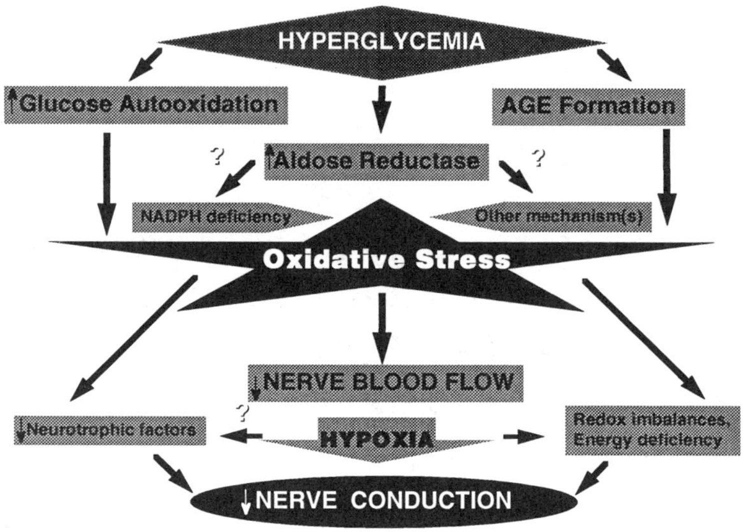

Figure 1 Mechanisms and pathogenetic consequences of oxidative stress in diabetic peripheral nerve.

(and no consensus has been reached so far) what the relative contribution of oxidative stress-linked defects in endoneurial blood flow, metabolism, and neurotrophic support to nerve conduction deficits is. It remains to be established whether ROS-induced neurovascular dysfunction and resulting endoneurial hypoxia mediate the diabetes-induced decrease in neurotrophic support as they, at least partially, mediate metabolic defects (10), considering that the levels of substance P (a product of nerve growth factor [NGF]-influenced gene in primary afferents) in the nerve are decreased under hypoxic conditions (11). Mechanisms leading from hyperglycemia to increased ROS formation require further studies as well. In particular, the relative contribution of the three aforementioned ROS-generating mechanisms to diabetes-induced nerve free radical damage remains to be identified. Little information is available on the changes in antioxidative defense enzymes (1) and mechanisms of their downregulation in diabetic peripheral nerve and a possibility of modulation of their activity with antioxidants and other pharmacological interventions. In addition, the role for AR in diabetes-induced changes in nerve antioxidant status needs further studies because reports (2,12) indicate an inconsistency between marked depletion of nerve total glutathione (TG) versus very minor increase in oxidized glutathione (GSSG) in diabetes and restoration of TG levels with

AR inhibitor (ARI) treatment, which points to the contribution of other AR-dependent mechanism(s) in addition to or instead of AR-mediated NADPH deficiency to nerve antioxidant deficit. Also, it remains to be established whether there is any role for the second enzyme of the sorbitol pathway, sorbitol dehydrogenase, in diabetes-induced nerve oxidative injury.

Some of the aforementioned questions were addressed in the present study, which was designed to identify diabetes-related deficits of peripheral nerve antioxidative defense enzymes; to evaluate a role of oxidative stress in impairment of protective mechanisms against superoxide, hydrogen peroxide, and semiquinone radical-induced oxidative injury by assessing a possibility of preventing downregulation of superoxide dismutase, catalase, and total quinone reductase by antioxidant DL-α-lipoic acid; and to compare the effects of ARI and sorbitol dehydrogenase inhibitor (SDI) on parameters of oxidative stress and antioxidative defense in diabetes and thus to identify the role for two enzymes of the sorbitol pathway in diabetes-induced nerve oxidative injury.

I. MATERIALS AND METHODS

Experiments were performed in accordance with regulations specified by the National Institutes of Health 1985 revised version of the principles of laboratory animal care and University of Michigan Protocol for Animal Studies.

A. Animals

Barrier-sustained cesarean-delivered male Wistar rats (Charles River, Wilmington, MA), body weight 250–300 g, were fed a standard rat chow diet (ICN Biomedicals, Cleveland, OH) and had ad libitum access to water. Diabetes was induced by a single intraperitoneal injection of streptozotocin (Upjohn, Kalamazoo, MI, 55 mg/kg body weight, IP, in 0.2 mL of 10 mM citrate buffer, pH 5.5) to animals that were fasted overnight. Blood samples for measurements of glucose were taken from the tail vein ~48 h after streptozotocin injection and the day before they were killed. The rats with blood glucose ≥250 mg/dL were considered diabetics, and the treatments were started ~48 h after streptozotocin injection. Three experiments were performed. In experiment 1, the experimental groups included control, 6-week diabetic, and 6-week diabetic rats treated with DL-α-lipoic acid (Sigma, 100 mg/kg body weight/day, IP, 5 days a week). Experiment 2 was performed in control, 3-week diabetic, and 3-week diabetic rats treated with the SDI-157 (Hoechst

Marion Roussel, 100 mg/kg body weight/day, in the drinking water). In experiment 3, the groups included control, 6-week diabetic, and 6-week diabetic rats treated with the ARI sorbinil (Pfizer, 65 mg/kg body weight/day, in the diet, for 2 weeks, after 4 weeks of untreated diabetes).

B. Reagents

Unless otherwise stated, all chemicals were of reagent-grade quality and were purchased from Sigma Chemical (St. Louis, MO). Methanol (high-performance liquid chromatography grade), perchloric acid, hydrochloric acid, and sodium hydroxide were purchased from Fisher Scientific (Pittsburgh, PA). Ethyl alcohol (200 proof dehydrated alcohol, U.S.P. punctilious) was purchased from Quantum Chemical Company (Tiscola, IL).

C. Experimental Procedure

Rats from each group were sedated with carbon dioxide and subsequently killed by cervical dislocation. Both nerves were rapidly dissected, carefully blotted with fine filter paper to remove any accompanying blood, and frozen in liquid nitrogen for subsequent biochemical analyses. In experiment 1, we measured levels of sorbitol pathway intermediates (glucose, sorbitol, fructose) and activities of antioxidative defense enzymes, including superoxide dismutase (SOD), catalase, glutathione reductase (GSSGRed), glutathione transferase (GSHTrans), total quinone reductase (TQR), and DT-diaphorase. In experiment 2 and 3, in addition to the above-mentioned sorbitol pathway intermediates and antioxidative defense enzyme activities (except DT-diaphorase), measurements of total MDA and 4-hydroxyalkenal and reduced glutathione (GSH) levels and glutathione peroxidase (GSH-Px) activities were performed.

D. Biochemical Measurements

1. Measurements of Sorbitol Pathway Intermediates

Nerve segments (~20 mg) were weighed and homogenized in 0.8 mL 0.9% NaCl. A 100-µL volume of 0.3 M zinc sulfate, followed by an equivalent of barium hydroxide, was then added to homogenate for protein precipitation. The samples were centrifuged at 4000 × *g* for 10 min (Sorvall MC 12V), and aliquots of the supernatant were taken for spectrofluorometric measurements of glucose, sorbitol, and fructose by enzymatic procedures, using hexokinase/glucose 6-phosphate dehydrogenase (13), sorbitol dehydrogenase

(14), and fructose dehydrogenase (15). In brief, the analytical mixture for glucose contained 0.9 mL of 1 mM $MgCl_2$, 0.5 mM dithiothreitol, 300 μM ATP, 5 μM NADP, and 0.02 U/mL glucose 6-phosphate dehydrogenase in 25 mM Tris-HCl buffer, pH 8.1, and deproteinized extract (0.1 mL for control and 0.02 plus 0.08 mL H_2O for diabetic nerves). The reaction was initiated by addition of ~0.14 U of hexokinase. Initial and final readings were taken at λ excitation 340 nm, λ emission 460 nm, slits 20 and 15 (spectrofluorometer Perkin-Elmer LS-5B), and were compared with the corresponding glucose standards (0.5–10 × 10^{-9} M) processed in the same run. The analytical mixture for sorbitol contained 0.8 mL 0.5 mM NAD in 0.1 M glycine-NaOH buffer (pH 9.5) and deproteinized extract (0.2 mL for control and 0.05 mL plus 0.15 mL H_2O for diabetic nerves). The reaction was started by addition of ~0.8 U of sorbitol dehydrogenase. Initial and final readings were taken at λ excitation 340 nm, λ emission 460 nm, slits 20 and 15. The analytical mixture for fructose contained 0.9 mL of rezasurin-containing 150 mM citrate buffer, pH 4.5 (1 aliquot of rezasurin [5 mg–10 mL H_2O] was mixed with 100 aliquots of citrate buffer), and deproteinized extract (0.1 mL for control and 0.05 mL plus 0.05 mL H_2O for diabetic nerves). The reaction was started by addition of ~0.5 U of fructose dehydrogenase. Initial and final readings were taken at λ excitation 572 nm, λ emission 585, slits 5 and 5. The differences in initial and final readings for tested samples were compared with those with corresponding sets of standards for glucose, sorbitol, and fructose (0.1–10 × 10^{-9} M) processed in the same run.

2. *Measurements of GSH*

Nerve segments (~15–20 mg) were weighed, homogenized in 1 mL of ice-cold 6% $HClO_4$, and centrifuged at 4000 × *g* for 10 min. After centrifugation, the samples were immediately neutralized with 5M K_2CO_3 to pH 6–7 and were centrifuged again at 4000 × *g* for 5 min to precipitate insoluble $KClO_4$. A total of 0.1 mL of extract was mixed with 0.89 mL of 20 mM EDTA in 1.0 M Tris-HCl buffer (pH 8.1), and the reaction was initiated by addition of 0.01 mL of *o*-phthaldialdehyde (10 mg–1 mL methanol). Initial and final readings were taken at λ excitation 345 nm, λ emission 425 nm, slits 5 and 5. The differences in initial and final readings were compared with those in corresponding GSH standards (1–10 × 10^{-9} M) processed in the same run.

3. *Measurements of Total MDA and 4-Hydroxyalkenal*

Measurements of total malondialdehyde (MDA) and 4-hydroxyalkenal levels were performed using kits from Oxis International, Inc. (LPO-586 assay). The method is based on the reaction of a chromogenic reagent, *N*-methyl-2-phenylindole, with MDA and 4-hydroxyalkenals at 45 °C. The samples were prepared by homogenization of preweighed nerve segments (~40 mg) in 1 mL of 20 mM Tris buffer, pH 7.4, containing 5 mM butylated hydroxytoluene a total of 200 μL of homogenate was used for measurements of total MDA and 4-hydroxyalkenal levels according to the procedure described in detail in the kit. The absorbance of chromogenic product was measured at 586 nm (spectrophotometer Beckman DU 640) and was compared with the absorbance in corresponding 4-hydroxyalkenal standards.

4. *Measurements of Antioxidative Defense Enzyme Activities*

For measurements of antioxidative defense enzyme activities, ~30 mg of frozen sciatic nerves were homogenized in 2 mL of ice-cold 0.1 M sodium-phosphate buffer, pH 6.5 (16). Homogenates were centrifuged at 20,000 × *g*, and supernatant fraction was used for assays of enzymatic activities and protein content. Protein levels were quantified with the Pierce BCA protein assay kits (Rockford, IL). SOD activity was measured by following spectrophotometrically (at 480 nm) the autooxidation of (−)-epinephrine at pH 10.4 (17). The reaction mixture contained 0.8 mL 50 mM glycine buffer, pH 10.4, and 0.2 mL supernatant. The reaction was started by addition of 0.02 ml of (−)-epinephrine (due to poor solubility of (−)-epinephrine in water, the solution was prepared by suspending 40 mg of the compound in 2 mL water and then by adding two to three drops of 2 N HCl). SOD activity was expressed as nmol of (−)-epinephrine protected from oxidation after addition of the sample compared with the corresponding readings in the blank cuvette. The molar extinction coefficient of 4.02 mM^{-1} cm^{-1} was used for calculations. Catalase activity was measured by following spectrophotometrically (at 240 nm) for 5 min the decrease in absorbance of hydrogen peroxide after addition of 0.1 mL of supernatant to 0.9 mL of H_2O_2-containing 50 mM phosphate buffer, pH 6.8. The enzyme activity was calculated using 2.04 mM^{-1} cm^{-1} as molar extinction coefficient. GSHTrans activity toward 1-chloro-2,4-dinitrobenzene (CDNB) was measured according to Habig et al. (18). A total of 0.8 mL of the reaction mixture contained 0.1 M sodium-phosphate buffer, pH 6.5, 1 mM GSH, 1 mM CDNB (preliminary dissolved in ethanol), and 1 mM EDTA. The reaction was started by addition of 0.2 mL supernatant and was monitored spectrophotometrically at 340 nm for 5 min. Calculations were performed using extinction coefficient of 9.6 mM^{-1} cm^{-1}. GSSGRed activity was measured spectrophotometrically at 340 nm by monitoring NADPH oxidation coupled to reduction of GSSG to GSH; 0.8 mL of the reaction mixture contained 0.1 M potassium-phosphate buffer, pH 7.0, 2.5 mM GSSG, and 125 μM NADPH. The reaction was started by addition of 0.2 mL of the sample and was monitored for 5 min. The calculations were performed by using a molar extinction coefficient of 6.22 mM^{-1} cm^{-1}. Total quinone reductase and DT-diaphorase activities were measured with ρ-benzoquinone as a substrate and Twin-20 as an activator as described in detail by Ernster et al. (19).

E. Statistical Analysis

The results are expressed as means ± SD. In experiment 1, differences among experimental groups were determined by ANOVA, and the significance of differences between these groups assessed by the Student-Newman-Keuls multiple range test. Significance was defined at $p = 0.05$. In experiments 2 and 3, analysis of the parameters was performed (on natural logarithm transformed data) with the SAS general linear models procedure. Overall differences among experimental groups for each parameter were first assessed by the Van der Waerden test; individual pairwise comparisons were evaluated by least-square means analysis only if the Van der Waerden test was significant at $p < 0.05$ for a given parameter. A nonparametric Blom transformation of all data was performed before assessment of individual pairwise group differences. Uncorrected p values based on two-tailed tests of significance are shown for the relevant comparisons.

II. RESULTS

The body weights were lower in diabetic rats compared with those in controls (experiment 1, 327.3 ± 50.9 vs. 420.4 ± 27.0 g, $p < 0.01$; experiment 2, 313.6 ± 25.7 vs. 372.8 ± 20.8 g, $p < 0.05$; and experiment 3, 300.1 ± 44.1 vs. 428.3 ± 17.9 g, $p < 0.01$). The initial body weights were similar in control and diabetic groups in all three experiments (not shown). No statistically significant difference was found between body weights in diabetic rats treated with DL-α-lipoic acid (305.5 ± 32.0 g), SDI (308.5 ± 32.6 g), or ARI (307.8 ± 65.2 g) and the corresponding untreated groups.

Blood glucose levels were markedly increased in diabetic rats compared with those in controls (experiment 1, 340.0 ± 60.3 vs. 66.8 ± 9.3 mg/dL; experiment 2, 334.1 ± 62.3 vs. 71.4 ± 10.5 mg/dL; and experiment 3, 326.3 ± 42.7 vs. 58.2 ± 5.0; $p < 0.001$ for all three comparisons). Blood glucose levels in diabetic rats were not affected by DL-α-lipoic acid (322.6 ± 43.5 mg/dL), SDI (348.5 ± 87.0 mg/dL), or ARI (332.7 ± 38.5 mg/dL).

Table 1 The Levels of Glucose, Sorbitol, and Fructose (μmol/g wet weight) in the Sciatic Nerve of Control and Diabetic Rats Treated With/Without DL-α-Lipoic Acid (LA) (n = 7–8)

	Control	Diabetic	Diabetic + LA
Glucose	3.54 ± 0.69	10.46 ± 2.32*	19.44 ± 3.79†
Sorbitol	0.260 ± 0.091	1.34 ± 0.51*	2.14 ± 0.88‡
Fructose	2.00 ± 0.42	7.47 ± 1.23*	10.12 ± 1.20‡

* Significantly different compared with those in controls ($p < 0.0001$).

†‡ Significantly different compared with those in untreated diabetics ($p < 0.01$ and 0.001, respectively).

Nerve glucose, sorbitol, and fructose levels in control and diabetic rats treated with/without DL-α-lipoic acid are presented in Table 1. Glucose, sorbitol, and fructose levels in diabetic rats were increased 3.9-, 19.6-, and 6.4-fold, respectively, compared with those in controls. DL-α-Lipoic acid treatment further increased levels of glucose, sorbitol, and fructose (1.9-, 1.6-, and 1.4-fold, respectively, compared with those in untreated diabetics).

Nerve glucose, sorbitol, and fructose levels in control and diabetic rats treated with/without SDI are presented in Table 2. Glucose, sorbitol, and fructose levels in diabetic rats were increased 3.6-, 11.1-, and 5.5-fold, respectively, compared with those in controls. Glucose levels were indistinguishable in diabetic rats treated with/without SDI. Sorbitol levels in the SDI-treated diabetic rats were increased 4.4-fold compared with those in untreated diabetics, whereas fructose levels were markedly reduced but not completely normalized.

Table 2 The Levels of Glucose, Sorbitol, and Fructose (μmol/g wet weight) in the Sciatic Nerve of Control and 3-Week Diabetic Rats Treated With/Without SDI (n = 7–8)

	Control	Diabetic	Diabetic + SDI
Glucose	3.24 ± 0.94	11.78 ± 4.17*	11.32 ± 2.78†
Sorbitol	0.149 ± 0.034	1.65 ± 0.36*	7.34 ± 1.77‡
Fructose	1.22 ± 0.15	6.66 ± 2.10*	1.73 ± 0.77‡

* Significantly different compared with those in controls ($p < 0.0001$).

†‡ Significantly different compared with those in untreated diabetics ($p < 0.01$ and 0.001, respectively).

Table 3 The Levels of Glucose, Sorbitol, and Fructose (μmol/g wet weight) in the Sciatic Nerve of Control and 6-Week Diabetic Rats Treated With/Without ARI (n = 7–8)

	Control	Diabetic	Diabetic + ARI
Glucose	3.58 ± 0.44	13.43 ± 2.44*	13.54 ± 1.78†
Sorbitol	0.128 ± 0.045	1.36 ± 0.37*	0.062 ± 0.042‡
Fructose	1.29 ± 0.40	6.54 ± 0.19*	1.21 ± 0.33‡

* Significantly different compared with those in controls ($p < 0.0001$).
‡ Significantly different compared with those in untreated diabetics ($p < 0.01$ and 0.001, respectively).

Nerve glucose, sorbitol, and fructose levels in control and diabetic rats treated with/without ARI are presented in Table 3. Glucose, sorbitol, and fructose levels in diabetic rats were increased 3.8-, 10.6-, and 5.1-fold over those in controls. Glucose levels in diabetic rats were not affected by the ARI treatment, whereas sorbitol levels were decreased below those in nondiabetic controls and fructose levels were normalized.

Nerve total MDA and 4-hydroxyalkenal levels in control and diabetic rats treated with/without ARI and SDI are presented in Fig. 2, A and B. Total MDA and 4-hydroxyalkenal levels were increased in both 3-week diabetic rats and 6-week diabetic rats vs. controls ($p < 0.02$ and <0.001, respectively). The increase in 6-week diabetic rats was completely corrected by the ARI treatment ($p < 0.001$ vs. untreated diabetics), whereas the increase in 3-week

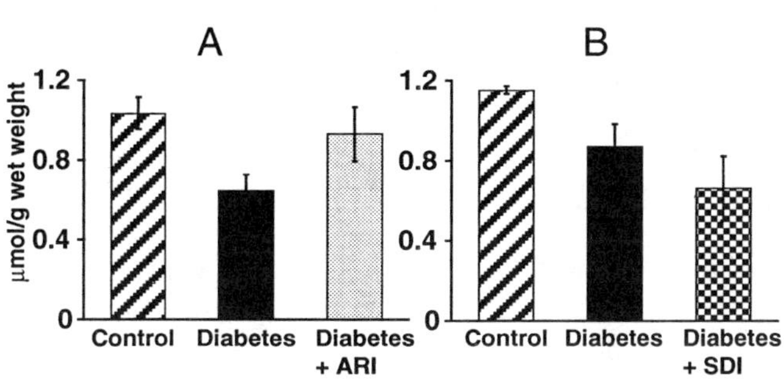

Figure 2 Total MDA and 4-hydroxyalkenal levels in sciatic nerve of control and diabetic rats treated with or without ARI (A) or SDI (B) (mean ± SD, n = 8–12).

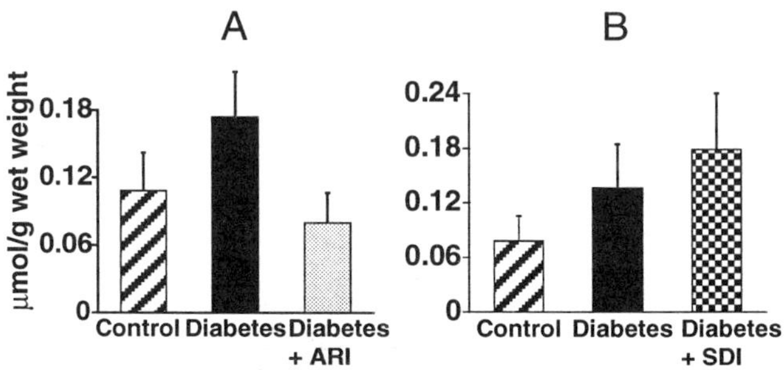

Figure 3 GSH levels in sciatic nerve of control and diabetic rats treated with or without ARI (A) or SDI (B) (mean ± SD, n = 8–12).

diabetic rats further progressed with the SDI treatment ($p < 0.03$ vs. untreated diabetics)

Nerve GSH levels in control and diabetic rats treated with/without ARI and SDI are presented in Fig. 3, A and B. GSH levels were decreased by 23.4% and 37.6% in 3-week and 6-week diabetic rats vs. corresponding controls ($p < 0.002$ and <0.001, respectively). The decrease in 6-week diabetic rats was completely corrected by the ARI treatment ($p < 0.001$ vs. untreated diabetics), whereas the decrease in 3-week diabetic rats further progressed with the SDI treatment ($p < 0.02$ vs. untreated diabetics).

Antioxidative defense enzyme activities in control and diabetic rats treated with/without DL-α-lipoic acid are presented in Table 4. SOD, catalase,

Table 4 Antioxidative Enzyme Activities in the Sciatic Nerve of Control and 6-Week Diabetic Rats Treated With/Without DL-α-Lipoic Acid (LA) (nmol/mg protein per min, n = 5–8).

	Control	Diabetic	Diabetic + LA
SOD	95.9 ± 18.9	70.5 ± 9.8*	136.8 ± 55.8†
Catalase	109.7 ± 28.6	77.4 ± 19.8*	122.9 ± 31.5‡
GSHTrans	39.6 ± 15.9	57.7 ± 12.9	56.3 ± 19.8
GSSGRed	9.0 ± 2.6	10.5 ± 3.0	12.0 ± 3.6
TQRed	174.9 ± 29.7	131.2 ± 32.8*	170.4 ± 44.2†
DT-diaphorase	119.7 ± 25.8	123.8 ± 30.8	119.7 ± 30.9

* Significantly different compared with those in controls ($p < 0.05$).
†‡ Significantly different compared with those in untreated diabetics ($p < 0.05$ and <0.01).

Table 5 Antioxidative Enzyme Activities in the Sciatic Nerve of Control and 3-Week Diabetic Rats Treated With/Without SDI (nmol/mg protein per min, n = 8–10)

	Control	Diabetic	Diabetic + SDI
SOD	50.8 ± 17.8	73.0 ± 26.4	93.0 ± 31.8*
Catalase	194.6 ± 56.6	195.2 ± 50.2	300.1 ± 82.3*†
GSHTrans	39.3 ± 4.9	31.5 ± 2.8‡	30.4 ± 3.6§
GSSGRed	21.6 ± 3.5	18.3 ± 2.6	16.5 ± 2.5‡
GSH-Px	13.7 ± 3.6	9.8 ± 4.6	17.1 ± 8.6†
TQRed	313.9 ± 52.3	236.8 ± 22.5‖	193.5 ± 39.2‡¶

*‡§‖ Significantly different compared with those in controls (p < 0.05, <0.01, <0.001, and <0.0001, respectively).

†¶ Significantly different compared with those in untreated diabetics (p < 0.05 and <0.01, respectively).

and TQRed activities were decreased in 6-week diabetic rats vs. controls, whereas GSHTrans, GSSGRed, and DT-diaphorase activities were indistinguishable between the two groups. DL-α-Lipoic acid treatment prevented diabetes-induced downregulation of SOD, catalase, and TQRed and did not affect GSHTrans, GSSGRed, and DT-diaphorase.

Antioxidative defense enzyme activities in control and 3-week diabetic rats treated with/without SDI are presented in Table 5. SOD, catalase, GSH-

Table 6 Antioxidative Enzyme Activities in the Sciatic Nerve of Control and 6-Week Diabetic Rats Treated With/Without ARI (nmol/mg protein per min, n = 8–10)

	Control	Diabetic	Diabetic + ARI
SOD	89.7 ± 22.5	64.7 ± 8.5*	76.9 ± 11.6†‡
Catalase	102.0 ± 37.1	71.6 ± 13.4*	76.8 ± 17.5*
GSHTrans	33.8 ± 4.5	44.5 ± 10.8	36.2 ± 4.4
GSSGRed	13.1 ± 1.9	12.2 ± 2.5	12.1 ± 2.5
GSH-Px	11.2 ± 2.2	13.0 ± 4.8	11.3 ± 1.7
TQRed	197.8 ± 64.4	134.6 ± 38.2*	160.4 ± 25.3§‖

*†§ Significantly different compared with those in controls (p < 0.05, <0.01, and <0.001, respectively).

‡‖ Significantly different compared with those in untreated diabetics (p < 0.05 and <0.01, respectively).

Px, and GSSGRed activities were similar in control and 3-week diabetic rats. SOD, catalase, and GSH-Px were increased in SDI-treated diabetic rats compared with untreated diabetic group, whereas GSSGRed activity was slightly decreased. TQRed and GSHTrans were decreased in 3-week diabetic rats vs. controls, and TQRed but not GSHTrans activity was further decreased by the SDI treatment.

Antioxidative defense enzyme activities in control and 6-week diabetic rats treated with/without ARI are presented in Table 6. Similar to experiment 1, SOD, catalase, and TQRed activities were decreased in the diabetic group vs. controls, whereas GSH-Px, GSSGRed, and GSHTrans remained unaffected. The ARI treatment partially corrected SOD and TQRed but not catalase activity. GSH-Px, GSSGRed, and GSHTrans activities were indistinguishable between the SDI-treated and untreated diabetic groups.

III. DISCUSSION

The findings of the present study are indicative of increased vulnerability of diabetic peripheral nerve to free radical-induced oxidative damage and are consistent with the studies of Low and colleagues (1,20,21), demonstrating accumulation of conjugated dienes and lipid peroxide, reduction of GSH levels and Cu,Zn-SOD activity, and changes of other markers of oxidative stress in nerve in the model of streptozotocin-induced diabetes. Comparison of Tables 5 and 6 suggests that antioxidative defense enzyme activities, especially those of SOD, catalase, GSSGRed, and TQRed, are age-dependent [consistent with observations of age dependence for other parameters related to oxidative stress (20)]. Also, it is important to point out that diabetes-induced changes in most parameters in the present study revealed strong dependence on the duration of diabetes. For example, depletion of GSH, the major biological antioxidant, progressed with the duration of diabetes, being more advanced in 6-week than in 3-week diabetic model. SOD, catalase, and TQRed activities remained within the normal range in 3-week diabetic rats but were markedly reduced in 6-week diabetic rats, whereas, on the contrary, GSHTrans deficit appeared to be transient and was present in the 3-week but not in the 6-week model of streptozotocin diabetes. Another important characteristic of diabetes-induced impairment of antioxidative defense is its selectivity, manifested by deficits in SOD, catalase, and TQRed coexisting (in 6-week diabetes) with normal GSSGRed, GSHTrans, and diaphorase activities. Although the significance of these changes for diabetes-induced increased ROS production and antioxidative defense against certain free radical species still remains to be established, the finding of the diabetes-induced deficit in TQRed together with normal DT-diaphorase activity [DT-diaphorase represents a cytoplasmic component of TQRed [19)] is probably indicative of increased attack of semiquinone free radicals (16) (very strong reducing agents that can also rapidly react with molecular oxygen generating the superoxide anion radical, O_2) in mitochondria and is consistent with the concept that mitochondria are a primary target for oxidative damage (1). It is also interesting that only those enzymes that are affected by diabetes respond to antioxidant (DL-α-lipoic acid) treatment.

The latter observation is consistent with the report of Maitra et al. (22) that demonstrated restoration of buthionine sulfoximine-induced catalase and GSH-Px deficits with α-lipoic acid treatment and with studies in other models of oxidative stress (23,24), suggesting a possibility of posttranslational down-regulation of some antioxidative defense enzymes by oxidative modification of their proteins. The concept of posttranslational regulation of antioxidative defense enzymes in diabetic peripheral nerve is supported by recent unpublished findings of Phillip Low's laboratory demonstrating the lack of any effect of streptozotocin-diabetes of different duration on Cu,Zn-SOD, Mn-SOD, GSSGRed, and GSH-Px mRNAs. The finding of a marked upregulation of SOD by α-lipoic acid in diabetic peripheral nerve in the present study is different from reports for other tissues in other models of oxidative stress (22,25), demonstrating the lack of correcting effect of α-lipoic acid on SOD activity. Based on this apparent discrepancy, it is possible to suggest the indirect modulation of SOD by α-lipoic acid in diabetic peripheral nerve, probably via NGF, which is known to both upregulate and replace SOD in some types of oxidative injury (26,27). This assumption is supported by the findings of decreased NGF levels in diabetic peripheral nerve and of partial prevention of diabetes-induced deficit in neurotrophic support with DL-α-lipoic acid treatment (28).

The elevated levels of total MDA and 4-hydroxyalkenals (products of lipid peroxidation) are consistent with the presence of peripheral nerve oxidative injury in both 3-week and 6-week streptozotocin-diabetic rat models. As MDA levels were reported (20) to be similar in control and diabetic rats (regardless of duration of diabetes), the increase in lipid aldehyde level in the present study probably reflects the accumulation of 4-hydroxy-2,3-transnonenal (HNE), a major toxic product of lipid peroxidation (29). Interestingly and surprisingly, the lipid aldehyde level is normalized by ARI despite the fact that AR has been reported to be involved in HNE metabolism (29). A possible explanation can be derived from a comparison of the results of the present study with the recent report of Srivastava et al. (30) for isolated perfused hearts from nondiabetic rats, indicating that the major metabolic transformations of HNE involve conjugation with glutathione and oxidation to 4-hydroxy-2-nonenoic acid and providing evidence that sorbinil does not affect formation of glutathione-HNE conjugates (at the same time, preventing their further AR-mediated reduction to glutathione-1,4-dihydroxy-2-nonene) and stimulates HNE oxidation to 4-hydroxy-*trans*-2-nonenoic acid. Based on these findings and assuming that the pathways of HNE metabolism are similar in heart and peripheral nerve, one would expect to find an accumulation of HNE in peripheral nerve under diabetic conditions [characterized by depletion of GSH (2, and in the present study) and by a decrease in the free cytosolic $NAD^+/NADH$ ratio (9,31) that may affect NAD-dependent oxidation of HNE to 4-hydroxy-*trans*-2-nonenoic acid by aldehyde dehydrogenase], which is consistent with the results of the present study. Also, taking into consideration that ARI treatment corrects both GSH levels (12, and in the present study) and the redox state of free cytosolic NAD-couple (31), the metabolic basis for prevention of total MDA and 4-hydroxyalkenal accumulation by sorbinil treatment becomes understandable.

The importance of GSH for neutralization of toxic products of lipid peroxidation is confirmed by the experiments with SDI, which effectively (by ~90.8%) inhibited increased flux through sorbitol dehydrogenase in the 3-week streptozotocin-diabetic rat model. GSH depletion in 3-week streptozotocin-diabetic rats was further exacerbated by the SDI treatment, which is consistent with a further accumulation of HNE over the level in the untreated diabetic group. A more advanced GSH depletion in the SDI-treated diabetic rats compared with the corresponding untreated group is consistent with the findings of Geisen et al. (32) for diabetic lens. These findings implicate sorbitol accumulation-linked osmotic stress in the mechanisms underlying increased vulnerability of diabetic peripheral nerve to oxidative injury and are in accordance with other reports demonstrating the inconsistency between a substantial (~40%) depletion of GSH versus a very minor (2) or an absent (12) depletion of GSSG, which calls into question the importance of glutathione redox cycling mechanism in diabetes-induced GSH depletion. In addition, total glutathione depletion in the diabetic nerve and correction of both total and reduced glutathione levels by ARIs (12, and in the present study) points to the involvement of other AR mediated mechanisms in addition to (or instead of) NADPH deficiency to nerve GSH deficit. It is important to point out that involvement of the osmotic factor in GSH depletion in the diabetic nerve does not necessarily mean increased GSH leakage from the endoneurium (although some studies for the lens (33) implicated decreased amino acid uptake and increased GSH efflux under hypersmotic conditions in the GSH deficit). We suggest that osmotic stress can be involved in diabetes-induced energy deficiency

(9,10) and, considering that ATP is required for both γ-glutamyl cysteine synthetase and glutathione synthetase reactions, contributes to diabetes-related GSH deficit through the impairment of cofactor supply of GSH biosynthesis. The assumption regarding the link between sorbitol accumulation-linked osmotic stress and energy deficiency in diabetic peripheral nerve is supported by observations in DL-α-lipoic acid-treated diabetic rats, demonstrating an increased sorbitol accumulation and the lack of prevention of nerve energy deficiency despite correction of both mitochondrial and cytosolic redox state of NAD couple (9,34) and by the findings of exacerbated decrease of nerve phosphocreatine/creatine ratio (a marker of free cytosolic ATP/ADP ratio) in diabetic rats treated with SDI (CP-166,572, Pfizer, 200 mg/kg/day in the drinking water), which had nerve sorbitol levels exceeding those in untreated diabetics ~6.3-fold (Obrosova, 1996, unpublished observations).

It has been suggested (35) that diabetes-induced increase in flux through sorbitol dehydrogenase causes increase in free cytosolic NADH/NAD^+ ratio (so called ''pseudohypoxia''), which in turn contributes to increased ROS formation due to activation of NADH oxidase, a superoxide generating enzyme [studies of NADH oxidase in diabetic tissues reported contradictory results (36–38)]. If this was true, one would expect the SDI treatment to be beneficial on parameters of oxidative injury and antioxidative defense. However, the present study demonstrates that the SDI treatment resulted in an opposite effect, because total MDA and 4-hydroxyalkenal accumulation, GSH depletion, and total quinone reductase deficit in the diabetic nerve were exacerbated with the SDI treatment. Interestingly, nerve SOD, catalase, and GSH-Px activities (which were similar in control and 3-week streptozotocin-diabetic rats) were increased in 3-week streptozotocin-diabetic rats treated with SDI, a phenomenon probably indicative of a compensatory response to the increased attack of ROS of superoxide and hydrogen peroxide due to exacerbated GSH and total quinone reductase deficits.

In conclusion, the increased vulnerability of diabetic peripheral nerve to oxidative injury results from impairment of antioxidative defense mechanisms manifested by decreased GSH levels and SOD, catalase, and total quinone reductase activities. Downregulation of these enzymes under diabetic conditions is caused by ROS (probably posttranslational regulation) and is prevented by antioxidant DL-α-lipoic acid treatment. AR is an important, although not the only, mechanism of diabetes-induced oxidative injury, whereas sorbitol dehydrogenase has a protective role, and its inhibition exacerbates oxidative damage. These findings implicate sorbitol accumulation-linked osmotic stress in nerve antioxidant deficit in diabetes.

REFERENCES

1. Low PA, Nickander KK, Tritschler HJ. The roles of oxidative stress and antioxidant treatment in experimental diabetic neuropathy. Diabetes 1997; 46(2S):38S–42S.
2. Nagamatsu M, Nickander KK, Schmelzer JD, Raya A, Wittrock DA, Tritschler H, Low PA. Lipoic acid improves nerve blood flow, reduces oxidative stress, and improves distal nerve conduction in experimental diabetic neuropathy. Diabetes Care 1995; 18:1160–1167.
3. Cameron NE, Cotter MA, Archibald V, et al. Anti-oxidant and pro-oxidant effects on nerve conduction velocity, endoneurial blood flow and oxygen tension in non-diabetic and streptozotocin-diabetic rats. Diabetologia 1994; 37:449–459.
4. Cotter MA, Love A, Watt MJ, et al. Effects of natural free radical scavengers on peripheral nerve and neurovascular function in diabetic rats. Diabetologia 1995; 38:1285–1294.
5. Karaso C, Dewhurst M, Stevens EJ, Tomlinson DR. Effects of anti-oxidant treatment on sciatic nerve dysfunction in streptozotocin-diabetic rats; comparison with essential fatty acids. Diabetologia 1995; 38:129–134.
6. Cameron NE, Cotter MA, Horrobin DH, Tritschler HJ. Effects of alpha-lipoic acid on neuro-vascular function in diabetic rats: interaction with essential fatty acids. Diabetologia 1998; 41:390–399.
7. Love A, Cotter MA, Cameron NE. Nerve function and regeneration in diabetic and galactosemic rats: antioxidant and metal chelator effects. Eur J Pharmacol 1996; 31:433–439.
8. Hounsom L, Horrobin DR, Tritschler H, et al. A lipoic acid-gamma linolenic acid conjugate is effective against multiple indices of experimental diabetic neuropathy. Diabetologia 1998; 41:839–843.
9. Greene DA, Cao X, Van Huysen C, Obrosova I. Effects of DL-α-lipoic acid on diabetic nerve function, bioenergetics, and antioxidative defense (abstr). Diabetes 1998; 47(suppl 1): A136.
10. Obrosova I, VanHeyningen D, Cao X, et al. Metabolic compensation for diabetes-induced endoneurial hypoxia (abstr). J Periph Nerv Syst 1997; 2:290.
11. Smith WJ, Diemel LT, Leach RM, Tomlinson DR. Central hypoxaemia in rats provokes neurological defects similar to those seen in experimental diabetes mellitus: evidence for a partial role of endoneurial hypoxia in diabetic neuropathy. Neuroscience 1991; 45:255–259.
12. Hohman TC, Banis D, Basso M, et al. Resistance to increased oxidative stress is decreased in experimental diabetic neuropathy (abstr). J Periph Nerv Syst 1997; 2:272.
13. Lowry OH, Passonneau JV. A Flexible System of Enzymatic Analysis. Orlando: Academic Press, 1972.
14. Bergmeyer HU. Methods of Enzymatic Analysis. Weinheim: Verlag Chemie, 1974.

15. Holmes EW. Coupled enzymatic assay for the determination of sucrose. Anal Biochem 1997; 244:103–109.
16. Romero FJ, Monsalve E, Hermenegildo C, et al. Oxygen toxicity in the nervous tissue: comparison of the antioxidant defense of rat brain and sciatic nerve. Neurochem Res 1991; 16: 157–161.
17. Misra HP, Fridovich I. The role of superoxide anion in the autooxidation of epinephrine and a simple assay for superoxide dismutase. J Biol Chem 1972; 247:3170–3175.
18. Habig WH, Pabst MJ, Jacoby WB. Glutathione S-transferases. The first enzymatic step in mercapturic acid formation. J Biol Chem 1974; 249:7130–7139.
19. Ernster L, Danielson L, Ljunggren M. DT diaphorase. I. Purification from the soluble fraction of rat liver cytoplasm, and properties. Biochim Biophys Acta 1962; 58:171–188.
20. Low PA, Nickander KK. Oxygen free radical effects in sciatic nerve in experimental diabetes. Diabetes 1991; 40:873–877.
21. Nickander KK, Schmelzer JD, Rohwer DA, Low PA. Effect of alpha-tocopherol deficiency on indices of oxidative stress in normal and diabetic peripheral nerve. J Neurol Sci 1994; 126:6–14.
22. Maitra I, Serbinova E, Trischler H, Packer L. Alpha-lipoic acid prevents buthionine sulfo-ximine-induced cataract formation in newborn rats. Free Rad Biol Med 1995; 18:823–829.
23. Sumathi R, Jayanthi S, Kalpanadevi V, Varalakshmi P. Effect of DL alpha-lipoic acid on tissue lipid peroxidation and antioxidant systems in normal and glycollate treated rats. Pharm Res 1993; 27:309–318.
24. Sandhya P, Varalakshmi P. Effect of lipoic acid administration on gentamicin-induced lipid peroxidation in rats. J Appl Toxicol 1997; 17:405–408.
25. Seaton TA, Jenner P, Marsden CD. Mitochondrial respiratory enzyme function and superoxide dismutase activity following brain glutathione depletion in the rat. Biochem Pharmacol 1996; 52:1657–1663.
26. Nistico G, Ciriolo MR, Fiskin K, et al. NGF restores decrease in catalase activity and increases superoxide dismutase and glutathione peroxidase activity in the brain of aged rats. Free Rad Biol Med 1992; 12:177–181.
27. Santos FX, Escudero M, Perez L, et al. Comparison of the effects of nerve growth factor and superoxide dismutase on vascular extravasation in experimental burns. Burns 1995; 21:445–448.
28. Garrett NE, Malcangio M, Dewhurst M, Tomlinson DR. α-Lipoic acid corrects neuropeptide deficits in diabetic rats via induction of trophic support. Neurosci Lett 1997; 222:191–194.
29. Spycher SE, Tabataba-Vakili S, O'Donnell VB, et al. Aldose reductase induction: a novel response to oxidative stress of smooth muscle cells. FASEB 1997; 11:181–188.
30. Srivastava S, Chandra A, Wang LF, et al. Metabolism of the lipid peroxidation product, 4-hydroxy-*trans*-2-nonenal, in isolated perfused rat heart. J Biol Chem 1998; 273:10893–10900.

31. Obrosova I, Marvel J, Faller A, Williamson JR. Reductive stress is a very early metabolic imbalance in sciatic nerve in diabetic and galactose-fed rats (abstr). Diabetologia 1995; 38(suppl 1):A8.
32. Geisen K, Utz R, Grotsch H, Lang J, Nimmesgern H. Sorbitol-accumulating pyrimidine derivatives. Arzneim Forsch Drug Res 1994; 44:1032–1043.
33. Lou MF, Dickerson JE Jr, Garadi R, York BM Jr. Glutathione depletion in the lens of galactosemic and diabetic rats. Exp Eye Res 1988; 46:517–530.
34. Low PA, Yao JK, Kishi Y, et al. Peripheral nerve energy metabolism in experimental diabetic neuropathy. Neurosci Res Comm 1997; 21:49–56.
35. Williamson JR, Chang K, Frangos M, et al. Hyperglycemic pseudohypoxia and diabetic complications. Diabetes 1993; 42:801–813.
36. Kuo TH, Moore KH, Giacomelli F, Wiener J. Defective oxidative metabolism of heart mitochondria from genetically diabetic mice. Diabetes 1983; 32:781–787.
37. Askar MA, Baquer NZ. Changes in the activity of NADH oxidase in rat tissues during experimental diabetes. Biochem Mol Biol Int 1994; 34:909–914.
38. Ellis EA, Grant MB, Murray FT, et al. Increased NADH oxidase activity in the retina of the BBZ/Wor diabetic rat. Free Rad Biol Med 1998; 24:111–120.

8

Pathways of Glucose-Mediated Oxidative Stress in Diabetic Neuropathy

Douglas A. Greene, Irina G. Obrosova, Martin J. Stevens, and Eva L. Feldman
University of Michigan Medical Center, Ann Arbor, Michigan

Diabetic distal symmetric sensorimotor polyneuropathy (DPN), the most common peripheral neuropathy in developed countries (1–3), affects up to 60–70% of diabetic patients (4) and is the leading cause of foot amputation (5). The typical slowing of nerve conduction and the advancing distal symmetrical sensorimotor deficits are thought to reflect an underlying slowly progressive distal axonopathy of the dying-back type primarily affecting sensory nerve fibers (6). Improved blood glucose control substantially reduces the risk of developing DPN in insulin-dependent (type 1) diabetes (7,8), thereby strongly implicating hyperglycemia as a causative factor.

Animal and in vitro experiments have implicated a variety of enzymatic and nonenzymatic metabolic mechanisms in the initiation of glucose-induced neurotoxicity. These ''metabolic initiators'' include nonenzymatic glycation of proteins with subsequent chemical rearrangements, yielding complex protein adducts known as advanced glycation end products (AGEs) (9,10); autooxidation of glucose (11); increased aldose reductase (AR) activity leading to sorbitol and fructose accumulation, NADP-redox imbalances, and alterations in signal transduction (12–14); and activation of protein kinase C (PKC), perhaps due to increased de novo synthesis of diacylglycerol (DAG) from glucose and inhibition of DAG kinase (15–18). These metabolic initiators are compartmentalized within the rich anatomical complexity and cellular heterogeneity of the peripheral nervous system (PNS) and its supporting vasculature and connective tissue elements. This compartmentalization channels and shapes the physiological response to metabolic initiators into the specific nerve fiber damage and loss underlying DPN. The intervening physiological mediators include interruption of nerve blood flow (NBF) (19–22), mitochondrial dysfunction (19,23), impaired neurotropic support (24), osmolyte derangements (14), and induction of neuronal and/or Schwann cell apoptosis (25). Combinations and permutations of metabolic initiators, cellular and subcellular compartmentalization, and physiological mediators give rise to the current spectrum of pathogenetic hypotheses for DPN (Table 1).

The intellectual challenge to basic and clinical scientists exploring the pathogenesis of DPN is the identification and characterization of the important initiators, compartments, and mediators common to various pathogenetic hypotheses. These common elements may serve as a linchpins around which to array and perhaps unify otherwise competing pathogenetic mechanisms. Glucose-induced generation of reactive oxygen species (ROS) may subserve this purpose (Fig. 1). Autooxidation of glucose, catalyzed by trace amounts of free transition metals such as iron and copper (26), generate ROS in vitro (27), and metal chelating agents to preserve normal nerve conduction velocity

Table 1 Putative Metabolic Initiators and Physiological Mediators of Glucose Toxicity in Experimental Diabetic Neuropathy

Metabolic initiators	Tissue compartments	Physiological mediators
Nonenzymatic glycation	Endoneurial microcirculation	Interruption of nerve blood flow
Sorbitol pathway	Perineurial/epineurial vessels	Mitochondrial dysfunction
Glucose autooxidation	Dorsal root/anterior horn neurons	Reduced neurotrophic support
Protein kinase C activation	Myelinated/unmyelinated axons	Osmolyte derangements
	Schwann cells	
	Perineurial cells	
	Distal motor/sensory projections	

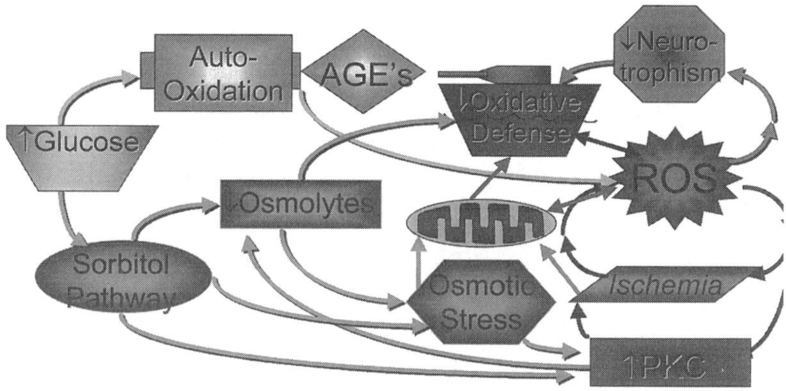

Figure 1 Generation of ROS from elevated levels of glucose may occur by multiple putative metabolic pathways: nonenzymatic glucose autooxidation and nonenzymatic formation of AGEs (yellow) and activation of the enzymes of the sorbitol pathway by mass action (red). Sorbitol pathway activation produces osmolyte and NADPH depletion that diminish antiooxidative defense and produce osmotic stress. Osmotic stress may trigger cellular stress-response mechanisms such as PKC that have been linked to endothelial dysfunction, vasoconstriction, and ischemia. Ischemia and osmotic stress impair mitochondrial function and integrity, which can limit mitochondrial contribution to oxidative defense. Ischemia/reperfusion and impaired oxidative defense further magnify ROS accumulation, vascular function, and mitochondrial integrity. Neurotrophic support that upregulates oxidative defense mechanisms may be impaired by ROS, further compromising oxidative defense.

and NBF in diabetic rats (28) [transition metal handling may be impaired in experimental diabetes (29)] (Fig. 1, yellow). Furthermore, ROS may interconnect autooxidation and AGE formation: ROS accelerate AGE formation and AGEs in turn supply ROS (''autooxidative glycosylation'') (30) (Fig. 1, yellow). AGEs generate ROS through a series of complex biochemical and molecular pathways (31–33). Binding of AGEs to their cell surface receptor (RAGE) is associated with activation and nuclear translocation of the transcription factor NF-κB (34), possibly contributing to endothelial dysfunction (35,36) impaired NBF and ischemia (Fig. 1, black).

Activation of the AR pathway has also been linked to ROS generation (Fig. 1, red). Reduction of glucose to sorbitol by AR oxidizes NADPH, directly impairing antioxidative defense (37). Sorbitol accumulation produces osmotic stress, which may promote oxidative stress through depletion of glutathione and other putative antioxidants such as taurine (38). The novel hypothesis that AR pathway activation produces mitochondrial dysfunction through osmotic stress is discussed in this volume. Mitochondrial dysfunction could impair antioxidative defense by diminishing ATP for the de novo synthesis of glutathione (39). AR pathway activation may also contribute to the activation of PKC reported in some (15,16) but not all tissues prone to diabetic complications (total PKC activity is reduced rather than increased by diabetes in rat sciatic nerve (40,41), but selective activation of specific isoforms in some tissue components has been described in diabetic kidney (42) and has not been excluded in diabetic PNS). Increased AR pathway activity could promote de novo DAG synthesis by diverting dihydroxyacetone phosphate toward formation of α-glycerophosphate or PKC activation through osmotic stimulation of the JNK-kinase cascade. PKC activation would further exacerbate reciprocal osmolyte depletion promoted by sorbitol accumulation by inhibiting the transport activity of the Na^+-myoinositol (43) and the Na^+-taurine (44) cotransporters. If activation of endoneurial or perineurial vascular PKC promoted vasoconstriction and nerve ischemia, then this would further exacerbate mitochondrial dysfunction through oxygen deprivation (ischemia). Mitochondrial dysfunction, impaired antioxidative defense, and ischemia would all contribute further to the generation of ROS (which would further exacerbate vasoconstriction (Fig. 1) (19).

ROS may interact with diminished neurotropic support, impaired energy metabolism, and ischemia in experimental DPN (neurotrophism). Oxidative stress induced by diabetes (45) would be particularly injurious to the PNS, which is particularly vulnerable to oxidative stress (46). Impaired neurotrophic support in diabetes (47) may be mediated by ROS (48). ROS contribute to inschemia-reperfusion injury (49). ROS-induced apoptosis may share similar cell death pathways with neurotrophic withdrawal (50,51), and neurotrophins may protect against ROS damage by inducing antioxidative defense mechanisms (52–54). Recent data suggest that antioxidant therapy may ameliorate some aspects of reduced neurotrophic support in experimental DPN (55).

Thus, oxidative stress and ROS link all of the potential intiators, encompass most of the cellular compartments in the PNS, and relate to virtually all physiological mediators implicated in the progressive nerve fiber dysfunction, damage, and loss in DPN (Table 1). In each of these pathogenetic elements, generation of ROS may initiate a feed-forward cycle, because oxidative stress itself impairs antioxidative defense mechanisms (Fig. 1, double-headed black arrow) (56), resulting in a ''viscous'' cycle of metabolic damage. The role of ROS and oxidative stress in DPN has only recently begun to emerge, and its potential as a therapeutic target for DPN holds great but as yet unfulfilled promise.

REFERENCES

1. The DCCT Research Group. Factors in the development of diabetic neuropathy: baseline analysis of the neuropathy in the feasibility phase of the Diabetes Control and Complication Trial (DCCT). Diabetes 1988; 37:476–481.
2. Pirart J. Diabetes mellitus and its degenerative complications: a prospective study of 4,400 patients observed between 1947 and 1973. Diabetes Care 1978; 1:168–188.
3. Young MJ, Boulton AJM, Macleod AF, Williams DRR, Sonksen PH. A multicentre study of the prevalence of diabetic peripheral neuropathy in the United Kingdom hospital clinic populations. Diabetologia 1993; 36:150–154.
4. Division of Diabetes Translation Center for Disease Control, American Diabetes Association, National Center for Health Statistics, The Bureau of the Census. Diabetes in America. 2nd ed. NIH Publication 95-1468. Bethesda, MD: National Institutes of Diabetes and Digestive and Kidney Diseases, 1995.
5. Brand PW. The diabetic foot. In: Ellenberg M, Rifkin H, eds. Diabetes Mellitus. New York: Medical Examination Publishing Co., Inc., 1982:829–849.
6. Thomas PK, Brown MJ. Diabetic polyneuropathy. In: Dyck PJ, Asbury AK, Winegrad AI, Porte D, eds. Diabetic Neuropathy. Philadelphia: W.B. Saunders, 1987:56–65.
7. The DCCT Research Group. The effect of intensive treatment of diabetes on the development and progression of long-term complications in insulin-dependent diabetes mellitus. N Engl J Med 1993; 329:977–986.
8. The DCCT Research Group. The effect of intensive diabetes therapy on the development and progression of neuropathy. Ann Intern Med 1995; 122:561–568.
9. Schmidt AM, Hasu M, Popov D, Zhang JH, Chen J, Yan SD, Brett J, Cao R, Kuwabara K, Costache G, Simionescu N, Simionescu M, Stern D. Receptor for advanced glycation end products (AGE's) has a central role in vessel wall interactions and gene activation in response to circulating AGE proteins. Proc Natl Acad Sci USA. 1994; 91:8807–8811.
10. Varma SD, Devamanoharan PS, Ali AH. Formation of advanced glycation end (AGE) products in diabetes: prevention by pyruvate and α-ketoglutarate. Mol Cell Biochem 1997; 171:23–28.
11. Love A, Cotter MA, Cameron NE. Nerve function and regeneration in diabetic and galactosemic rats: antioxidant and metal chelator effects. Eur J Pharmacol 1996; 31:433–439.
12. Greene DA, Sima AA, Stevens MJ, Feldman EL, Killen PD, Henry DN, Thomas

T, Dananberg J, Lattimer SA. Aldose reductase inhibitors: an approach to the treatment of diabetic nerve damage. Diabetes Metab Rev 1993; 9:189–217.

13. Stevens MJ, Dananberg J, Feldman EL, Lattimer SA, Kamijo M, Thomas TP, Shindo H, Sima AA, Greene DA. The linked roles of nitric oxide, aldose reductase and, (Na^+, K^+)-ATPase in the slowing of nerve conduction in the streptozotocin diabetic rat. J Clin Invest 1994; 94:853–859.
14. Cameron NE, Cotter MA, Basso M, Hohman TC. Comparison of the effects of inhibitors of aldose reductase and sorbitol dehydrogenase on neurovascular function, nerve conduction and tissue polyol pathway metabolites in streptozotocin-diabetic rats. Diabetologia 1997; 40:271–281.
15. Inoguchi T, Battan R, Handler E, Sportsman JR, Heath W, King GL. Preferential elevation of protein kinase C isoform beta II and diacylglycerol levels in the aorta and heart of diabetic rats: differential reversibility to glycemic control by islet cell transplantation. Proc Natl Acad Sci USA 1992; 89:11059–11063.
16. Bursell SE, Takagi C, Clermont AC, Takagi H, Mori F, Ishii H, King GL. Specific retinal diacylglycerol and protein kinase C beta isoform modulation mimics abnormal retinal hemodynamics in diabetic rat. Invest Ophthalmol Vis Sci 1997; 38:2711–2720.
17. Ishii H, Koya D, King GL. Protein kinase C activation and its role in the development of vascular complication in diabetes mellitus. J Mol Med 1998; 78:21–31.
18. Cameron NE, Cotter MA, Lai K, Hohman TC. Effects of protein kinase C inhibition on nerve function, blood flow and Na^+, K^+-ATP-ase defects in diabetic rats (abst). Diabetes 1997; 46(suppl 1):31A.
19. Low PA, Nickander KK, Tritschler HJ. The roles of oxidative stress and antioxidant treatment in experimental diabetic neuropathy. Diabetes 1997; 46(2S):38S–42S.
20. Nagamatsu M, Nickander KK, Schmelzer JD, Raya A, Wittrock DA, Tritschler H, Low PA. Lipoic acid improves nerve blood flow, reduces oxidative stress, and improves distal nerve conduction in experimental diabetic neuropathy. Diabetes Care 1995; 18:1160–1167.
21. Cameron NE, Cotter MA, Archibald V, Dines KC, Maxfield EK. Anti-oxidant and pro-oxidant effects on nerve conduction velocity, endoneurial blood flow and oxygen tension in non-diabetic and streptozotocin-diabetic rats. Diabetologia 1994; 37:449–459.
22. Cotter MA, Love A, Watt MJ, Cameron NE, Dines KC. Effects of natural free radical scavengers on peripheral nerve and neurovascular function in diabetic rats. Diabetologia 1995; 38:1285–1294.
23. Obrosova I, VanHeyningen D, Cao X, Stevens M, Greene D. Metabolic compensation for diabetes-induced endoneurial hypoxia. J Periph Nerv Syst 1997; 2: 290.
24. Fernyhough P, Diemel LT, Tomlinson DR. Target tissue production and axonal transport of neurotrophin-3 are reduced in streptozotocin-diabetic rats. Diabetologia 1998; 41:300–306.

25. Ekstrom PA. Neurones and glial cells of the mouse sciatic nerve undergo apoptosis after injury in vivo and in vitro. Neuroreport 1995; 6:1029–1032.
26. Wolf SP. Transition metals and oxidative stress in the complications of diabetes. In: Gries FA, Wessels K, eds. The Role of Anti-oxidants in Diabetes Mellitus. Frankfurt am Main: pmi Verlagsgrupe, 1993:82–101.
27. Jiang, Z-Y, Woollard ACS, Wolf SP. Hydrogen peroxide production during experimental protein glycation. FEBS Lett 1990; 268:69–71.
28. Cameron NE, Cotter MA. Neurovascular dysfunction in diabetic rats. Potential contribution of autoxidation and free radicals examined using transition metal chelating agents. J Clin Invest 1995; 96:1159–1163.
29. Cutler P. Deferoxamine therapy in high-ferritin diabetes. Diabetes 1989; 38: 1207–1210.
30. Baynes JW. Role of oxidative stress in the development of complications of diabetes. Diabetes 1991; 40:405–412.
31. Van SD, Schmidt AM, Anderson GM, Zhang J, Brett J, Zou YS, Pinsky D, Stern D. Enhanced cellular oxidant stress by the interaction of advanced glycation endproducts with their receptors/binding proteins. J Biol Chem 1994; 269:9889–9897.
32. Mullarkey CJ, Edelstein D, Brownlee M. Free radical generation by early glycation products: a mechanism for accelerated atherogenesis in diabetes. Biochem Biophys Res Commun 1990; 173:932–939.
33. Giardino I, Fard AK, Hatchell DL, Brownlee M. Aminoguanidine inhibits reactive oxygen species formation, lipid peroxidation, and oxidant-induced apoptosis. Diabetes 1998, 47:1114–1120.
34. Bierhaus A, Illmer T, Kasper M, Luther T, Quehenberger P, Tritschler H, Wahl P, Ziegler R, Muller M, Nawroth PP. Advanced glycation end product (AGE)-mediated induction of tissue factor in cultured endothelial cells is dependent on RAGE. Circulation, in press.
35. Amore A, Cirina P, Mitola S, Peruzzi L, Gianoglio B, Rabbone I, Sacchetti C, Cerutti F, Grillo C, Coppo R. Nonenzymatically glycated albumin (Amadori adducts) enhances nitric oxide synthase activity and gene expression in endothelial cells. Kidney Int 1997; 51:27–35.
36. Pieper GM, Riaz-ul-Haq. Activation of nuclear factor-kappaB in cultured endothelial cells by increased glucose concentration: prevention by calphostin C. J Cardiovasc Pharmacol 1997; 30:528–532.
37. Hohman TC, Banis D, Basso M, Cotter MA, Cameron NE. Resistance to inceased oxidative stress is decreased in experimental diabetic neuropathy. J Periph Nerv Syst 1997; 2:272.
38. Aruoma OI, Halliwell B, Hoey BM, Butler J. The antioxidant action of taurine, hypotaurine and their metabolic precursors. Biochem J 1988; 256:251–255.
39. Hothersall JS, Taylaur CE, McLean P. Antioxidant status in an in vitro model for hyperglycemic lens Cataract formation: effect of aldose reductase inhibitor statil. Biochem Med Metab Biol 1988; 40:109–117.

40. Kim J, Rushovich EH, Thomas TP, Ueda T, Agranoff BW, Greene DA. Diminished specific activity of cytosolic protein kinase C in sciatic nerve of streptozocin-induced diabetic rats and its correction by dietary myo-inositol. Diabetes 1991; 40:1545–1554.
41. Kowluru RA, Jirousek M, Stramm L, Farid N, Engerman RL, Kern TS. Abnormalities of retinal metabolism in diabetes or experimental galactosemia. V. Relationship between protein kinase C and ATPases. Diabetes 1998; 47:464–469.
42. Koya D, Lee IK, Ishii H, Kanoh H, King GL. Prevention of glomerular dysfunction in diabetic rats by treatment with d-alpha-tocopherol. J Am Soc Nephro 1997; 8:426–435.
43. Karihaloo A, Kato K, Greene DA, Thomas TP. Protein kinase and Ca^{2+} modulation of myo-inositol transport in cultured retinal pigment epithelial cells. Am J Physiol 1997; 273:C671–C678.
44. Brandsch M, Miyamoto Y, Ganapathy V, Leibach FH. Regulation of taurine transport in human colon carcinoma cell lines (HT-29 and Caco-2) by protein kinase C. Am J Physiol 1993; 264:G939–G946.
45. Low PA, Nickander KK. Oxygen free radical effects in sciatic nerve in experimental diabetes. Diabetes 1991; 40:873–877.
46. Romero FJ, Monsalve E, Hermenegildo C, Puertas FJ, Higueras V, Nies E, Segura-Aguilar J, Roma J. Oxygen toxicity in the nervous tissue: Comparison of the antioxidant defense of rat brain and sciatic nerve. Neurochem Res 1991; 16: 157–161.
47. Fernyhough P, Diemel LT, Brewster WJ, Tomlinson DR. Altered neurotrophin mRNA levels in peripheral nerve and skeletal muscle of experimentally diabetic rats. J Neurochem 1995; 64:1231–1237.
48. Hounsom L, Horrobin DR, Tritschler H, Corder R, Tomlinson DR. A lipoic acid-gamma linolenic acid conjugate is effective against multiple indices of experimental diabetic neuropathy. Diabetologia (in press).
49. Chan PH, Epstein CJ, Li Y, Huang TT, Carlson E, Kinouchi H, Yang G, Kamii H, Mikawa S, Kondo T. Transgenic mice and knockout mutants in the study of oxidative stress in brain injury. J Neurotrauma 1995; 12:815–824.
50. Park DS, Morris EJ, Stefanis L, Troy CM, Shelanski ML, Geller HM, Greene LA. Multiple pathways of neuronal death induced by DNA-damaging agents, NGF deprivation, and oxidative stress. J Neurosci 1998; 18:830–840.
51. Luo Y, Umegaki H, Wang X, Abe R, Roth GS. Dopamine induces apoptosis through an oxidation-involved SAPK/JNK activation pathway. J Biol Chem 1998; 273:3756–3764.
52. Jackson GR, Apffel L, Werrbach-Perez K, Perez-Polo JR. Role of nerve growth factor in oxidant-antioxidant balance and neuronal injury. I. Stimulation of hydrogen peroxide resistance. J Neurosci Res 1990; 25:360–368.
53. Jackson GR, Werrbach-Perez K, Perez-Polo JR. Role of nerve growth factor in oxidant-antioxidant balance and neuronal injury. II. A conditioning lesion paradigm. J Neurosci Res 1990; 25:369–374.
54. Nistico G, Ciriolo MR, Fiskin K, Iannone M, de Martino A, Rotilio G. NGF

restores decrease in catalase activity and increases superoxide dismutase and glutathione peroxidase activity in the brain of aged rats. Free Rad Biol Med 1992; 12:177–181.

55. Garrett NE, Malcangio M, Dewhurst M, Tomlinson DR. Alpha-lipoic acid corrects neuropeptide deficits in diabetic rats via induction of trophic support. Neurosci Lett 1997; 222:191–194.
56. Magwere T, Naik YS, Hasler JA. Primaquine alters antioxidant enzyme profiles in rat liver and kidney. Free Rad Res 1997; 27:173–179.

9

Experimental Diabetic Neuropathy: Oxidative Stress and Antioxidant Therapy

Hans J. Tritschler
ASTA Medica AWD GmbH, Frankfurt, Germany

James D. Schmelzer, Yutaka Kishi, Yoshiyuki Mitsui, Masaaki Nagamatsu, Kim K. Nickander, Paula J. Zollman, and Phillip A. Low
Mayo Foundation, Rochester, Minnesota

There is ample evidence of oxidative stress in both experimental (EDN) and human diabetic neuropathy. Most studies have been done on plasma, with limited study on neural tissues. We briefly review and update our studies.

I. MECHANISMS OF OXIDATIVE STRESS

A. Endoneurial Ischemia/Hypoxia

There is a perfusion deficit of approximately 50% that affects peripheral nerve endoneurium (1) and the parent cell bodies in relevant dorsal root and sympathetic ganglia (2). The onset of ischemia occurs within the first week (3) and is due to a reduction in nutritive rather than arteriovenous flow. There is attendant hypoxia, seen in both experimental (4) and human diabetes (5).

B. Hyperglycemic Glycation and Autooxidation

Glucose, by a process of autooxidation in the presence of decompartmentalized trace transitional metals, can cause lipid peroxidation (6). We have evaluated the role of hyperglycemia in lipid peroxidation in vitro, using an in vitro lipid peroxidation model, with an ascorbate-iron-EDTA system. The addition of 20 mM glucose to the incubation medium increased lipid peroxidation fourfold, confirming rapid and marked glucose-mediated autooxidative lipid peroxidation (7). Glucose autooxidation results in the production of protein reactive ketoaldehydes, hydrogen peroxide highly reactive oxidants, and the fragmentation of proteins (free radical mechanisms). Glycation and oxidation are simultaneous and inextricably linked (8).

II. ANTIOXIDANT ENZYMES

Free radical defenses of peripheral nerve are reduced relative to brain and liver, especially involving glutathione (GSH)-containing enzymes (9). Cuprozinc superoxide dismutase (SOD) is reduced in sciatic nerve of experimental diabetic neuropathy, and this reduction is improved by insulin treatment (10). Glutathione peroxidase (GSH-Px) is reported to be further reduced in experimental diabetic neuropathy in alloxan diabetic mice 7–21 days after induction of diabetes, and enzyme activity inversely regresses with glucose level (11). We recently evaluated the gene expression of the antioxidant enzymes, GSH-Px, SOD (cuprozinc [czSOD] and manganese [mnSOD] separately), and catalase (CAT) in L4-L6 dorsal root ganglia (DRG) and superior cervical ganglion (SCG) of rats that had been diabetic for 3 and 12 months (Kishi et al., unpublished data). cDNA fragments for rat GSH-Px, czSOD, mnSOD, CAT, and cyclophilin was obtained by reverse transcriptase polymerese chain reaction of rat DRG RNA using specific primers for each probe and evaluated by Northern blot analysis. We also evaluated GSH-Px activity in sciatic nerve, DRG, and superior cervical ganglion, of these animals. GSH-Px, CAT, czSOD, and mnSOD were not reduced in EDN at either 3 or 12 months. CAT mRNA was significantly increased in EDN more than 12 months. GSH-Px enzyme activity was normal in sciatic nerve. We conclude that gene expression is not reduced in peripheral nerve tissues in EDN. Changes in enzyme activity may be due to posttranslational modifications.

III. ANTIOXIDANT THERAPY WITH α-LIPOIC ACID IN EDN

Hyperglycemia causes lipid peroxidation of brain and sciatic nerve in vitro. We evaluated the effectiveness of the R(+)-, S(−)-enantiomers, and racemate of α-lipoic acid in reducing thiobarbituric acid reactive substances generation in rat brain and sciatic nerve. Studies were also done in an incubation medium containing 20 mM glucose, which increased lipid peroxidation up to fourfold. A dose-dependent and statistically significant reduction in lipid peroxidation was seen in both tissues with similar potencies for both enantiomers (7).

We also evaluated if lipoic acid will reduce oxidative stress in diabetic peripheral nerve and improve neuropathy in vivo, using the model of streptozotocin diabetic neuropathy. End points were nerve blood flow (NBF), electro-

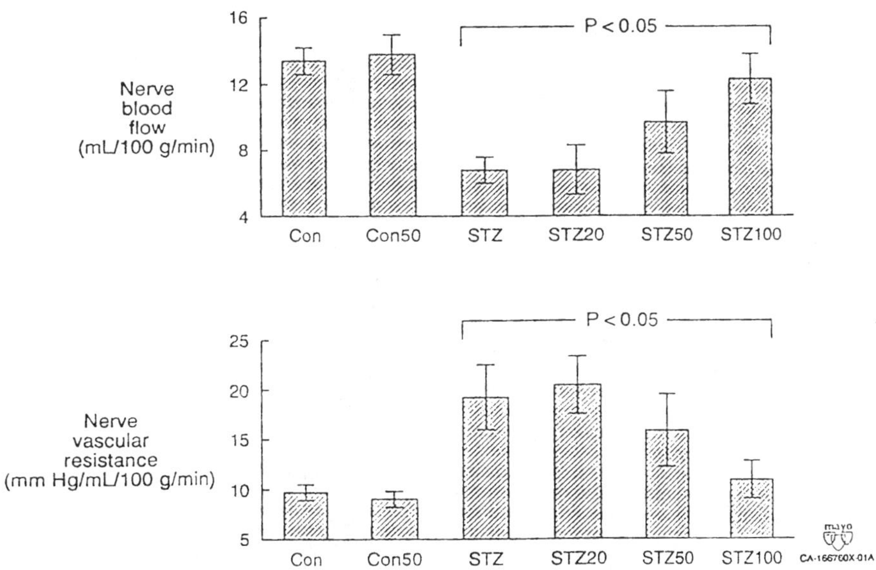

Figure 1 NBF and nerve vascular resistance of control (Con; $n = 8$), streptozotocin-diabetic neuropathy (STZ; $n = 5$), and animals given lipoic acid supplements at doses of 20 mg/kg (STZ20; $n = 6$), 50 mg/kg (Con50; STZ50; $n = 5$), and 100 mg/kg (STZ100; n 8). Lipoic acid supplementation results in normal flow and nerve vascular resistance. Significance of difference, STZ-supplemented vs. STZ. Bars, SE. (From Ref. 12.)

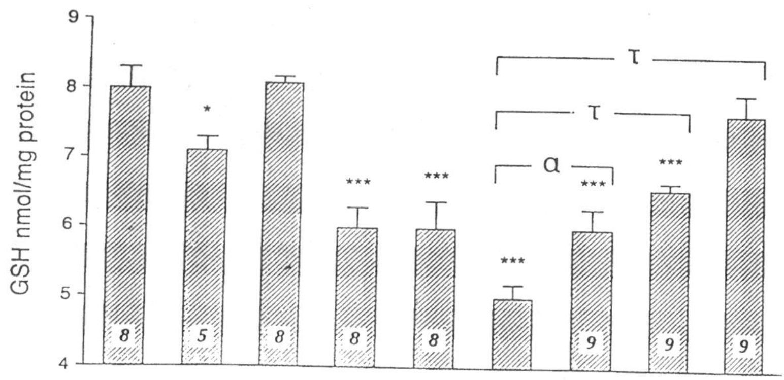

Figure 2 Sciatic nerve GSH concentrations in controls (Con) and on restricted caloric intake (Con[R]), streptozotocin diabetic (STZ), α-tocopherol-depleted (−), and supplemented with lipoic acid at 20, 50, and 100 mg/kg. Lipoic acid supplementation resulted in a dose-dependent prevention of GSH depletion. Significance of difference, vs. control, * $p < 0.05$; *** $p < 0.001$; vs. STZ: α, $p < 0.05$; τ, $p < 0.001$. (From Low et al., Diabetes 1997; 46 (suppl 2): S38–S42.

physiology, and indices of oxidative stress in peripheral nerve at 1 month after onset of diabetes and in age-matched control rats (12). Lipoic acid, in doses of 20, 50, and 100 mg/kg, was administered intraperitoneally five times per week after onset of diabetes. NBF in EDN was reduced by 50%; lipoic acid did not affect NBF of normal nerves but improved that of EDN in a dose-dependent fashion. After 1 month of treatment, lipoic acid-supplemented rats (100 mg/kg) had normal NBF (Fig. 1). The most sensitive and reliable indicator of oxidative stress was a reduction in GSH, which was significantly reduced in EDN; it was improved in a dose-dependent manner in lipoic acid-supplemented rats (Fig. 2). The conduction velocity of digital nerve was reduced in EDN and was significantly improved by lipoic acid.

IV. ANTIOXIDANT THERAPY WITH α-LIPOIC ACID IN ISCHEMIA-REPERFUSION INJURY

Reperfusion after peripheral nerve ischemia results in reduced reperfusion and a breakdown of the blood–nerve barrier (13). After 1 h of ischemia, the permeability-surface area product (PA) is unaltered but becomes significantly greater with reperfusion. After 3 h of ischemia, PA is increased and becomes further increased with reperfusion (13). Reperfusion results in a significant increase in endoneurial lipid hydroperoxides (14). Because α-lipoic acid is a powerful lipophilic antioxidant, we evaluated its efficacy in protecting peripheral nerve from reperfusion injury, using our established model of ischemia-reperfusion injury. We used male Sprague-Dawley rats, 300 ± 5 g. Surgical ligation of the supplying arteries to the sciatic-tibial nerve of the right hindlimb was performed for predetermined periods of ischemia (either 3 or 5 h), followed by the release of the ligatures. Lipoic acid (100 mg/kg/day) was given by intraperitoneal injection daily for 3 days pre- and postsurgery. The same dose of saline was given intraperitoneally to the control rats. A behavioral score of clinical neurological deficits and electrophysiology of motor and sensory nerves was analyzed at 1 week after the surgery. After the electrophysiological examination, the sciatic-tibial nerve was fixed in situ and embedded in epon. One-micron sections with toluidine blue staining were evaluated for ischemic fiber degeneration (IFD) and edema, using previously described methodology (15).

Distal sensory conduction (amplitude of sensory action potential and sensory conduction velocity of digital nerve) was significantly improved in 3-h ischemia treated with lipoic acid ($p < 0.05$). Lipoic acid also improved IFD and edema. The changes after a longer duration of ischemia (5 h) were fewer. These results suggest that the therapeutic window of α-lipoic acid might be relatively narrow but still has some protective effect on peripheral nerve against mild ischemia and reperfusion insults, especially on distal sensory nerves.

V. NEUROPATHOLOGY

Neuropathological alterations in sciatic nerve have been modest in EDN. However, with more recent focus on nerve root, marked alterations in the spinal roots have been reported in long-standing streptozotocin-diabetic rats (16). We recently undertook a study addressing the status of vascular perfusion and neuropathology of DRG (17). Vascular perfusion and neuropathologic evaluation of the lumbar spinal roots and DRG were studied in long-standing (duration of 12–18 months) streptozotocin-induced diabetic rats and age- and sex-matched control rats. We also undertook nerve conduction studies, including F wave recordings.

We have undertaken both perfusion-fixed and immersion-fixed ganglia. Light microscopically, changes of the myelin sheath in the dorsal and ventral roots and vacuolated cells in the DRG were the major findings, being significantly higher in diabetic rats than in control rats. The effects of the diabetic state on myelin splitting was greater in the dorsal than ventral roots. Electron microscopic studies revealed the consecutive changes of myelin from mild separation to severe ballooning of myelin with relative axonal sparing (Fig. 3). DRG cells showed vacuoles of all sizes with cristae-like residua, suggestive of mitochondria. These findings suggest that diabetes mellitus has a dual effect: It accelerates the normal age-related degenerative changes in the spinal roots and DRG and it also has a selective effect on the sensory neuron.

Nerve conduction studies showed markedly reduced conduction velocities in the distal nerve segments and prolonged F wave latency and proximal conduction time despite the shorter conduction pathway in diabetic rats. We suggest that the combination of hyperglycemia and ischemia results in oxidative stress and a predominantly sensory neuropathy.

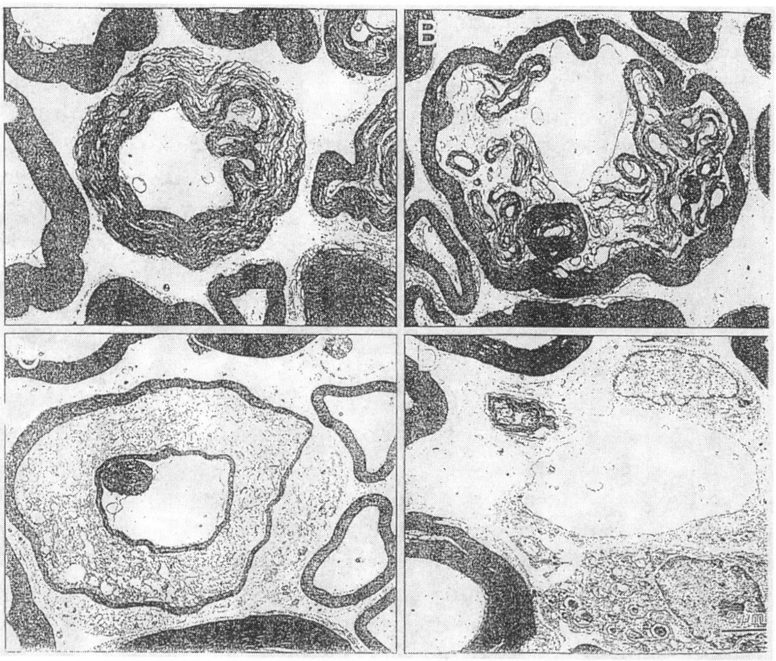

Figure 3 Electron micrographs of representative ventral root fibers showing a progression of myelinopathy in experimental diabetes. (A) Myelin decompaction. (B) A rim of intact myelin surrounds degenerating myelin with early myelin balls and a denuted atrophic axon. (C) An atrophic axon is surrounded by myelin, showing residual rims separated by myelin degeneration and assuming a prominent honeycombed appearance. (D) A completely demyelinated axon is seen. (From Ref. 17.)

VI. GLUCOSE UPTAKE AND ENERGY METABOLISM

α-Lipoic acid has a number of actions in addition to its antioxidant properties. These include its effect on glucose uptake. We therefore evaluated glucose uptake, nerve energy metabolism, and the polyol pathway in EDN induced by streptozotocin. Control and diabetic rats received lipoic acid at various doses (0, 10, 25, 50, and 100 mg/kg). Duration of diabetes was 1 month, and α-lipoic acid was administered intraperitoneally 5 times during the final week of the experiment. Nerve glucose uptake was reduced to 60%, 37% and 30% of control values in the sciatic nerve, L5 DRG, and superior cervical ganglion, respectively, in EDN. α-Lipoic acid supplementation had no effect on glucose uptake in normal nerves at any dose but reversed the deficit in EDN, with a threshold between 10 and 25 mg/kg.

Endoneurial glucose, fructose, sorbitol, and myo-inositol were measured in sciatic nerve and L5 DRG. ATP, creatine phosphate, and lactate were measured in sciatic nerve and superior cervical ganglion. α-Lipoic acid had no significant effect on either energy metabolism or polyol pathway of normal nerves. In contrast, it significantly increased glucose, fructose, and sorbitol but paradoxically increased, rather than reduced, endoneurial myo-inositol. α-Lipoic acid prevented the reduction in superior cervical ganglion creatine phosphate. We conclude that glucose uptake is reduced in EDN and that this deficit is dose-dependently reversed by α-lipoic acid, a change associated with an improvement in peripheral nerve function, possibly by improving energy metabolism in ischemic nerve and by increasing endoneurial myo-inositol.

VII. CONCLUSION

Oxidative stress occurs in EDN due to ischemic and autooxidative lipid peroxidation, with resultant neuropathy. Antioxidant therapy with lipoic acid will improve perfusion, electrophysiology, and indices of oxidative stress. The drug has additional effects, improving glucose uptake and energy metabolism.

REFERENCES

1. Low PA, Lagerlund TD, McManis PG. Nerve blood flow and oxygen delivery in normal, diabetic, and ischemic neuropathy. Int Rev Neurobiol 1989; 31:355–438.

2. Brook WH. Postural hypotension and the anti-gravity suit. Aust Fam Physician 1994; 23:1948, 1948–1949.
3. Cameron NE, Cotter MA, Low PA. Nerve blood flow in early experimental diabetes in rats: relation to conduction deficits. Am J Physiol 1991; 261:E1–E8.
4. Tuck RR, Schmelzer JD, Low PA. Endoneurial blood flow and oxygen tension in the sciatic nerves of rats with experimental diabetic neuropathy. Brain 1984; 107:935–950.
5. Newrick PG, Wilson AJ, Jakubowski J, Boulton AJ, Ward JD. Sural nerve oxygen tension in diabetes. Br Med J 1986; 293:1053–1054.
6. Wolff SP, Jiang ZY, Hunt JV. Protein glycation and oxidative stress in diabetes mellitus and ageing. Free Rad Biol Med 1991; 10:339–352.
7. Nickander KK, McPhee BR, Low PA, Tritschler H-J. α-Lipoic acid: antioxidant potency against lipid peroxidation of neural tissue in vitro and implications for diabetic neuropathy. Free Rad Biol Med 1996; 21:631–639.
8. Hunt JV, Wolff SP. Oxidative glycation and free radical production: a causal mechanism of diabetic complications. Free Rad Res Commun 1991; 1:115–123.
9. Romero FJ, Monsalve E, Hermenegildo C, Puertas FJ, Higueras V, Nies E, Segura-Aguilar J, Roma J. Oxygen toxicity in the nervous tissue: comparison of the antioxidant defense of rat brain and sciatic nerve. Neurochem Res 1991; 16:157–161.
10. Low PA, Nickander KK. Oxygen free radical effects in sciatic nerve in experimental diabetes. Diabetes 1991; 40:873–877.
11. Hermenegildo C, Raya A, Roma J, Romero FJ. Decreased glutathione peroxidase activity in sciatic nerve of alloxan-induced diabetic mice and its correlation with blood glucose levels. Neurochem Res 1993; 18:893–896.
12. Nagamatsu M, Nickander KK, Schmelzer JD, Raya A, Wittrock DA, Tritschler H, Low PA. Lipoic acid improves nerve blood flow, reduces oxidative stress, and improves distal nerve conduction in experimental diabetic neuropathy. Diabetes Care 1995; 18:1160–1167.
13. Schmelzer JD, Zochodne DW, Low PA. Ischemic and reperfusion injury of rat peripheral nerve. Proc Natl Acad Sci USA 1989; 86:1639–1642.
14. Nagamatsu M, Schmelzer JD, Zollman PJ, Smithson IL, Nickander KK, Low PA. Ischemic reperfusion causes lipid peroxidation and fiber degeneration. Muscle Nerve 1996; 19:37–47.
15. Kihara M, Zollman PJ, Schmelzer JD, Low PA. The influence of dose of microspheres on nerve blood flow, electrophysiology, and fiber degeneration of rat peripheral nerve. Muscle Nerve 1993; 16:1383–1389.
16. Tamura E, Parry GJ. Severe radicular pathology in rats with longstanding diabetes. J Neurol Sci 1994; 127:29–35.
17. Sasaki H, Schmelzer JD, Zollman PJ, Low PA. Neuropathology and blood flow of nerve, spinal roots and dorsal root ganglia in longstanding diabetic rats. Acta Neuropathol 1997; 93:118–128.

10

Antioxidants in the Treatment of Diabetic Polyneuropathy: Synergy with Essential Fatty Acids

Norman E. Cameron and Mary A. Cotter
University of Aberdeen, Aberdeen, Scotland

I. INTRODUCTION

A. Neuropathy and Nerve Blood Flow

Neuropathy is a common complication of diabetes mellitus. Studies in patients and animal models have shown that endoneurial hypoxia, caused by impaired nerve blood flow, is a major factor in the etiology of diabetic neuropathy (1–4). Changes in vascular function, particularly of the endothelium, occur early after diabetes induction in experimental models, and in some preparations, this may even be partially mimicked by acute exposure to hyperglycemia (5,6). In streptozotocin-induced diabetic rats, sciatic nerve blood flow is reduced by approximately 50% within a week of diabetes induction (7,8), and this precedes changes in nerve conduction velocity (NCV). Large diameter sensory and motor fibers are particularly susceptible to endoneurial hypoxia in experimental diabetes (9,10).

Several treatment strategies have been used to prevent or correct the blood flow deficit in diabetic rats, and, when achieved, this results in improvements of nerve function measures, such as sensory and motor NCV, and the increased resistance to hypoxic conduction failure (3). Powerful evidence for a direct link between impaired blood flow and nerve dysfunction in diabetes comes from studies using peripheral vasodilators. These do not change the hyperglycemic state or consequent alterations in nerve metabolism such as increased polyol pathway activity; however, they can completely correct reduced NCV and attenuate the development of resistance to hypoxic conduction failure (11–15). Vasodilator treatment has also been used to improve nerve function in diabetic patients (16). Other approaches, such as chronic electrical nerve stimulation (17), and drugs that correct metabolic changes in diabetes, including L-carnitine analogues, *n*-6 essential fatty acids, aldose reductase inhibitors (ARIs), protein kinase C (PKC) inhibitors, antiadvanced glycation agents, and antioxidants, ameliorate NCV defects via their effects on nerve blood flow (3,18). For several of these agents, the vascular endothelium nitric oxide (NO) system appears to be a primary target because their effects on NCV and blood flow are abolished by NO synthase inhibitor cotreatment, whereas many of their other direct biochemical effects on nerve remain unchanged, for example, ARI-mediated suppression of polyol pathway metabolite levels (19–22). Several studies have identified a diminished vasa nervorum NO system in experimental diabetes (23,24). Thus, impaired nerve perfusion lies at the heart of the etiology of diabetic neuropathy. The relationship between sciatic motor NCV and nutritive (capillary) endoneurial blood flow is shown in Figure 1 for groups of diabetic rats pooled from a large number of experiments in which various doses of these drugs were used (reviewed in Refs. 3 and 4). This includes antioxidants, which are the main subject of this review. It is clear that the results of these diverse treatments all fit the same relationship: NCV increases with increasing perfusion and reaches asymptote at blood flow levels within the normal range.

B. Sources of Reactive Oxygen Species in Diabetes, NO, and Vasorelaxation

Reactive oxygen species (ROS) are increased by diabetes. NO is an important vascular target for ROS; superoxide neutralizes NO (25), and the peroxynitrite formed is a source of hydroxyl radicals that can cause endothelial damage (26). Glucose-induced oxidative stress therefore diminishes vessel endothelium-dependent relaxation (27), which contributes to impaired vasa nervorum function (3,4). There are several sources of ROS in diabetes, including those derived from altered metabolism such as autoxidation of glucose and its metabolites, the advanced glycation/glycoxidation process, altered prostanoid production, inefficient mitochondrial function, and upregulation of the vascular NAD(P)H oxidase system (28–30). ROS are also produced as a result of

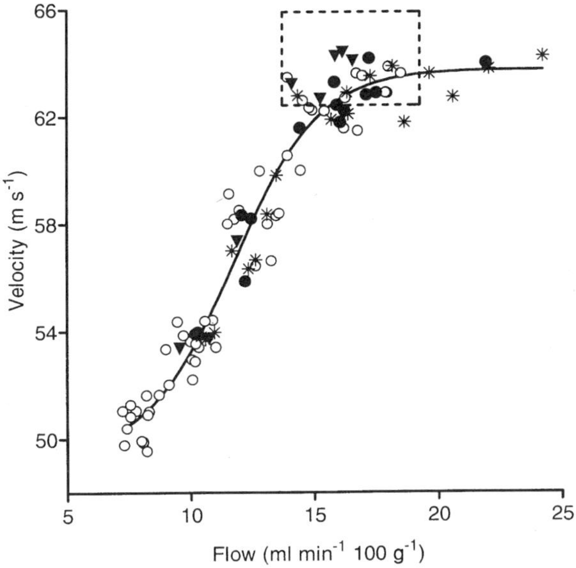

Figure 1 Relationship between sciatic nutritive endoneurial blood flow and motor conduction velocity in groups of streptozotocin-diabetic rats (n = 6–16) given different drug treatments in our laboratory. Diabetes duration was 1–3 months, and treatment was preventive or corrective. Groups treated with various vasodilators (*); groups treated with essential fatty acids, miscellaneous metabolically active compounds such as L-carnitine derivatives, aminoguanidine, sorbitol dehydrogenase inhibitors, PKC inhibitors, and myo-inositol (○); groups treated with different antioxidants (●); and data from aldose reductase inhibitor studies (▼). The solid curve is the best-fitting Boltzmann sigmoid curve (r^2 = 0.95 for df = 97). The dashed rectangle denotes the nondiabetic range (± 1 SD; n = 40). All treatment effects appear to follow a similar relationship; conduction velocity is low at low flow rates and reaches an asymptote that approximates the nondiabetic level as perfusion increases.

the blood flow problems they cause during episodes of ischemia-reperfusion by the xanthine oxidase mechanism (31). Another potential source that may be relevant during infection and inflammatory disease is the macrophage respiratory burst. The degree of oxidative stress seen in diabetic patients is inversely proportional to the degree of metabolic regulation (32), and very tight metabolic control is necessary to slow the development of the major diabetic complications, including neuropathy (33). Because strict glycemic control is difficult to achieve and carries with it the risk of hypoglycemic episodes, there is a strong case for supplementary treatment with antioxidants to further reduce ROS activity.

II. OXIDATIVE STRESS AND ANTIOXIDANT TREATMENT EFFECTS ON NEUROVASCULAR FUNCTION IN EXPERIMENTAL DIABETES

Antioxidant protection mechanisms are compromised in nerves of diabetic rats; lipid peroxidation is increased, and the levels of superoxide dismutase and reduced glutathione (GSH) are decreased, although glutathione peroxidase and reductase remain unchanged (34–37). Long-term exposure to elevated ROS, coupled with diminished endogenous antioxidant protection, could lead to cumulative neurodegenerative changes involving axonopathy and demyelination, and damage to dorsal root ganglion cell bodies and their mitochondria has been observed (37,38). However, in the short term, ROS effects on vasa nervorum are more important, being responsible for the earliest defects in nerve function in diabetic rats.

A. Antioxidant Treatment, Vascular Endothelium, and Nerve Function

Defective endothelium-dependent relaxation has been found in diabetic animals and in type 1 and type 2 patients (39–47) and is an important target for antioxidant treatment. An example is shown in Figure 2, where the lipophilic ROS scavenger, α-tocopherol, protected rat aorta against a diabetic deficit in NO-mediated endothelium-dependent relaxation to acetylcholine (39). A similar protective effect of ROS scavengers has been noted for vasa nervorum blood flow and NCV. The magnitude of effects possible by this approach is illustrated in Figure 3, where a high dose of the probucol analogue, BM 150639, completely corrected motor NCV and blood flow deficits in diabetic rats. These effects were attenuated by cotreatment with a NO synthase inhibitor, emphasizing the importance of the vasa nervorum NO system (19). The effectiveness of a variety of scavengers has been assessed over the last 5 years, including lipophilic drugs like butylated hydroxytoluene, α-tocopherol (vitamin E), β-carotene, and probucol, and the hydrophilic scavengers, *N*-acetyl-L-cysteine and ascorbic acid (vitamin C) (48–54).

α-Lipoic acid is the subject of considerable current interest and is both lipid and water soluble (55). In experiments on diabetic rats, α-lipoic acid has been shown to improve nerve antioxidant protection by increasing GSH con-

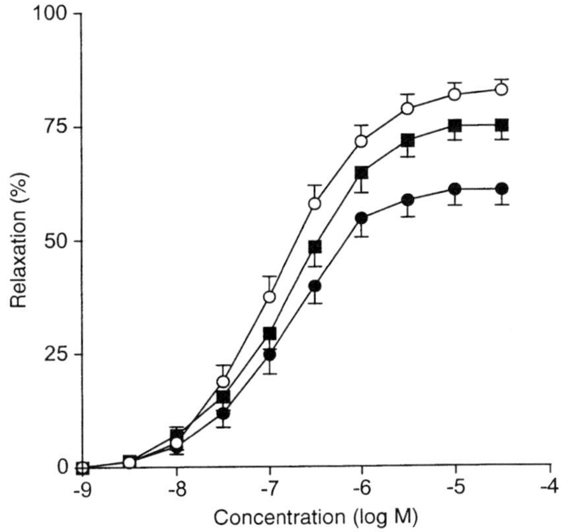

Figure 2 Effects of diabetes and antioxidant treatment with α-tocopherol on endothelium-dependent relaxation of phenylephrine-precontracted aortas to acetylcholine in vitro. Groups (n = 14–17); nondiabetic control (○); 8-week streptozotocin-diabetic (●); α-tocopherol (1 g / kg/day) treated from diabetes induction (■). (From Ref. 39.)

tent and to correct blood flow and motor and sensory NCV deficits (36,56,57). R and S enantiomers of α-lipoic acid had similar efficacy on impaired nerve function and perfusion (57) and for the inhibition of lipid peroxidation of neural tissues in vitro (56). α-Lipoic acid was found to be approximately 10 times more potent than α-tocopherol in correcting motor NCV deficits in diabetic rats (50,57). Clinical trials of symptomatic and cardiac autonomic neuropathy revealed beneficial effects of α-lipoic acid treatment (58,59).

In rats, the diabetes-induced decrease in sciatic nutritive blood flow was accompanied by a reduction in mean endoneurial oxygen tension, which was prevented by probucol treatment (49). In nondiabetic rats, prooxidant treatment with the antimalarial drug primaquine mimicked the reductions in blood flow, endoneurial oxygen tension, and NCV found in experimental diabetes while having no effect on plasma glucose levels. These effects were blocked by probucol, which stresses the importance of ROS to neurovascular dysfunction. Furthermore, both diabetes and primaquine treatment caused an increase in plasma angiotensin-converting enzyme activity, a marker of endothelial damage, which was attenuated by probucol treatment (49). Effects on plasma

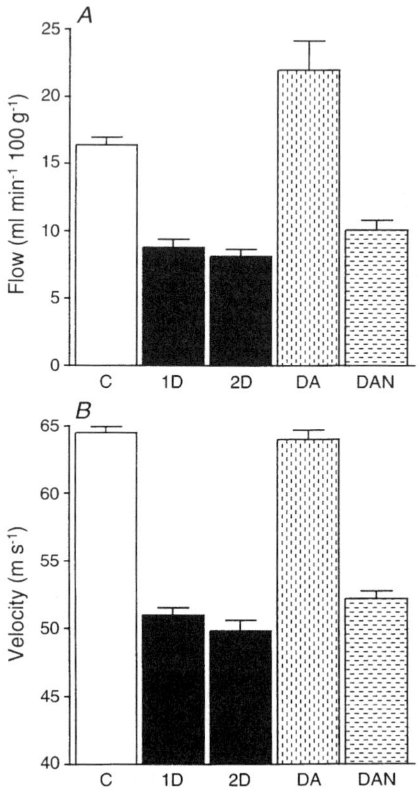

Figure 3 Reversal of sciatic nutritive endoneurial blood flow (A) and motor conduction velocity (B) deficits in diabetic rats by treatment with the probucol analogue BM 150639. Groups (n = 9–10); C, nondiabetic control; 1D, 2D, 1-month, and 2-month streptozotocin-diabetic; DA, 1-month untreated diabetes followed by 1-month BM 150639 (400 mg/kg/day) treatment; DAN, as for DA but cotreated with the nitric oxide synthase inhibitor, N^G-nitro-L-arginine (10 mg/kg/day) during the second month. Data are mean ± SEM. The diabetic deficits in blood flow and motor conduction velocity were well developed after 1 month. BM 150639 treatment was highly effective in reversing these defects, blood flow being approximately 33% supranormal and conduction velocity in the nondiabetic range. The effects of BM 150639 on blood flow and conduction velocity were almost completely blocked by N^G-nitro-L-arginine, which suggests that blood flow modulates conduction velocity and that antioxidant treatment corrects a diabetic deficit in the vasa nervorum nitric oxide mechanism. (See Ref. 24 for further details.)

angiotensin-converting enzyme activity suggest increased activation of the vasoconstrictor renin-angiotensin system in diabetes, and studies with angiotensin-converting enzyme inhibitors and angiotensin AT_1 receptor antagonists have shown that this is important for vasa nervorum; these inhibitors correct blood flow, endoneurial hypoxia, and NCV defects in diabetic rats (60). Increased local angiotensin II also causes upregulation of endothelial NADH oxidase, which may exacerbate dysfunction by increasing ROS production (30). Furthermore, oxidative stress also stimulates endothelial endothelin-1 synthesis, and this interacts with the angiotensin II system to increase vasa nervorum vasoconstriction (61). Thus, ROS cause a self-reinforcing cycle that compromises vasodilation by NO and increases local vasoconstrictor mechanisms. This cycle may be interrupted by antioxidant treatment.

B. Antioxidant Dose Considerations

The normal dietary intake of natural antioxidants could in theory influence NCV and blood flow in diabetic rats. However, high doses that far exceed normal availability are required in practice; for example, 0.62 g/kg/day of α-tocopherol was necessary to give ~50% protection of sciatic motor NCV in diabetic rats (50). For ascorbic acid, 150 mg/kg/day gave an optimal level of protection that was relatively modest (~35%). At high doses (500 mg/kg/day), protection was less, probably because ascorbic acid is susceptible to autoxidation, acting as a prooxidant (50,62). Under physiological conditions, ascorbic acid may aid the recycling of α-tocopherol from its tocopheroxyl radical form (63); however, with the pharmacological doses used in diabetic rats, there was no evidence of a synergy between ascorbic acid and α-tocopherol cotreatment on NCV. Instead, their effects were simply additive, as if they were acting independently in lipid and aqueous phases (50).

C. Studies Using Transition Metal Chelators

As an alternative to scavenging ROS, it may be therapeutically preferable to prevent their formation by autoxidation, the Fenton reaction, and the advanced glycation process, all of which are catalyzed by free transition metal ions. This can be accomplished using transition metal chelators. Low doses of deferoxamine (relatively specific for iron) and trientine (relatively specific for copper) completely corrected sciatic nerve blood flow and motor and sensory NCV deficits in diabetic rats (64). In vessels such as aorta, chronic trientine and deferoxamine treatment prevented the development of defective NO-mediated, endothelium-dependent relaxation (65,66). For diabetic rat vasa nerv-

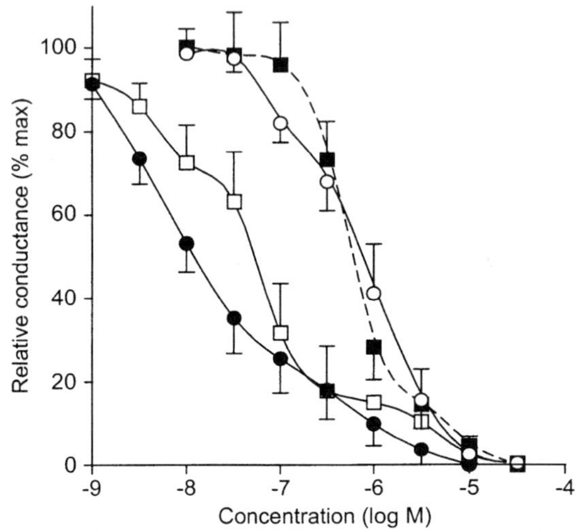

Figure 4 Cumulative dose-response curves for changes in sciatic vasa nervorum vascular conductance after suffusion of saline containing increasing concentrations of norepinephrine. Blood flow in epi- and perineurial vessels was monitored by laser-Doppler flowmetry, and the results are expressed as a percentage of the maximum vascular conductance. Groups (n = 8–12): nondiabetic control (○); 8-week duration diabetic control (●); 8-week diabetic rats treated with deferoxamine (8 mg/kg/day) for the last 2 weeks (■). Data are mean ± SEM. Diabetes caused a leftward shift of the dose-response curve, indicating greatly enhanced sensitivity to vasoconstriction by norepinephrine. In nondiabetic rats, cosuffusion with the nitric oxide synthase inhibitor N^G-nitro-L-arginine (100 μM) caused a similar leftward shift (□). Treatment of diabetic rats with deferoxamine completely restored norepinephrine sensitivity, the interpretation being that it corrected a vasa nervorum NO deficit. (See Refs. 52 and 67 for further details.)

orum, the NO deficit markedly increases reactivity to norepinephrine (Fig. 4), and this was corrected by deferoxamine treatment (24,67). The relatively high potency of α-lipoic acid compared with other natural scavengers such as α-tocopherol could be due to the additional property of transition metal chelation (55). Thus, transition metal-catalyzed ROS production makes an important contribution to nerve and vascular dysfunction in experimental diabetes.

D. Nerve Growth, Regeneration, and Small Fiber Function

In addition to effects on NCV and blood flow, antioxidant treatment improves other aspects of nerve function, including growth and regenerative responses and the performance of small fibers (which do not normally contribute to NCV measurements). Thus, the hydrophilic scavenger *N*-acetyl-L-cysteine allowed normal nerve maturation in young diabetic rats, preventing a reduction in mean nerve fiber size caused by impaired growth. *N*-acetyl-L-cysteine improved the regenerative response to nerve trauma, which is blunted by diabetes (Fig. 5), inhibited an increase in plasma tumor necrosis factor activity, and prevented red cell lipid peroxidation (51,52). The lipophilic scavengers α-tocopherol and butylated hydroxytoluene and the metal chelator trientine also prevent blunted nerve growth and regeneration in young diabetic rats (53,54). Recently, improved regeneration, remyelination, and muscle reinnervation have been noted for α-lipoic acid treatment (Flint H, Cotter MA, and Cameron NE, unpublished observations, 1998). Interestingly, butylated hydroxytoluene and trientine also prevented nerve regeneration and growth deficits in the galactosemic rat model of enhanced polyol pathway and PKC activity (54). Vasodilator treatment had similar effects on these nerve growth parameters in diabetic rats (60); therefore, it is likely that antioxidant-mediated improvements in perfusion and their consequences for the supply of energy and nutrients to nerve fibers and cell

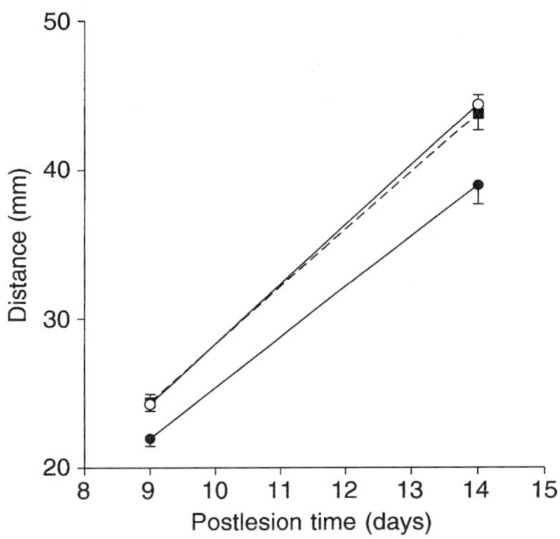

Figure 5 Effects of 4 weeks of diabetes and *N*-acetyl-L-cysteine treatment on sciatic nerve myelinated fiber regeneration distance 9 and 14 days after a freeze lesion. Groups (n = 7–10): nondiabetic control (○); diabetic control (●); diabetic rats treated with 250 mg/kg/day *N*-acetyl-L-cysteine from diabetes induction (■). Data are mean ± SEM. At both time points there was a significant regeneration deficit ($p < 0.01$) with untreated diabetes, which was completely prevented by *N*-acetyl-L-cysteine treatment. (See Ref. 52 for further details.)

bodies are primarily responsible for their growth and regeneration-promoting actions.

The effects of antioxidant treatment on small fiber function has not been examined in as much detail as large fibers. However, in the isolated corpus cavernosum preparation from diabetic rats, a deficit in vasorelaxation to nitrergic nerve fiber stimulation was completely prevented by chronic α-lipoic acid treatment and partially prevented by trientine (68).

E. Polyol Pathway, Oxidative Stress, and Neurovascular Dysfunction

Polyol pathway activity also contributes to oxidative stress; therefore, ARIs have an indirect antioxidant action. The reductions in nerve GSH content found in experimental diabetes and galactosemia were rapidly corrected by ARI treatment (69), which also prevented the elevation of nerve malondialdehyde, a marker of lipid peroxidation, in diabetic rats (70). ARIs correct nerve blood flow and NCV defects in diabetic rats (71,72). They improve defective NO-mediated endothelium-dependent relaxation in vessels from diabetic animals and similar dysfunction resulting from acute hyperglycemic exposure of vessels from nondiabetic animals (3,6). The first half of the polyol pathway, catalyzed by aldose reductase, is much more important than the second half, catalyzed by sorbitol dehydrogenase, because sorbitol dehydrogenase inhibitors did not correct blood flow or NCV in diabetic rats (73) and did not rectify the nerve GSH deficit (Hohman TC, personal communication, 1997).

Aldose reductase requires NADPH as a cofactor, and NADPH is also used by glutathione reductase for maintaining GSH concentrations. Therefore, competition for NADPH in diabetes probably contributes to diminished GSH levels. A further potential polyol pathway action is to increase the formation of advanced glycation end products (AGEs). ARI treatment reduces tissue AGE accumulation, perhaps by inhibiting the synthesis of fructose or by decreasing elevated flux through the pentose phosphate pathway, processes that produce sugars that are considerably more potent glycating agents than glucose (74). Alternatively, the ARI-induced increases in tissue GSH and antioxidant capacity may be sufficient to oppose AGE formation by glycoxidation (75). AGE reactions are an important source of ROS; therefore, their reduction would decrease oxidative stress. Aminoguanidine, although not [directly] an antioxidant, irreversibly binds to reactive carbonyl intermediates, thus blocking AGE formation. Aminoguanidine treatment of diabetic rats has similar functional effects to ARIs and antioxidants in preventing and correcting NCV, nerve blood flow, and NO-mediated endothelium-dependent vasorelax-

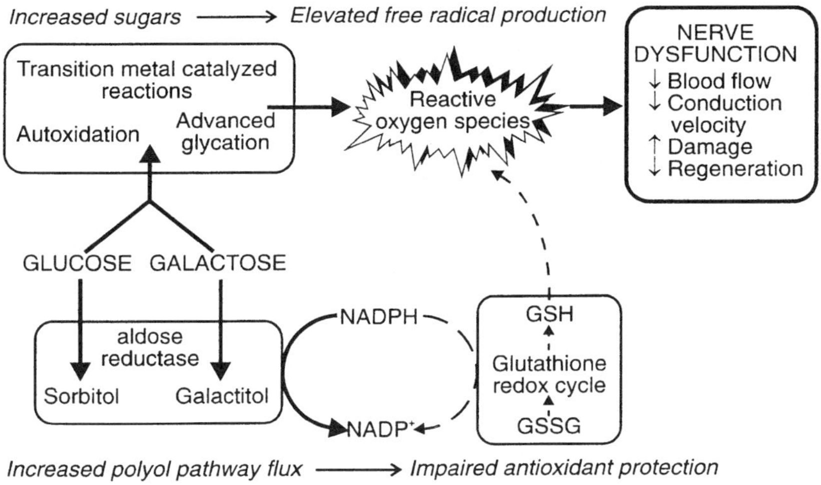

Figure 6 Relation of oxidative stress and nerve dysfunction to elevated polyol pathway activity and transition metal-catalyzed reactions in diabetes or galactosemia. The increased autoxidation and advanced glycation reactions produce ROS, and flux through the first half of the polyol pathway consumes NADPH. This impairs the glutathione redox cycle so that endogenous antioxidant protection is reduced.

ation deficits (3,4,40,76). The putative interrelations between the polyol pathway, advanced glycation, and autoxidation processes in the production of oxidative stress under hyperglycemic conditions are summarized in Figure 6.

F. Antioxidants, NF-κB, and PKC

One of the cellular events stimulated by oxidative stress-related biochemical changes in hyperglycemia, either directly or via AGE receptors, oxidized low-density lipoprotein, or cytokine receptors, is the activation of NF-κB, an effect that may be prevented by antioxidant treatment with α-lipoic acid (77). This transcription factor is responsible for changes in gene expression that have important effects on vascular function relevant to diabetes, including elevated endothelin-1 synthesis and upregulation of intercellular and vascular cell adhesion molecules. It has also been linked to increased NADH oxidase activity (30,78).

PKC is another cell-signaling mechanism activated by diabetes, particularly in vascular tissue (79) although not in the nerve itself (80). In the retina of diabetic rats, there is an early reduction in blood flow paralleling that for nerve. In both retina and nerve, flow was restored by PKC inhibitor treatment (18,81), and nerve NCV deficits were corrected. Diabetes activates PKC via increased de novo synthesis of diacylglycerol from glucose; however, even in the absence of hyperglycemia, PKC is also stimulated by oxidative stress (82). Antioxidants such as α-tocopherol inhibit PKC both directly and via stimulation of diacylglycerol kinase, which breaks down diacylglycerol (79,82). When activated, PKC can modulate several important vascular systems. For example, it is involved in cell signaling mechanisms for endothelin-1 action and can also stimulate NF-κB, which increases endothelin-1 gene expression in endothelial cells (83). Phosphorylation by PKC controls endothelial constitutive NO synthase, reducing its activity (84). Furthermore, phosphorylation of vascular smooth muscle contractile proteins promotes vasoconstriction (85). Thus, PKC is at the heart of altered vascular responses in experimental diabetes and forms a major component of the dysfunctional mechanisms targeted by antioxidant treatment.

G. Therapeutic Implications

From this brief literature review, it is clear that antioxidant strategies based on the use of ROS scavengers and transition metal chelators can be very effective against experimental models of diabetic neuropathy and vasculopathy. The drawback with the scavenger approach is that very large doses of drug are required, one-two orders of magnitude greater than necessary if using transition metal chelators. However, it is possible that with lower blood glucose concentrations than normally found in the experimental models, more physiological doses, for example, of α-tocopherol, could be effective as an adjunct to tight metabolic control in patients. The use of agents with both scavenger and chelator properties, such as α-lipoic acid, or combined therapy with drugs that improve endogenous antioxidant protection mechanisms, such as ARIs, or drugs that target key cell signaling events, such as PKC inhibitors, could provide exciting future strategic approaches to the therapy of diabetic complications including neuropathy.

III. INTERACTIONS BETWEEN ANTIOXIDANTS AND ESSENTIAL FATTY ACIDS

Most of the preceding discussion has dealt with effects of ROS on the NO system and cell-signaling pathways. Another major ROS target is the polyunsaturated fatty acids, including the essential fatty acids necessary for eicosanoid production and normal membrane structure and fluidity. ROS subject these important molecules to self-propagating destructive chain reactions initiated by lipid peroxidation.

A. Essential Fatty Acids, Diabetes, and Neurovascular Dysfunction

The most common dietary essential fatty acids are *n*-6 linoleic acid and *n*-3 α-linolenic acid. They are metabolized by an alternating series of desaturation and elongation steps to produce *n*-6 arachidonic acid and *n*-3 eicosapentaenoic acid, which are important precursors of prostanoids, leukotrienes, and other mediators. In addition to being subjected to destruction by the elevated ROS in diabetes, metabolism of these essential fatty acids is rate limited by the desaturation steps that are inhibited by diabetes. Depressed hepatic Δ-6 desaturation results in lower plasma levels of the *n*-6 metabolites γ-linolenic acid (GLA) and arachidonic acid. This reduces synthesis of the vasodilator, prostacyclin (PGI_2), by vasa nervorum (86). The desaturation deficit may be bypassed by GLA or arachidonic acid treatments, which improve vasa nervorum prostacyclin production, nerve blood flow, and NCV (3,4,87). In contrast to the *n*-6 essential fatty acids, *n*-3 metabolites, such as eicosapentaenoic and docosahexaenoic acids, have relatively little effect on nerve function in experimental diabetes (88).

B. Multiple Endothelial Dysfunction in Diabetes and the Potential for Synergistic Therapies

There are multiple defects of vasa nervorum endothelium and possibly smooth muscle in diabetes that cause reduced nerve blood flow and function. The NO deficit is compounded by diminished PGI_2 synthesis and increases in endothelin-1 and angiotensin II. Recently, it was shown that relaxation mediated by endothelium-derived hyperpolarizing factor (EDHF) is also affected by diabetes. In the rat mesenteric vascular bed, EDHF was 76% reduced after 8 weeks of diabetes. In common with the NO defect, the EDHF deficit was attenuated by antioxidant treatment with α-lipoic acid (89). Vasodilator prostanoid synthesis is also deleteriously affected by oxidative stress; high levels of lipid peroxides inhibit cyclooxygenase (90), and α-tocopherol treatment corrected the lowering of the PGI_2/thromboxane A_2 ratio found in diabetic rats (91).

Normally, these different mechanisms provide an integrated local system for nerve blood flow control; however, by disrupting several mechanisms simultaneously, diabetes disintegrates control, and markedly shifts the balance toward vasoconstriction. These individual mechanisms do not exist in isolation but are mutually interactive (92); therefore, changes in one will affect the others. In experiments on nondiabetic rats designed to mimic some of the vasa nervorum changes in diabetes and assess the consequences for nerve function, chronic treatment with a low dose of a cyclooxygenase inhibitor to reduce PGI_2 synthesis or a NO synthase inhibitor caused modest NCV reductions. However, with combined treatment, there was a fivefold amplification of drug effects on NCV compared with that expected for simple summation (93). This demonstrates a marked synergism between blockade of the prostanoid and the NO systems, suggesting that they normally act in a mutually compensatory manner to limit nerve perfusion changes. The converse effect, joint treatment of diabetes with drugs that target the NO and prostanoid mechanisms, as schematized in Figure 7, could potentially offer a marked therapeutic advantage.

C. Synergy Between Antioxidant and *n*-6 Essential Fatty Acid Treatments

Low doses of an ARI or evening primrose oil (which contains GLA) had modest effects on NCV and blood flow in diabetic rats; however, in combination, improvements matching those obtained by an eightfold increase in the dose of either drug alone were noted (20). A similar magnitude of synergistic interaction was seen for joint treatment with low-dose GLA and the lipophilic scavenger, BM 150639 (94). The notion of antioxidant–*n*-6 essential fatty acid combination therapy has led to the synthesis of hybrid drugs, such as ascorbyl-6-GLA. Although ascorbic acid alone is not particularly effective against NCV deficits in diabetic rats, its combination with GLA increases lipid solubility and therefore the ability to enter cell membranes. It also places the ascorbate moiety in a good physical position to protect the GLA component from ROS damage. Compared with GLA alone, ascorbyl-6-GLA was 4.4-fold more efficacious in correcting NCV and nerve blood flow deficits in diabetic rats (95).

Recent attention has focused on GLA–α-lipoic acid combinations because both drugs have similar dose-response relationships for correcting NCV deficits and because of the greater effective antioxidant power of α-lipoic acid than ascorbate in experimental diabetic neuropathy. Effects on motor NCV and nerve blood flow are shown in Figure 8. Low doses of GLA or α-lipoic

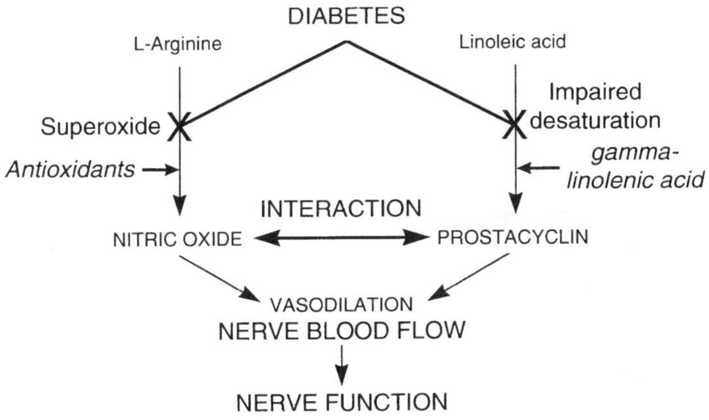

Figure 7 Schematic for the synergistic interaction between NO and prostacyclin pathways. Increased oxidative stress in diabetes and the generation of superoxide neutralizes endothelial NO production, which impairs vasa nervorum vasodilation. Diabetes also reduces hepatic *n*-6 essential fatty acid metabolism, particularly the rate-limiting desaturation steps in the conversion of dietary linoleic acid to γ-linolenic acid. In turn this reduces vasa nervorum prostacyclin production and vasodilation. Normally, at the level of the endothelial cell, and possibly vascular smooth muscle, there is a mutual facilitatory interaction between NO and prostacyclin systems. This may give a therapeutic advantage for the use of joint treatment with antioxidant, which corrects the NO defect, and γ-linolenic acid, which bypasses the desaturation block to boost prostacyclin production.

acid alone had modest effects on NCV and no statistically significant effects on blood flow. However, when the drugs were combined, NCV and blood flow were in the nondiabetic range, showing a greater than additive effect (57). Synergy was found for GLA–α-lipoic acid mixtures in ratios between 1:3 and 3:1, the greatest amplification of drug action being for ratios near 1:1 or with GLA slightly in excess. Similar interactive effects were noted for the novel orally active drug, SOC0150, which contains equimolar amounts of GLA and α-lipoic acid (Fig. 9). The dose-response curve for correction of sciatic motor NCV showed that SOC0150 had an ED_{50} of 9.3 mg/kg/day (giving 3.5 mg/kg/day α-lipoic acid and 4.5 mg/kg/day GLA). This compares very favorably with the ED_{50} of α-lipoic acid alone (38 mg/kg/day). In contrast to SOC0150, α-lipoic acid-containing compounds in which the GLA was substituted by the *n*-3 essential fatty acids docosahexaenoic acid (57) or eico-

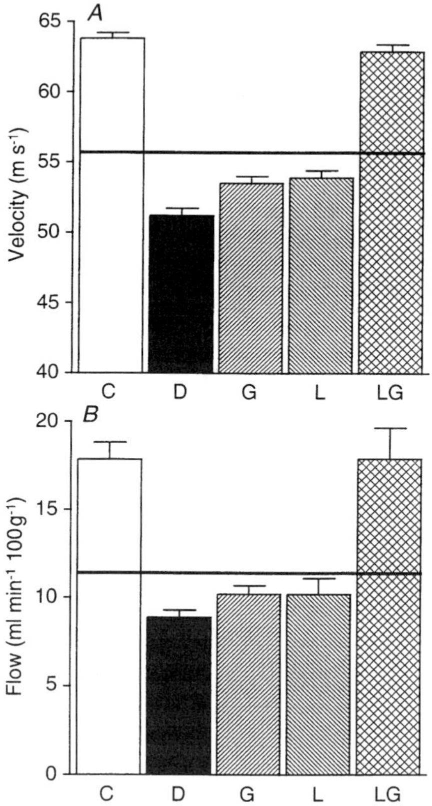

Figure 8 Effects of low-dose γ-linolenic acid and α-lipoic acid treatment, alone and in combination, on (A) sciatic motor conduction velocity and (B) sciatic endoneurial blood flow in streptozotocin-diabetic rats. Groups (n = 8–12): C, nondiabetic control; D, 8-week diabetic control; G or L, 8-week diabetic treated for the final 2 weeks with γ-linolenic acid (20 mg/kg/day) as the monoester or α-lipoic acid (20 mg/kg/day); LG, 8-week diabetic given combined γ-linolenic acid and α-lipoic acid treatment for the final 2 weeks. Data are mean ± SEM. The horizontal lines show the predicted conduction velocity and blood flow values for additive drug effects. The LG group greatly exceeded this level for both measures, indicating a marked synergistic drug interaction. (See Ref. 57 for further details.)

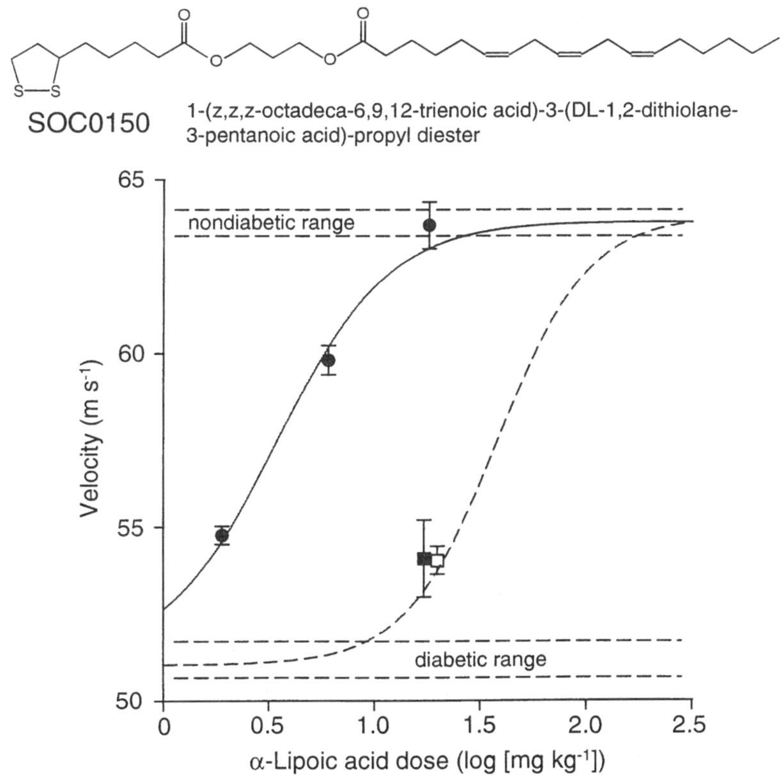

Figure 9 Dose-response relationship for the correction of sciatic motor conduction velocity by the novel drug SOC0150 containing equimolar amounts of γ-linolenic acid and α-lipoic acid. The chemical name and structure of SOC0150 are shown at the top of the figure. Diabetes duration was 8 weeks, and oral treatment was given for the final 2 weeks. The graph shows data points (± SEM; n = 7–10) for SOC0150 (●), plotted in terms of α-lipoic acid content, and the best-fitting sigmoid dose-response relationship (solid curve) for comparison with the dose-response relationship for α-lipoic acid (dashed curve). The SOC0150 curve is displaced approximately 1 log unit to the left of that for α-lipoic acid, indicating an approximately 10-fold increase in efficacy. Also shown are data points for similar drugs in which the γ-linolenic acid moiety was replaced with the n-3 components, eicosapentaenoic acid (■, n = 6), or docosahexaenoic acid (□, n = 8). Conduction velocity was not significantly different from that predicted from their α-lipoic acid content alone, showing that synergistic interactions with antioxidants are specific to n-6 essential fatty acids. (From Ref. 57 and Cameron NE, Cotter MA, unpublished observations, 1998).

sapentaenoic acid (Cameron NE, Cotter MA, unpublished observations, 1998) were no more effective than their α-lipoic acid component alone (Fig. 9). This suggests that synergistic actions are relatively specific to the *n*-6 series.

IV. SUMMARY AND CONCLUSIONS

Studies on antioxidant treatment have shown that ROS makes a marked contribution to the etiology of nerve dysfunction in experimental diabetes. Effects on vasa nervorum predominate in the short term; ROS cause dysfunction of vascular endothelium which at the very least reduces NO-mediated vasodilation and increases local vasoconstrictor production and reactivity. The effects of oxidative stress are crucial, complex, and far reaching, causing basic changes in cell signaling such as PKC and NF-κB that affect a plethora of systems involved in the maintenance of vascular control and integrity. ROS effects also impinge on prostanoid and EDHF systems, further exacerbating a diabetic deficit of substrate availability in the former. The result is reduced nerve perfusion, causing endoneurial hypoxia, which in turn is responsible for NCV and other functional deficits. Autooxidation of glucose and its metabolites and other transition metal-catalyzed reactions such as advanced glycation are important sources of ROS. Polyol pathway activity contributes to oxidative stress by compromising the glutathione redox cycle. Antioxidant treatment strategies, in combination with good metabolic control, offer a potential way forward in the prevention or control of diabetic neuropathy and other vascular complications. The powerful synergistic interactions between ROS–NO and *n*-6 essential fatty acid–prostanoid mechanisms on nerve perfusion offer a potential therapeutic advantage for the use of antioxidant–GLA mixtures and novel compounds.

REFERENCES

1. Low PA, Lagerlund TD, McManis PG. Nerve blood flow and oxygen delivery in normal, diabetic and ischemic neuropathy. Int Rev Neurobiol 1989; 31:355–438.
2. Tesfaye S, Malik R, Ward JD. Vascular factors in diabetic neuropathy. Diabetologia 1994; 37:847–854.
3. Cameron NE, Cotter MA. The relationship of vascular changes to metabolic factors in diabetes mellitus and their role in the development of peripheral nerve complications. Diabetes Metab Rev 1994; 10:189–224.

4. Cameron NE, Cotter MA. Metabolic and vascular factors in the pathogenesis of diabetic neuropathy. Diabetes 1997; 46(suppl 2):S31–S37.
5. Mayhan WG, Patel KP. Acute effects of glucose on reactivity of cerebral microcirculation: role of activation of protein kinase C. Am J Physiol 1995; 269: H1297–H1302.
6. Cohen RA. Dysfunction of vascular endothelium in diabetes mellitus. Circulation 1993; 87(suppl V):V67–V76.
7. Cameron NE, Cotter MA, Low PA. Nerve blood flow in early experimental diabetes in rats: relation to conduction deficits. Am J Physiol 1991; 261:E1–E8.
8. Wright RA, Nukada H. Vascular and metabolic factors in the pathogenesis of experimental diabetic neuropathy in mature rats. Brain 1994; 117:1395–1407.
9. Cameron NE, Cotter MA, Harrison J. The effects of diabetes on motor nerve conduction velocity in different branches of the rat sciatic nerve. Exp Neurol 1986; 92:757–761.
10. Cameron NE, Cotter MA, Robertson S. The effect of aldose reductase inhibition on the pattern of nerve conduction deficits in diabetic rats. Q J Exp Physiol 1989; 74:917–926.
11. Cameron NE, Cotter MA, Ferguson K, Robertson S, Radcliffe MA. Effects of chronic α-adrenergic receptor blockade on peripheral nerve conduction, hypoxic resistance, polyols, Na^+-K^+-ATPase activity, and vascular supply in STZ-D rats. Diabetes 1991; 40:1652–1658.
12. Cotter MA, Cameron NE. Correction of neurovascular deficits in diabetic rats by β_2 agonist and α_1 adrenoceptor antagonist treatment: interactions with the nitric oxide system. Eur J Pharmacol 1988; 343:217–223.
13. Kihara M, Schmelzer JD, Low PA. Effect of cilostazol on experimental diabetic neuropathy in the rat. Diabetologia 1995; 38:914–918.
14. Hotta N, Koh N, Sakakibara F, Nakamura J, Kakuta H, Fukasawa H, Sakamoto N. Effects of beraprost sodium and insulin on the electroretinogram, nerve conduction and nerve blood flow in rats with streptozotocin-induced diabetes. Diabetes 1996; 45:361–366.
15. Cameron NE, Cotter MA, Robertson S. Angiotensin converting enzyme inhibition prevents the development of muscle and nerve dysfunction and stimulates angiogenesis in streptozotocin-diabetic rats. Diabetologia 1992; 35:12–18.
16. Reja A, Tesfaye S, Harris ND, Ward JD. Is ACE inhibition with lisinopril helpful in diabetic neuropathy? Diabet Med 1995; 12:307–309.
17. Cameron NE, Cotter MA, Robertson S, Maxfield EK. Nerve function in experimental diabetes in rats: effects of electrical stimulation. Am J Physiol 1993; 264: E161–E166.
18. Cameron NE, Cotter MA, Jack A, Hohman TC. Inhibition of protein kinase C corrects nerve conduction and blood flow deficits in diabetic rats (abstr). Diabetologia 1997; 40(suppl 1):A31.
19. Cameron NE, Cotter MA. Reversal of peripheral nerve conduction and perfusion deficits by the free radical scavenger, BM15.0639, in diabetic rats. Naunyn Schmiedeberg's Arch Pharmacol 1995; 321:685–690.

20. Cameron NE, Cotter MA, Hohman TC. Interactions between essential fatty acid, prostanoid, polyol pathway and nitric oxide mechanisms in the neurovascular deficit of diabetic rats. Diabetologia 1996; 39:172–182.
21. Cameron NE, Cotter MA. Rapid reversal by aminoguanidine of the neurovascular effects of diabetes in rats: modulation by nitric oxide synthase inhibition. Metabolism 1996; 45:1147–1152.
22. Cameron NE, Cotter MA. Neurovascular effects of L-carnitine treatment in diabetic rats. Eur J Pharmacol 1997; 319:239–244.
23. Kihara M, Low PA. Impaired vasoreactivity to nitric oxide in experimental diabetic neuropathy. Exp Neurol 1995; 132:180–185.
24. Maxfield EK, Cameron NE, Cotter MA. Effects of diabetes on reactivity of sciatic vasa nervorum in rats. J Diabet Complications 1997; 11:47–55.
25. Gryglewski RJ, Palmer RMJ, Moncado S. Superoxide anion is involved in the breakdown of endothelium-derived vascular relaxing factor. Nature 1986; 320: 454–456.
26. Beckman JS, Beckman TW, Chen J, Marshall PA, Freeman BA. Apparent hydroxyl radical production by peroxynitrite: implications for endothelial injury from nitric oxide and superoxide. Proc Natl Acad Sci USA 1990; 87:1620–1624.
27. Tesfamariam B, Cohen RA. Free radicals mediate endothelial cell dysfunction caused by elevated glucose. Am J Physiol 1992; 263:H321–H326.
28. Baynes JW. Role of oxidative stress in the development of complications in diabetes. Diabetes 1991; 40:405–412.
29. Wolff SP. Diabetes mellitus and free radicals. Br Med Bull 1993; 49:642–652.
30. Harrison DG. Endothelial function and oxidant stress. Clin Cardiol 1997; 20(suppl 2):11–17.
31. McCord JM. Oxygen-derived free radicals in postischemic tissue injury. N Engl J Med 1985; 312:159–163.
32. Wieruszwysocka B, Wysocki H, Byks H, Zozulinska D, Wykretowicz A, Kazierczak M. Metabolic control quality and free radical activity in diabetic patients. Diabetes Res Clin Pract 1995; 27:193–197.
33. Diabetes Control and Complications Trial Research Group. The effect of intensive diabetes therapy on the development and progression of neuropathy. Ann Intern Med 1995; 122:561–568.
34. Low PA, Nickander KK. Oxygen free radical effects in sciatic nerve in experimental diabetes. Diabetes 1991; 40:873–877.
35. Nickander KK, Schmelzer JD, Rohwer D, Low PA. Effects of α-tocopherol-deficiency on indices of oxidative stress in normal and diabetic peripheral nerve. J Neurol Sci 1994; 126:6–14.
36. Nagamatsu M, Nickander KK, Schmelzer JD, Raya A, Wittrock A, Tritschler H, Low PA. Lipoic acid improves nerve blood flow, reduces oxidative stress and improves distal nerve conduction in experimental diabetic neuropathy. Diabetes Care 1995; 18:1160–1167.

37. Low PA, Nickander KK, Tritschler HJ. The roles of oxidative stress and antioxidant treatment in experimental diabetic neuropathy. Diabetes 1997; 46(suppl 2): S38–S42.
38. Sasaki H, Schmelzer JD, Zollman PJ, Low PA. Neuropathology and blood flow of nerve, spinal roots and dorsal root ganglia in longstanding diabetic rats. Acta Neuropathol 1997; 93:118–128.
39. Keegan A, Walbank H, Cotter MA, Cameron NE. Chronic vitamin E treatment prevents defective endothelium-dependent relaxation in diabetic rat aorta. Diabetologia 1995; 38:1475–1478.
40. Archibald V, Cotter MA, Keegan A, Cameron NE. Contraction and relaxation of aortas from diabetic rats: effects of chronic anti-oxidant and aminoguanidine treatments. Naunyn Schmiedeberg's Arch Pharmacol 1996; 353:584–591.
41. Rösen P, Ballhausen T, Bloch W, Addicks K. Endothelial relaxation is disturbed by oxidative stress in the diabetic rat heart: influence of tocopherol as antioxidant. Diabetologia 1995; 38:1157–1168.
42. Pieper GM, Gross GJ. Oxygen free radicals abolish endothelium-dependent relaxation in diabetic rat aorta. Am J Physiol 1988; 255:H825–H833.
43. Kamata K, Miyata N, Kasuya Y. Impairment of endothelium-dependent relaxation and changes in levels of cyclic GMP in aorta from streptozotocin-induced diabetic rats. Br J Pharmacol 1989; 97:614–618.
44. McVeigh GE, Brennan GM, Johnston GD, McDermott BJ, McGrath LT, Henry WR, Andrews JW, Hayes JR. Impaired endothelium -dependent and independent vasodilation in patients with type 2 (non-insulin-dependent) diabetes mellitus. Diabetologia 1992; 35:771–776.
45. Johnstone MT, Creager SJ, Scales KM, Cusco JA, Lee BK, Creager MA. Impaired endothelium-dependent vasodilation in patients with insulin-dependent diabetes mellitus. Circulation 1993; 88:2510–2516.
46. Nitenberg A, Valensi P, Sachs R, Dali M, Aptecar E, Attali JR. Impairment of coronary vascular reserve and ACh-induced coronary vasodilation in diabetic patients with angiographically normal coronary arteries and normal left ventricular systolic function. Diabetes 1993; 42:1017–1025.
47. Morris SJ, Shore AC, Tooke JE. Responses of the skin microcirculation to acetylcholine and sodium nitroprusside in patients with NIDDM. Diabetologia 1995; 38:1337–1344.
48. Cameron NE, Cotter MA, Maxfield EK. Antioxidant treatment prevents the development of peripheral nerve dysfunction in streptozotocin-diabetic rats. Diabetologia 1993; 36:299–304.
49. Cameron NE, Cotter MA, Archibald V, Dines KC, Maxfield EK. Anti-oxidant and pro-oxidant effects on nerve conduction velocity, endoneurial blood flow and oxygen tension in non-diabetic and streptozotocin-diabetic rats. Diabetologia 1994; 37:449–459.
50. Cotter MA, Love A, Watt MJ, Cameron NE, Dines KC. Effects of natural free radical scavengers on peripheral nerve and neurovascular function in diabetic rats. Diabetologia 1995; 38:1285–1294.

51. Sagara M, Satoh J, Wada R, Yagihashi S, Takahashi K, Fukuzawa M, Muto G, Muto Y, Toyota T. Inhibition of development of peripheral neuropathy in streptozotocin-induced diabetic rats with *N*-acetylcysteine. Diabetologia 1996; 39:263–269.
52. Love A, Cotter MA, Cameron NE. Effects of the sulphydryl donor, *N*-acetyl-L-cysteine, on nerve conduction, perfusion, maturation, and regeneration following freeze-damage in diabetic rats. Eur J Clin Invest 1996; 26:698–706.
53. Love A, Cotter MA, Cameron NE. Effects of α-tocopherol on nerve conduction velocity and regeneration following a freeze lesion in immature diabetic rats. Naunyn Schmeideberg's Arch Pharmacol 1997; 355:126–130.
54. Love A, Cotter MA, Cameron NE. Nerve function and regeneration in diabetic and galactosaemic rats: antioxidant and metal chelator effects. Eur J Pharmacol 1996; 314:33–39.
55. Packer L, Tritschler HJ, Wessel K. Neuroprotection by the metabolic antioxidant α-lipoic acid. Free Rad Biol Med 1996; 22:359–378.
56. Nickander KK, McPhee BR, Low PA, Tritschler H. Alpha-lipoic acid: antioxidant potency against lipid peroxidation of neural tissues in vitro and implications for diabetic neuropathy. Free Rad Biol Med 1996; 21:631–639.
57. Cameron NE, Cotter MA, Horrobin DH, Tritschler HJ. Effects of α-lipoic acid on neurovascular function in diabetic rats: interaction with essential fatty acids. Diabetologia 1998; 41:390–399.
58. Ziegler D, Hanefeld M, Ruhnau KJ, Meißner HP, Lobisch M, Schütte K, Gries FA, The ALADIN Study Group. Treatment of symptomatic diabetic peripheral neuropathy with the anti-oxidant α-lipoic acid. A 3-week multicentre randomized controlled trial (ALADIN Study). Diabetologia 1995; 38:1425–1433.
59. Ziegler D, Schatz H, Gries FA, Ulrich H, Reichel G. Effects of treatment with the antioxidant α-lipoic acid on cardiac autonomic neuropathy in NIDDM patients. A 4-month randomized controlled multicenter trial (DEKAN Study). Diabetes Care 1997; 20:369–373.
60. Maxfield EK, Love A, Cotter MA, Cameron NE. Nerve function and regeneration in diabetic rats: effects of ZD-7155, an AT_1 receptor antagonist. Am J Physiol 1995; 269:E530–E537.
61. Cameron NE, Cotter MA. Effects of a nonpeptide endothelin-1 ET_A antagonist on neurovascular function in diabetic rats: interaction with the renin-angiotensin system. J Pharmacol Exp Ther 1996; 278:1262–1268.
62. Hunt JV, Bottoms MA, Mitchison MJ. Ascorbic acid oxidation: a potential cause of the elevated severity of atherosclerosis in diabetes mellitus. FEBS Lett 1992; 311:161–164.
63. Packer LE, Slater TF, Wilson RL. Direct observation of a free radical interaction between vitamin E and vitamin C. Nature 1979; 278:737–738.
64. Cameron NE, Cotter MA. Neurovascular dysfunction in diabetic rats: potential contribution of autoxidation and free radicals examined using transition metal chelating agents. J Clin Invest 1995; 96:1159–1163.
65. Pieper GM, Siebeneich W. Diabetes-induced endothelial dysfunction is pre-

vented by long-term treatment with the modified iron chelator, hydroxyethyl starch conjugated-deferoxamine. J Cardiovasc Pharmacol 1997; 30:734–738

66. Keegan A, Cotter MA, Archibald V, Cameron NE. Metal chelator and free radical scavenger treatments prevent chronic aorta relaxation defects in diabetic rats (abstr). Diabetologia 1996; 39(suppl 1):A240.
67. Cameron NE, Cotter MA, Maxfield EK. Correction of impaired neurovascular function by desferrioxamine in anaesthetized diabetic rats (abstr). J Physiol 1995; 487:84P–85P.
68. Keegan A, Cotter MA, Cameron NE. Impaired endothelial and autonomic relaxation of the corpus cavernosum in diabetic rats: effects of antioxidants (abstr). Diabetic Med 1998; 15(suppl 1):S7.
69. Hohman TC, Banas D, Basso M, Cotter MA, Cameron NE. Increased oxidative stress in experimental diabetic neuropathy (abstr). Diabetologia 1997; 40(suppl 1):A549.
70. Lowitt S, Malone JI, Salem AF, Korthals J, Benford S. Acetyl-L-carnitine corrects altered peripheral nerve function in experimental diabetes. Metabolism 1995; 44:677–680.
71. Cameron NE, Cotter MA, Dines KC, Maxfield EK, Carey F, Mirrlees DJ. Aldose reductase inhibition, nerve perfusion, oxygenation and function in streptozotocin-diabetic rats: dose-response considerations and independence from a myo-inositol mechanism. Diabetologia 1994; 37:651–663.
72. Hotta N, Kaskuta H, Fukasawa H, Koh N, Sakakibara F, Nakamura J, Hamada Y, Wakao T, Hara T, Mori K, Naruse K, Nakashima E, Inukai S, Sakamoto N. Effect of a potent new aldose reductase inhibitor (5-(3-thienyl)tetrazol-1-yl)-acetic acid (TAT), on diabetic neuropathy in rats. Diabetes Res Clin Pract 1995; 27:107–117.
73. Cameron NE, Cotter MA, Basso M, Hohman TC. Comparison of the effects of inhibitors of aldose reductase and sorbitol dehydrogenase on neurovascular function, nerve conduction and tissue polyol pathway metabolites in streptozotocin-diabetic rats. Diabetologia 1997; 40:271–281.
74. Hamada Y, Araki N, Horiuchi S, Hotta N. Role of polyol pathway in nonenzymatic glycation. Nephrol Dial Transplant 1996; 11:95–98.
75. Fu MX, Wells-Knecht KJ, Blackledge JA, Lyons TJ, Thorpe SR, Baynes JW. Glycation, glycoxidation and cross-linking of collagen by glucose: kinetics, mechanisms, and inhibition of late stages of the Maillard reaction. Diabetes 1994; 43:676–683.
76. Cameron NE, Cotter MA. Rapid reversal by aminoguanidine of the neurovascular effects of diabetes in rats: modulation by nitric oxide synthase inhibition. Metabolism 1996; 45:1147–1152.
77. Bierhaus A, Chevion S, Chevion M, Hofmann M, Quehenberger P, Illmer T, Luther Y, Berentshtein E, Tritschler H, Müller M, Wahl P, Ziegler R, Nawroth PP. Advanced glycation end product-induced activation of NF-κB is suppressed by α-lipoic acid in cultured endothelial cells. Diabetes 1997; 46:1481–1490.

78. Collins T. Endothelial nuclear factor-κB and the initiation of the atherosclerotic lesion. Lab Invest 1993; 68:499–508.
79. Kunisaki M, Bursell S, Umeda F, Nawata H, King GL. Normalization of diacylglycerol-protein kinase C activation by vitamin E in aorta of diabetic rats and cultured rat smooth muscle cells exposed to elevated glucose levels. Diabetes 1994; 43:1372–1377.
80. Borghini I, Ania-Lahuerta A, Regazzi R, Ferrari G, Gjinovci A, Wollheim CB, Pralong W-F. α, βI, βII, δ, and ε protein kinase C isoforms and compound activity in the sciatic nerve of normal and diabetic rats. J Neurochem 1994; 62:686–696.
81. Ishii H, Jirousek MR, Koya D, Takagi C, Xia P, Clermont A, Bursell S-E, Kern TS, Ballas LM, Heath WF, Stramm LE, Feener EP, King GL. Amelioration of vascular dysfunctions in diabetic rats by an oral PKC β inhibitor. Science 1996; 272:728–731.
82. Keaney JF Jr, Guo Y, Cunningham D, Shwaery GT, Xu A, Vita JA. Vascular incorporation of alpha-tocopherol prevents endothelial dysfunction due to oxidized LDL by inhibiting protein kinase C stimulation. J Clin Invest 1996; 98: 386–394.
83. Rubanyi GM, Polokoff MA. Endothelins: molecular biology, biochemistry, pharmacology, physiology and pathophysiology. Pharmacol Rev 1994; 46:325–415.
84. Davda RK, Chandler LJ, Guzman NJ. Protein kinase C modulates receptor-independent activation of endothelial nitric oxide synthase. Eur J Pharmacol 1994; 266:237–244.
85. Shimamoto Y, Shimamoto H, Kwan C, Daniel EE. Differential effects of putative protein kinase C inhibitors on contraction of rat aortic smooth muscle. Am J Physiol 1993; 264:H1300–H1306.
86. Ward KK, Low PA, Schmelzer JD, Zochodne DW. Prostacyclin and noradrenaline in peripheral nerve of chronic experimental diabetes in rats. Brain 1989; 112:197–208.
87. Cotter MA, Cameron NE. Effects of dietary supplementation with arachidonic acid rich oils on nerve conduction and blood flow in streptozotocin-diabetic rats. Prostaglandins Leukot Essent Fatty Acids 1997; 56:337–343.
88. Dines KC, Cotter MA, Cameron NE. Contrasting effects of treatment with ω-3 and ω-6 essential fatty acids on peripheral nerve function and capillarization in streptozotocin-diabetic rats. Diabetologia 1993; 36:1132–1138.
89. Jack A, Cotter MA, Cameron NE. Impaired endothelium-derived hyperpolarizing factor in the mesenteric vasculature of diabetic rats: effects of antioxidant treatment (abstr). Diabetic Med 1998; 15(suppl 1):S31.
90. Moncada S, Gryglewski RJ, Bunting S, Vane JR. A lipid peroxide inhibits the enzyme in blood vessel microsomes that generates from prostaglandin endoperoxides the substance (prostaglandin X) which prevents platelet aggregation. Prostaglandins 1976; 12:715–737.
91. Karpen CW, Pritchard KA, Arnold JH, Cornwell DG, Pangonamala RV. Restora-

tion of the prostacyclin/thromboxane A_2 balance in the diabetic rat: influence of vitamin E. Diabetes 1982; 31:947–951.

92. De Nucci G, Gryglewski RJ, Warner TD, Vane JR. Receptor mediated release of endothelium-derived relaxing factor and prostacyclin from bovine aortic endothelial cells is coupled. Proc Natl Acad Sci USA 1988; 85:2334–2338.
93. Cameron NE, Cotter MA, Dines KC, Maxfield EK. Pharmacological manipulation of vascular endothelium in non-diabetic and streptozotocin-diabetic rats: effects on nerve conduction, hypoxic resistance and endoneurial capillarization. Diabetologia 1993; 36:516–522.
94. Cameron NE, Cotter MA. Interaction between oxidative stress and γ-linolenic acid in the impaired neurovascular function of diabetic rats. Am J Physiol 1996; 271:E471–E476.
95. Cameron NE, Cotter MA. Comparison of the effects of ascorbyl γ-linolenic acid and γ-linolenic acid in the correction of neurovascular deficits in diabetic rats. Diabetologia 1996; 39:1047–1054.

11

A Thioctic Acid–Gamma-Linolenic Acid Conjugate Protects Neurotrophic Support in Experimental Diabetic Neuropathy

Luke Hounsom
Queen Mary and Westfield College, London, England

David R. Tomlinson
University of Manchester, Manchester, England

Defects of the peripheral nervous system are common in patients with diabetes mellitus, and a large fraction of patients will develop a form of diabetic neuropathy within 25 years after diagnosis (1). Although a rigid classification of diabetic neuropathy is difficult, at least three major syndromes are recognized: symmetrical distal polyneuropathy, symmetrical proximal motor neuropathies, and focal asymmetrical neuropathies (2–4). As in most polyneuropathies, sensory, motor, and autonomic nerves are concomitantly involved although sensory dysfunction usually predominates.

Recent attempts to rationalize the etiology of diabetic neuropathy have focused initially on the identification of the biochemical defects that follow directly from hyperglycemia, in this case, the polyol pathway, protein glycation, and oxidative stress (for recent reviews, see Refs. 5 and 6). Second, there is the issue of the importance of reduced nerve blood flow and possible consequent ischemic damage (7–9). Related to this is the proposition that defective metabolism of essential fatty acids, resulting in reduced levels of γ-linolenic acid and subsequently arachidonic acid and vasoactive prostanoids, also has a large part to play in the pathogenesis of diabetic neuropathy (see

Ref. 10 for review). A chain of consequences comprising hyperglycemia, exaggerated polyol pathway flux, oxidative stress, impaired endoneurial nitric oxide production, reduced nerve blood flow, endoneurial hypoxia, and impaired nerve conduction has been suggested (11–13). Impaired neurotrophic support from nerve growth factor (NGF) and neurotrophin 3 (NT-3) (14–17) is also important, because a failure of neurotrophic factors to regulate neuronal phenotype might be expected to result in such a clinical picture as presents in symptomatic diabetic neuropathy.

Recently, the antioxidant thioctic (α-lipoic) acid has been found to protect against a broad range of defects in diabetic rats, (18–20) including both those related to nerve blood flow and those related to neurotrophins.

I. NEUROTROPHIC FACTORS

Neurotrophic factors were discovered as agents with the capacity to stimulate neurite outgrowth in culture systems of embryonic sensory or sympathetic neurons. Some of these factors, such as ciliary neurotrophic factor (a member of the interleukin-6 cytokine family) and basic fibroblast growth factor (a member of the fibroblast growth factor family), are quite distinct from NGF, the archetypal neurotrophic factor. It has now been established that NGF belongs to a family of neurotrophic factors known as the neurotrophins that now includes NT-3, brain-derived neurotrophic factor (BDNF), and neurotrophin-4/5 (see Ref. 21 for review).

NGF undergoes retrograde transport in sensory and sympathetic neurons in adult rats (22,23), and about 50% of adult lumbar sensory neurons can bind NGF with high affinity (24). BDNF and NT-3 also undergo retrograde transport from an injection site in the sciatic nerve to the dorsal root ganglia (DRG) and motor neurons of adult rats (25).

The neurotrophins bind to two distinct sites on responsive neurons. Low-affinity binding is associated with the p75 neurotrophin receptor (p75NTR) and shows no selectivity between the neurotrophins. High-affinity binding is provided by a family of trk proto-oncogene receptors that have intrinsic tyrosine kinase activity. trkA is specific for NGF (26,27), trkB for BDNF and NT-4/5 (28,29), and trkC for NT-3 (30). However, NT-3 is promiscuous and will also bind to trkB and trkA at increasing concentrations.

There is a large body of evidence suggesting that NGF and the other neurotrophins are involved, not just in the survival of neurons during embryonic development but also in the regulation of neuronal phenotype in the adult. Deprivation of trophic support by nerve transection provokes a pattern of change in the nerve cell body that is prevented by the administration of exogenous neurotrophin. Direct evidence for modulation of adult phenotype was provided when it was demonstrated that NGF can regulate the expression of substance P (SP) and calcitonin gene-related peptide (CGRP) in primary cultures of adult rat DRG neurons (31). Additionally, deprivation of NGF has been found to cause a proportional reduction in the expression of these neuropeptides (32,33).

II. NEUROTROPHINS IN DIABETIC NEUROPATHY

Decreased capture and retrograde transport of iodinated NGF in the sciatic nerve was observed in diabetic rats many years ago (34). Reduced retrograde transport of iodinated NGF in ileal mesenteric nerves has also been demonstrated (35). These observations imply that even in the absence of any deficit in production of NGF in diabetes, a deficit in the amount delivered to the cell body might be expected. In diabetic rats, there are reduced levels of NGF in the submandibular gland, superior cervical ganglion, and sciatic nerve (36–38). NGF levels have also been shown to be decreased in the serum of diabetic patients with symptomatic peripheral neuropathy (39).

Work in our laboratory has shown that with increasing duration of diabetes, progressive reductions in NGF mRNA appear in leg muscle and sciatic nerve followed by reductions in skin. There is a profound reduction in the retrograde transport of NGF in the sciatic nerve, which can be reversed by intensive insulin treatment, and dose-related increases in sciatic nerve NGF retrograde transport were seen with recombinant human NGF (rhNGF) treatment (33). Additionally, it is clear that there are also deficits in the production of NGF target genes, and deficits in expression of SP and CGRP are easily demonstrable in experimental diabetic neuropathy (32).

It is quite apparent that there are deficits in NGF expiation in experimental diabetes, but this does not explain the earlier observation of reduced capture and transport of exogenous NGF. Recent work in our laboratory has revealed a marked decrease in the retrograde transport of the p75NTR, which closely follows the changes seen with NGF transport in diabetes (40). No changes in transport of trkA were observed, but it is not yet possible to suggest which are the precedent changes because NGF availability is known to affect the expression of the p75NTR (41).

NT-3 mRNA levels are reduced in leg muscle from diabetic rats, but an assessment of NT-3 neurotrophic support is difficult because gene targets of NT-3 have yet to be identified. Work in our laboratory showed that treatment of diabetic rats with rhNT-3 for the last 4 weeks of a 12-week period of diabetes could completely normalize the reduced sensory nerve conduction velocity, which is characteristic of diabetic rats (16). This implies that NT-3 may be even more instrumental than NGF in the development of important functional deficits in diabetic neuropathy. However, although treatment of animals with NGF or NT-3 prevents some of the deficits characteristic of experimental neuropathy (14,16), these agents do not influence reduced nerve blood flow or motor nerve conduction velocity (42), other classic hallmarks of experimental neuropathy.

III. NEUROTROPHINS AND OXIDATIVE STRESS

Shifts in cellular redox balance due to increased levels of free radicals may cause or result from neuronal injury (43,44). Oxygen free radicals are generated as a consequence of ischemia-reperfusion, inflammation, traumatic, and oxidative injury and are associated with neuronal cell death (45,46).

Peripheral nerves, including the sciatic nerve, have inherent low antioxidant defenses compared with the central nervous system, because total reduced glutathione (GSH) content and activities of GSH utilizing enzymes like glutathione peroxidase (GSH-Px) are about 10-fold lower than they are in brain (47).

NGF stimulates cellular resistance to oxidative stress in PC12 cells (48). In particular, NGF protects from oxidative injury induced by hydrogen peroxide and 6-hydroxydopamine, (48–50) both of which generate hydroxyl radicals. From these observations, it might be expected that NGF regulates cellular oxidant-antioxidant equilibrium.

NGF has been found to regulate the expression of the antioxidant enzymes, catalase (Cat), and GSH-Px. Application of NGF to PC12 cells in culture results in an increase in the transcription of the mRNA for Cat and GSH-Px and, in addition, appears to stabilize the transcript for Cat (51). This is associated with an increase in the activities of both enzymes (52). Furthermore, newborn rat astrocytes in culture synthesise NGF in a dose-dependent fashion in response to superoxide anion, as generated by xanthine/xanthine oxidase and to hydrogen peroxide (53).

IV. OXIDATIVE STRESS IN DIABETES

Diabetes is associated with increases in oxidative stress in humans and in experimental animal models. Chronic hyperglycemia *per se* results in autoxidative glycation/oxidation and lipid peroxidation (54–56), and hyperglycemia alone will cause lipid peroxidation of peripheral nerve in vitro (57).

Diabetic peripheral nerve has increased levels of conjugated dienes (end products from peroxidation of polyunsaturated fatty acids) (57,58), decreased levels of GSH (19), and reduced activity of copper/zinc-superoxide dismutase that is reversible with reinstatement of moderate glycemic control (58).

Further support for the role of oxidative stress in the pathogenesis of diabetic neuropathy come from the effectiveness of antioxidant treatment in reversing some of the functional neurological deficits observed in experimental animal models.

Probucol, a powerful free radical scavenger, normalizes both decreases in endoneurial nerve blood flow and motor nerve conduction velocity (59,60). Dietary treatment with 1% butylated hydroxytoluene or α-tocopherol also has similar effects (61,62). Intravenous administration of GSH can also partially prevent motor nerve conduction velocity slowing in diabetic rats (63). Beneficial effects on conduction velocity have also been reported using the metal chelator deferoxamine (64).

V. THIOCTIC ACID

Thioctic acid (TA) was first isolated in 1951 (65) and is now known by a variety of different names, including α-lipoic acid, 1,2-dithiolane-3-pentanoic acid, 1,2-dithiolane valenic acid, and 6,8-thioctic acid. As lipoamide, it functions as a cofactor in the multienzyme complexes that catalyze the oxidative decarboxylations of α-keto acids such as pyruvate, α-ketoglutarate, and branched chain α-keto acids (66). In addition, TA is a powerful antioxidant (67) and a potent free radical scavenger in peripheral nerve (57,68) that would appear to act by substituting for α-tocopherol (57). Interestingly, endogenous TA is depleted in diabetes (69,70).

A study carried out by Kahler et al. (71) confirmed the association of long-term diabetic complications with increased lipid peroxidation and enhanced lipid peroxidation. Treatment with TA decreased peroxidation rate, improved thermal and vibration sensibilities, and improved patellar and Achilles tendon reflexes. Furthermore, results from the α-Lipoic Acid in Diabetic Neuropathy study (72) revealed that TA at a dose of 600 or 1200 mg administered intravenously significantly reduced the incidence of burning sensation, parasthesiae, and numbness in patients with symptomatic diabetic neuropathy.

TA has effects beyond that of a simple antioxidant. TA stimulates glucose utilization by tissues (73,74) and may also act as a chelator of transition metal ions, which are thought to contribute to oxidative stress (75–77). Furthermore, TA also inhibits nonenzymatic glycation/glycosylation, which is now thought to play a role in the pathogenesis of diabetic late complications (see Ref. 78 for review).

Unrelated to this, TA is also able to induce neurite outgrowth (79) and promote nerve regeneration (80). TA can also stimulate NGF synthesis and secretion (81).

VI. IN VIVO STUDIES WITH THIOCTYL-γ-LINOLENIC ACID

γ-Linolenic acid (GLA) is an Ω-6 essential fatty acid that is thought to be the active ingredient of evening primrose oil (EPO). Previous studies using EPO as a dietary supplement have shown complete reversal of motor nerve conduction deficits in diabetic rats (82,83). EPO has also been found to increase prostacyclin release in diabetic sciatic nerve (84), increase nerve blood flow, reduce subsequent nerve trunk ischemia (85), and reduce resistance to ischemic conduction failure (86,87).

Given the known effects of TA in experimental diabetes (19,20) and the ability of EPO to reverse some of the deficits seen in experimental diabetes, the rationale for use of a TA-γ-linolenic acid conjugate (thioctyl γ-linolenic acid; GLA^^TATA) are not difficult to realize. However, in the search for compounds that are active against a broad spectrum of defects encountered in diabetes, no such compound has fit that bill. Therefore, in vivo studies with the conjugate were designed to reflect two classes of defect, with motor and sensory nerve conduction velocities indicating the polyol-nerve blood flow pathway and NGF and neuropeptides as markers of neurotrophic support.

In vivo studies evaluated the efficacy of dietary supplementation with 2.5% GLA^^TA (see Fig. 1 for structural representation), 100 mg/kg TA IP five times per week, and dietary supplementation with 1.5% butylated hydroxytoluene (BHT) in 8-week streptozotocin-induced diabetic rats.

Untreated diabetic animals showed both motor and sensory nerve conduction velocity deficits (Fig. 2A) and reduced levels of NGF, neuropeptide Y (NPY), and SP (Fig. 2B) in their sciatic nerves. Treatment with BHT was without effect on any of these variables. Treatment with TA increased the NGF content of sciatic nerve and produced small arithmetic increases in both SP and NPY, which did not attain significance. There was no effect on either sensory or motor nerve conduction velocity. Treatment with the GLA^^TA conjugate increased sciatic nerve levels of both SP and NPY, so that they were significantly higher than those measured in nerves from untreated diabetic rats ($p < 0.05$), although they remained significantly lower than those of controls

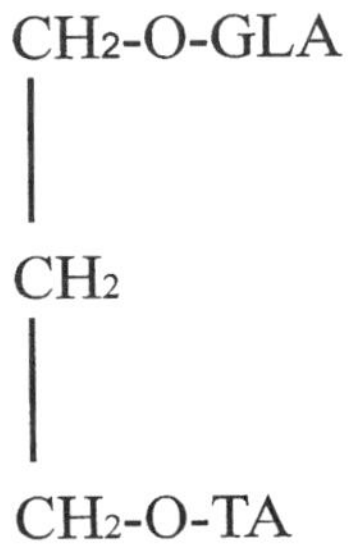

Figure 1 Structure of thioctyl-γ-linolenic acid (GLA^^TA). The molecule is a 1,2,3-propanediol diester with one molecule of GLA and one molecule of TA joined to the propanediol backbone by ester linkages.

($p < 0.05$ and 0.01 respectively) (Fig. 2B). GLA^^TA also increased NGF levels (Fig. 2B) and both motor and sensuous nerve conduction velocities (Fig. 2A), so that these values were not significantly different from those of control rats. The potential dependence of the neuropeptide changes on NGF levels was examined by regression analyses. For the dependence of SP on NGF, r^2 was 0.257 ($p < 0.005$), but the levels of NPY were less closely related to those of NGF, where r^2 was 0.145 and the regression was barely significant ($p < 0.05$).

NPY in the sciatic nerve may derive from mixed fiber populations—some must be in sympathetic postganglionic fibers (88,89), but there may also be some in somatic sensory fibers. However, the level of expression in somatic afferents is low unless they are damaged, when it increases (90); after axotomy, this increased expression may be reduced by either NT-3 or NGF (91,92). Expression of NPY by the sympathetic phenotype is clearly stimulated by NGF (93), and NGF-responsive elements have been identified on the NPY promoter (94). Thus, the findings reported here might be most easily explained by the proposition that the NPY deficit in sciatic nerves of diabetic rats is also derived from reduced NGF neurotrophic support. However, our previous study showed that treatment of diabetic rats with NGF, although normalizing the SP levels in sciatic nerve, did not affect the NPY deficit (20). Thus, there may be control of NPY expression in these fibers by another neurotrophin, and the NGF response elements become functional only when other influences are removed. This might explain the NGF effects on NPY in vitro (93,95) and increases in NPY after axotomy in vivo (90,96). Thus, the evolution of the decrease in NPY expression in our diabetic rats cannot be explained as yet, though the deficit clearly responds to treatment with the GLA^^TA conjugate and, in our previous study, also responded to TA (20).

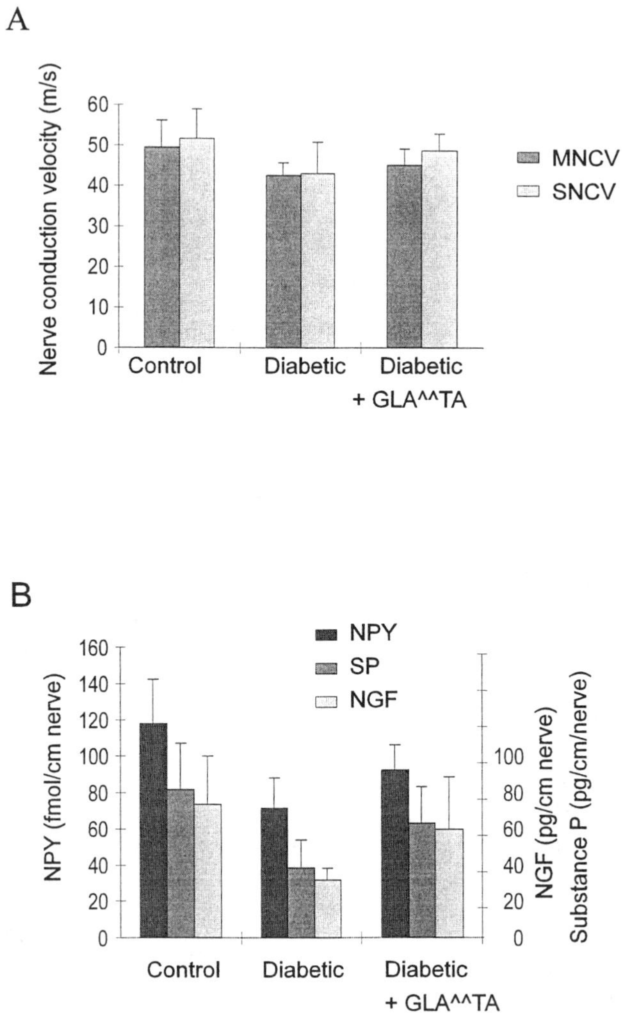

Figure 2 (A) Bar chart showing nerve conduction velocities in control, diabetic, and 2.5% GLA^^TA-treated diabetic rats. Control versus diabetic $p < 0.01$ for both motor and sensory nerve conduction velocity; 2.5% GLA^^TA treated animals were not statistically different from controls or untreated diabetic rats by ANOVA with Duncan's multiple range tests. (B) Bar chart showing sciatic nerve levels of SP, NPY, and NGF. Control versus diabetic $p < 0.01$ for SP, NPY, and NGF; 2.5% GLA^^TA increased sciatic nerve levels of SP and NPY ($p < 0.05$), although they remained significantly different from controls, $p < 0.05$ and $p < 0.01$, respectively. GLA^^TA 2.5% also increased NGF levels, so that these values were not different from controls.

EFFECT OF THIOCTYL-γ-LINOLENIC ACID ON THE ACTIVATION OF STRESS-ACTIVATED PROTEIN KINASES

Mitogen-activated protein (MAP) kinases are proline-directed serine/threonine kinases that are activated by dual phosphorylation in response to a wide variety of extracellular stimuli. Three distinct groups of MAP kinases have been identified in mammalian cells; extracellular signal-regulated kinase (ERK), c-*jun* N-terminal kinase (JNK), and p38MAP kinase (p38) (see Refs. 97 and 98 for review). MAP kinase activation is achieved through kinase cascades, which serve as information relays connecting cell surface receptors to specific transcription factors and other regulatory proteins, thus allowing extracellular signals to regulate the expression of specific genes (99).

Recently, among this large family of MAP kinases, a family of stress-activated protein kinases (SAPKs), including JNK and p38, have been delineated and characterized (see Ref. 100 for review). JNK exits in three forms in mammalian cells: JNK1, JNK2, and JNK3 of 46, 54, and 56 kDa molecular weight, respectively. JNK has been found to be activated by a variety of different stimuli, including inflammatory cytokines such as interleukin-1 and tumor necrosis factor α, γ-irradiation, ultraviolet irradiation, and oxidative stress (101). Once activated, JNK phosphorylates a number of different substrates, including c-*jun* and ATF2. Both of these transcription factors can form part of the AP-1 transcription factor complex, which is known to regulate the transcription of many different genes (reviewed in Ref. 98). Because oxidative stress, as part of the dysmetabolism of diabetes mellitus, seemed an excellent candidate for activation of SAPKs, we included measurement of activation of these molecules in the present study.

The expression of the subtypes of JNK was investigated using antibodies raised against either the native protein (JNK-FL) of the phosphorylated (activated) form (pJNK) in the DRG from 8-week diabetic rats and diabetic rats treated with 2.5% GLA$^{\wedge\wedge}$TA. Western blots were analyzed by densitometry and levels of protein compared by normalizing to controls.

Eight weeks of diabetes resulted in a significant increase in the level of the p54 form of activated JNK ($p < 0.05$ compared with controls). This increase in activation of p54 JNK as measured by Western blotting with phospho-specific antibodies was reversed by 2.5% GLA$^{\wedge\wedge}$TA (Fig. 3) Total levels of the full-length JNK protein were unchanged by diabetes or GLA$^{\wedge\wedge}$TA treatment.

Levels of the phosphorylated transcription factors, ATF2, and c-*jun* were investigated using antibodies specific to the phosphorylated forms of these transcription factors and were also unchanged by diabetes or GLA$^{\wedge\wedge}$TA treatment.

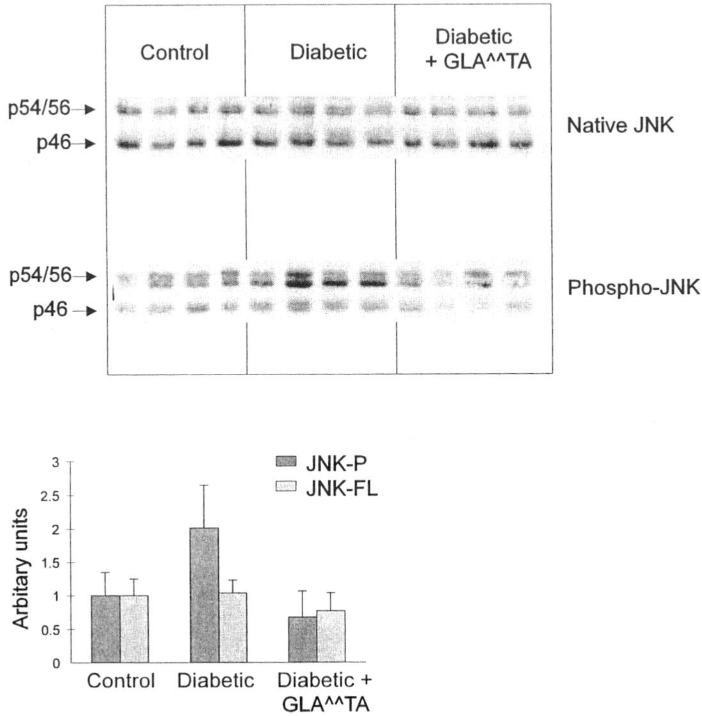

Figure 3 Western blots from lumbar DRG exposed to antibodies against a nonphosphorylated epitope of JNK (JNK-FL) or a phosphorylated epitope (pJNK). Bar chart shows diabetes-induced increase in p54/p56 JNK phosphorylation ($p < 0.05$ controls) can be reversed by GLA^^TA. There were no changes in the levels of the native protein, JNK-FL.

The reduction in the activation of JNK by GLA^^TA may reflect a reduction in neuronal stress. TA treatment is known to increase levels of GSH in diabetic sciatic nerve (19), and GSH is a critical regulator for the induction of SAPKs, including JNK (102). However, it is not yet known whether the conjugate has similar effects on glutathione metabolism, but this warrants closer investigation.

VIII. ROLE FOR GLA^^TA IN THE TREATMENT OF DIABETIC NEUROPATHY

This is the first instance of a treatment that is capable of attenuating both electrophysiological and neurochemical deficits in the nerves of diabetic rats. The effect of the GLA^^TA conjugate is also remarkable when related to the current effects of TA and previously reported effects of EPO. Approximate calculations suggest that the dose of GLA^^TA used here could deliver about 14 mg/kg/day TA and 18 mg/kg/day GLA. TA must be given at doses of at least 50 mg/kg/day to influence nerve conduction (19), and in the present and in previous (20) studies had little effect on sciatic nerve NGF levels at 100 mg/kg/day. Assuming an approximate content of 10% GLA in EPO (83), a daily consumption of about 180 mg oil would be required to match the current dose of the conjugate. A previous study demonstrated no effect of EPO at about 3.5 g/day per rat (equivalent to about 10 g/kg/day) on the deficit in sciatic nerve SP in diabetic rats (82). It is therefore clear that the properties of the conjugate are significantly greater than those of its constituent molecules. We suspected that a membrane localization might be important and that was why BHT, a lipid-soluble antioxidant, was included in this study, but it showed no efficacy, indicating that simple membrane sequestration of TA does not provide an explanation for the efficacy of the conjugate. Furthermore, although NGF treatment of diabetic rats does not affect nerve conduction deficits, the conjugate had multiple protective effects on different fiber groups—*viz*, increasing nerve NGF levels, stimulating NPY expression by a different mechanism, and boosting deficient conduction velocities. Clearly, this molecule shows clinical potential.

REFERENCES

1. Diabetes Control and Complications Trial Research Group. The effect of intensive treatment of diabetes on the development and progression of long-term complications in insulin-dependent diabetes mellitus. N Engl J Med 1993; 329: 977–986.
2. Brown MJ, Asbury AK. Diabetic neuropathy. Ann Neurol 1984; 15:2–12.
3. Dyck PJ, Bushek W, Spring EM, Karnes JL, Litchy WJ, O'Brien PC, Service FJ. Vibratory and cooling detection thresholds compared with other tests in diagnosing and staging diabetic neuropathy. Diabetes Care 1987; 10:432–440.

4. Thomas PK, Tomlinson DR. Diabetic and hypoglycaemic neuropathy. In: Dyck PJ, Thomas PK, Griffin JW, Low PA, Poduslo JF, ed. Peripheral Neuropathy. 3rd ed. Philadelphia: W.B. Saunders, 1992:1219–1250.
5. Biessels GJ, Van Dam PS. Diabetic neuropathy pathogenesis and current treatment perspectives. Neurosci Res Commun 1997; 20:1–10.
6. Yagihashi S. Pathology and pathogenetic mechanisms of diabetic neuropathy. Diabetes Metab Rev 1996; 11:193–225.
7. Dyck PJ, Giannini C. Pathologic alterations in the diabetic neuropathies of humans: a review. J Neuropathol Exp Neurol 1996; 55:1181–1193.
8. Tesfaye S, Malik R, Ward JD. Vascular factors in diabetic neuropathy. Diabetologia 1994; 37:847–854.
9. Williamson JR, Chang K, Frangos M, Hasan KS, Ido Y, Kawamura T, et al. Hyperglycemic pseudohypoxia and diabetic complications. Diabetes 1993; 42: 801–813.
10. Horrobin DF. The roles of essential fatty acids in the development of diabetic neuropathy and other complications of diabetes mellitus. Prostaglandins Leukot Essent Fatty Acids 1988; 31:181–197.
11. Cameron NE, Cotter MA, Basso M, Hohman TC. Comparison of the effects of inhibitors of aldose reductase and sorbitol dehydrogenase on neurovascular function, nerve conduction and tissue polyol pathway metabolites in streptozotocin-diabetic rats. Diabetologia 1997; 40:271–281.
12. Sasaki H, Schmelzer JD, Zollman PJ, Low PA. Neuropathology and blood flow of nerve, spinal roots and dorsal root ganglia in longstanding diabetic rats. Acta Neuropathol (Berl) 1997; 93:118–128.
13. Kihara M, Low PA. Impaired vasoreactivity to nitric oxide in experimental diabetic neuropathy. Exp Neurol 1995; 132:180–185.
14. Tomlinson DR, Fernyhough P, Diemel LT. Role of neurotrophins in diabetic neuropathy and treatment with nerve growth factors. Diabetes 1997; 46:S43–S49.
15. Dyck PJ. Nerve growth factor and diabetic neuropathy. Lancet 1996; 348: 1044–1045.
16. Tomlinson DR, Fernyhough P, Diemel LT. Neurotrophins and peripheral neuropathy. Philos Trans R Soc Lond B 1996; 351:455–462.
17. Thomas PK. Growth factors and diabetic neuropathy. Diabet Med 1994; 11: 732–739.
18. Packer L. Antioxidant properties of lipoic acid and its therapeutic effects in prevention of diabetes complications and cataracts. Ann NY Acad Sci 1994; 738:257–264.
19. Nagamatsu M, Nickander KK, Schmelzer JD, Raya A, Wittrock DA, Tritschler H, et al. Lipoic acid improves nerve blood flow, reduces oxidative stress, and improves distal nerve conduction in experimental diabetic neuropathy. Diabetes Care 1995; 18:1160–1167.

20. Garrett NE, Malcangio M, Dewhurst M, Tomlinson DR. α-Lipoic acid corrects neuropeptide deficits in diabetic rats via induction of trophic support. Neurosci Lett 1997; 222:191–194.
21. Ebendal T. Function and evolution in the NGF family and its receptors. J Neurosci Res 1992; 32:461–470.
22. Hendry IA, Stoeckel K, Thoenen H, Iversen LL. The retrograde axonal transport of nerve growth factor. Brain Res 1974; 68:103–121.
23. Schmidt RE, Plurad SB, Saffitz JE, Grabau GG, Yip HK. Retrograde axonal transport of [^{125}I]-nerve growth factor in rat Ileal mesentric nerves—effect of streptozocin diabetes. Diabetes 1985; 34:1230–1240.
24. Richardson PM, Verge Issa VMK, Riopelle RJ. Distribution of neuronal receptors for nerve growth factor in the rat. J Neurosci 1986; 6:2312–2321.
25. DiStefano PS, Friedman B, Radziejewski C, Alexander C, Boland P, Schick CM, et al. The neurotrophins BDNF, NT-3, and NGF display distinct patterns of retrograde axonal transport in peripheral and central neurons. Neuron 1992; 8:983–993.
26. Meakin SO, Suter U, Drinkwater CC, Welcher AA, Shooter EM. The rat trk protooncogene product exhibits properties characteristic of the slow nerve growth factor receptor. Proc Natl Acad Sci USA 1992; 89:2374–2378.
27. Martin-Zanca D, Oskam R, Mitra G, Copeland T, Barbacid M. Molecular and biochemical characterization of the human trk proto-oncogene. Mol Cell Biol 1989; 9:24–33.
28. Klein R, Nanduri V, Jing SA, Lamballe F, Tapley P, Bryant S, et al. The trkB tyrosine protein kinase is a receptor for brain-derived neurotrophic factor and neurotrophin-3. Cell 1991; 66:395–403.
29. Klein R, Lamballe F, Bryant S, Barbacid M. The *trk*B tyrosine protein kinase is a receptor for neurotrophin-4. Neuron 1992; 8:947–956.
30. Lamballe F, Tapley P, Barbacid M. *trk*C encodes multiple neurotrophin-3 receptors with distinct biological properties and substrate specificities. EMBO J 1993; 12:3083–3094.
31. Lindsay RM, Harmar AJ. Nerve growth factor regulates expression of neuropeptide genes in adult sensory neurons. Nature 1989;337:362–364.
32. Fernyhough P, Diemel LT, Brewster WJ, Tomlinson DR. Deficits in sciatic nerve neuropeptide content coincide with a reduction in target tissue nerve growth factor mRNA in streptozotocin-diabetic rats; effects of insulin treatment. Neuroscience 1994; 62:337–344.
33. Fernyhough P, Diemel LT, Hardy J, Brewster WJ, Mohiuddin L, Tomlinson DR. Human recombinant nerve growth factor replaces deficient neurotrophic support in the diabetic rat. Eur J Neurosci 1995; 7:1107–1110.
34. Jakobsen J, Brimijoin S, Skau K, Sidenius P, Wells D. Retrograde axonal transport of transmitter enzymes, fucose-labeled protein, and nerve growth factor in streptozotocin-diabetic rats. Diabetes 1981; 30:797–803.

35. Schmidt RE, Grabau GG, Yip HK. Retrograde axonal transport of [^{125}I]nerve growth factor in ileal mesenteric nerves in vitro: effect of streptozotocin diabetes. Brain Res 1986; 378:325–336.
36. Hellweg R, Hartung H-D. Endogenous levels of nerve growth factor (NGF) are altered in experimental diabetes mellitus: a possible role for NGF in the pathogenesis of diabetic neuropathy. J Neurosci Res 1990; 26:258–267.
37. Hellweg R, Wöhrle M, Hartung H-D, Stracke H, Hock C, Federlin K. Diabetes mellitus-associated decrease in nerve growth factor levels is reversed by allogeneic pancreatic islet transplantation. Neurosci Lett 1991; 125:1–4.
38. Hanaoka Y, Ohi T, Furukawa S, Furukawa Y, Hayashi K, Matsukura S. Effect of 4-methylcatechol on sciatic nerve growth factor level and motor nerve conduction velocity in experimental diabetic neuropathic process in rats. Exp Neurol 1992; 115:292–296.
39. Faradji V, Sotelo J. Low serum levels of nerve growth factor in diabetic neuropathy. Acta Neurol Scand 1990; 81:402–406.
40. Delcroix J, Tomlinson DR, Fernyhough P. Diabetes and axotomy-induced deficits in retrograde axonal transport of nerve growth factor correlate with decreased levels of p^{75LNTR} protein in lumbar dorsal root ganglia. Mol Brain Res 1997; 51:82–90.
41. Doherty P, Seaton P, Flanigan TP, Walsh FS. Factors controlling the expression of the NGF receptor in PC12 cells. Neurosci Lett 1988; 92:222–227.
42. Maeda K, Fernyhough P, Tomlinson DR. Effects of treatment of diabetic rats with human recombinant nerve growth factor on sciatic nerve conduction, Doppler flux and substance P levels. Diabet Nutr Metab 1997; 10:3–8.
43. Perez-Polo JR. The nerve growth factor receptor. In: Horrocks LA, Neff NH, Yates AJ, Handjiconstantinou M, eds. Trophic Factors and the Nervous System. New York: Raven Press, 1990:107–118.
44. Gaetani P, Lombardi D. Brain damage following subarachnoid hemorrhage: the imbalance between anti-oxidant systems and lipid peroxidative processes. J Neurosurg Sci 1992; 36:1–10.
45. Kitagawa K, Matsumoto M, Oda T, Niinobe M, Hata R, Handa N, et al. Free radical generation during brief period of cerebral ischemia may trigger delayed neuronal death. Neuroscience 1990; 35:551–558.
46. Jenner P, Dexter DT, Sian J, Schapira AH, Marsden CD. Oxidative stress as a cause of nigral cell death in Parkinson's disease and incidental Lewy body disease. Ann Neurol 1992; 32(suppl):S82–S87.
47. Romero FJ, Monsalve E, Hermenegildo C, Puertas FJ, Higueras V, Nies E, et al. Oxygen toxicity in the nervous tissue: comparison of the antioxidant defense of rat brain and sciatic nerve. Neurochem Res 1991; 16:157–161.
48. Jackson GR, Apffel L, Werrbach-Perez K, Perez-Polo JK. Role of nerve growth factor in oxidant-antioxidant balance and neuronal injury. I. Stimulation of hydrogen peroxide resistance. J Neurosci Res 1990; 25:360–368.
49. Tiffany-Castiglioni E, Perez-Polo JR. Stimulation of resistance to 6-hydroxy-

dopamine in a human neuroblastoma cell line by nerve growth factor. Neurosci Lett 1981; 26:157–161.
50. Tiffany-Castiglioni E, Perez-Polo JR. The role of nerve growth factor in vitro in cell resistance to 6-hydroxydopamine toxicity. Exp Cell Res 1979; 121:179–189.
51. Sampath D, Perez-Polo R. Regulation of antioxidant enzyme expression by NGF. Neurochem Res 1997; 22:351–362.
52. Sampath D, Jackson GR, Werrbach-Perez K, Perez-Polo JR. Effects of nerve growth factor on glutathione peroxidase and catalase in PC12 cells. J Neurochem 1994; 62:2476–2479.
53. Naveilhan P, Neveu I, Jehan F, Baudet C, Wion D, Brachet P. Reactive oxygen species influence nerve growth factor synthesis in primary rat astrocytes. J Neurochem 1994; 62:2178–2186.
54. Wolff SP. Diabetes mellitus and free radicals. Br Med Bull 1993; 49:642–652.
55. Wolff SP, Jiang ZY, Hunt JV. Protein glycation and oxidative stress in diabetes mellitus and ageing. Free Rad Biol Med 1991; 10:339–352.
56. Stith BJ, Proctor WR. Microinjection of inositol 1,2-(cyclic)-4,5-trisphosphate, inositol 1,3,4,5,-tetrakisphosphate, and inositol 1,4,5-trisphosphate into intact *Xenopus* oocytes can induce membrane currents independent of extracellular calcium. J Cell Biochem 1989; 40:321–330.
57. Nickander KK, McPhee BR, Low PA, Tritschler H. Alpha-lipoic acid: antioxidant potency against lipid peroxidation of neural tissues in vitro and implications for diabetic neuropathy. Free Rad Biol Med 1996; 21:631–639.
58. Low PA, Nickander KK. Oxygen free radical effects in sciatic nerve in experimental diabetes. Diabetes 1991; 40:873–877.
59. Cameron NE, Cotter MA, Archibald V, Dines KC, Maxfield EK. Anti-oxidant and pro-oxidant effects on nerve conduction velocity, endoneurial blood flow and oxygen tension in non-diabetic and streptozotocin-diabetic rats. Diabetologia 1994; 37:449–459.
60. Karasu Ç, Dewhurst M, Stevens EJ, Tomlinson DR. Effects of anti-oxidant treatment on sciatic nerve dysfunction in streptozotocin-diabetic rats; comparison with essential fatty acids. Diabetologia 1995; 38:129–134.
61. Cameron NE, Cotter MA, Maxfield EK. Anti-oxidant treatment prevents the development of peripheral nerve dysfunction in streptozotocin-diabetic rats. Diabetologia 1993; 36:299–304.
62. Love A, Cotter MA, Cameron NE. Effects of a-tocopherol on nerve conduction velocity and regeneration following a freeze lesion in immature diabetic rats. Naunyn Schmiedebergs Arch Pharmacol 1997; 355:126–130.
63. Bravenboer B, Kappelle AC, Hamers FPT, Van Buren T, Erkelens DW, Gispen WH. Potential use of glutathione for the prevention and treatment of diabetic neuropathy in the streptozotocin-induced diabetic rat. Diabetologia 1992; 35:813–817.
64. Cameron NE, Cotter MA. Neurovascular dysfunction in diabetic rats. Potential

contribution of autoxidation and free radicals examined using transition metal chelating agents. J Clin Invest 1995; 96:1159–1163.

65. Reed LJ, DeBusk BG, Gunsalius IC, Hornberger CSJ. Crystalline alpha-lipoic acid: a catalytic agent associated with pyruvate dehydrogenase. Science 1951; 114:93–94.
66. Reed LJ. Multienzyme complex. Acc Chem Res 1974; 7:40–46.
67. Packer L, Witt EH, Tritschler HJ. α-Lipoic acid as a biological antioxidant. Free Rad Biol Med 1995; 19:227–250.
68. Busse E, Zimmer G, Schopohl B, Kornhuber B. Influence of alpha-lipoic acid on intracellular glutathione in vitro and in vivo. Arzneimittelforschung 1992; 42:829–831.
69. Natraj CV, Gandhi VM, Menon KKG. Lipoic acid and diabetes: effects of dihydrolipoic acid administration in diabetic rats and rabbits. J Biosci 1984; 6:37–46.
70. Wagh SS, Natraj CV, Menon KKG. Mode of action of lipoic acid in diabetes. J Biosci 1987; 11:59–74.
71. Kahler W, Kuklinski B, Ruhlmann C, Plotz C. Diabetes mellitus—a free radical-associated disease. Results of adjuvant antioxidant supplementation. Z Gesamte Inn Med 1993; 48:223–232. In German.
72. Ziegler D, Hanefeld M, Ruhnau KJ, Meissner HP, Lobisch M, Schütte K, et al. Treatment of symptomatic diabetic peripheral neuropathy with the antioxidant a-lipoic acid—a 3-week multicentre randomized controlled trial (ALADIN study). Diabetologia 1995; 38:1425–1433.
73. Haugaard N, Haugaard ES. Stimulation of glucose utilization by thioctic acid in rat diaphragm incubated in vitro. Biochim Biophys Acta 1970; 222:583–586.
74. Bashan N, Burdett E, Klip A. Effect of thioctic acid on glucose transport. 3rd Int Thoctic Acid Workshop 1993; 3:218–223.
75. Grunert R. The effect of D L-alpha-lipoic acid on heavy metal intoxication in mice and dogs. Arch Biochem Biophys 1960; 86:190–195.
76. Matsugo S, Yan LJ, Han D, Trischler HJ, Packer L. Elucidation of antioxidant activity of alpha-lipoic acid toward hydroxyl radical. Biochem Biophys Res Commun 1995; 208:161–167.
77. Ou P, Tritschler HJ, Wolff SP. Thioctic (lipoic) acid: a therapeutic metal-chelating antioxidant? Biochem Pharmacol 1995; 50:123–126.
78. Brownlee M. Glycation products and the pathogenesis of diabetic complications. Diabetes Care 1992; 15:1835–1843.
79. Dimpfel W, Spuler M, Pierau FK, Ulrich H. Thioctic acid induces dose-dependent sprouting of neurites in cultured rat neuroblastoma cells. Dev Pharmacol Ther 1990; 14:193–199.
80. Kemplay S, Martin P, Wilson S. The effects of thioctic acid on motor nerve terminals in acrylamide-poisoned rats. Neuropathol Appl Neurobiol 1988; 14:275–288.
81. Murase K, Hattori A, Kohno M, Hayashi K. Stimulation of nerve growth factor

synthesis/secretion in mouse astroglial cells by coenzymes. Biochem Mol Biol Int 1993; 30:615–621.
82. Tomlinson DR, Robinson JP, Compton AM, Keen P. Essential fatty acid treatment—effects on nerve conduction, polyol pathway and axonal transport in streptozotocin diabetic rats. Diabetologia 1989; 32:655–659.
83. Lockett MJ, Tomlinson DR. The effects of dietary treatment with essential fatty acids on sciatic nerve conduction and activity of the Na^{+}/K^{+} pump in streptozotocin-diabetic rats. Br J Pharmacol 1992; 105:355–360.
84. Stevens EJ, Carrington AL, Tomlinson DR. Prostacyclin release in experimental diabetes: effects of evening primrose oil. Prostaglandins Leukot Essent Fatty Acids 1993; 49:699–706.
85. Stevens EJ, Lockett MJ, Carrington AL, Tomlinson DR. Essential fatty acid treatment prevents nerve ischaemia and associated conduction anomalies in rats with experimental diabetes mellitus. Diabetologia 1993; 36:397–401.
86. Carrington AL, Lockett MJ, Tomlinson DR. The effects of dietary supplementation with evening primrose oil on resistance to anoxic conduction block in nerves from control and streptozotocin-diabetic rats (abstr). Diabet Med 1992; 9(suppl 1):35A.
87. Stevens EJ, Lockett MJ, Carrington AL, Tomlinson DR. Essential fatty acid treatment prevents nerve ischaemia and associated conduction anomalies in experimental diabetes (abst). Br J Pharmacol 1993; 108:38P.
88. Lundberg JM, Terenius L, Hökfelt T, Martling CR, Tatemoto K, Mutt V, et al. Neuropeptide Y (NPY)-like immunoreactivity in peripheral noradrenergic neurons and effects of NPY on sympathetic function. Acta Physiol Scand 1982; 116:477–480.
89. Tatemoto K, Carlquist M, Mutt V. Neuropeptide Y—a novel brain peptide with structural similarities to peptide YY and pancreatic polypeptide. Nature 1982; 296:659–660.
90. Wakisaka S, Kajander KC, Bennett GJ. Increased neuropeptide Y (NPY)-like immunoreactivity in rat sensory neurons following peripheral axotomy. Neurosci Lett 1991; 124:200–203.
91. Ohara S, Tantuwaya V, DiStefano PS, Schmidt RE. Exogenous NT-3 mitigates the transganglionic neuropeptide Y response to sciatic nerve injury. Brain Res 1995; 699:143–148.
92. Verge VMK, Richardson PM, Wiesenfeld-Hallin Z, Hökfelt T. Differential influence of nerve growth factor on neuropeptide expression in vivo: a novel role in peptide suppression in adult sensory neurons. J Neurosci 1995; 15:2081–2096.
93. Allen JM, Tischler AS, Lee YC, Bloom SR. Neuropeptide Y (NPY) in PC12 phaeochromocytoma cultures: responses to dexamethasone and nerve growth factor. Neurosci Lett 1984; 46:291–296.
94. Higuchi H, Nakano K, Miki N. Identification of NGF-response element in the rat neuropeptide Y gene and induction of the binding proteins. Biochem Biophys Res Commun 1992; 189:1553–1560.

95. Balbi D, Allen JM. Role of protein kinase C in mediating NGF effect on neuropeptide Y expression in PC12 cells. Brain Res Mol Brain Res 1994; 23:310–316.
96. Zhang X, Wiesenfeld-Hallin Z, Hökfelt T. Effect of peripheral axotomy on expression of neuropeptide Y receptor mRNA in rat lumbar dorsal root ganglia. Eur J Neurosci 1994; 6:43–57.
97. Kiefer F, Tibbles LA, Lassam N, Zanke B, Iscove N, Woodgett JR. Novel components of mammalian stress-activated protein kinase cascades. Biochem Soc Trans 1997; 25:491–498.
98. Whitmarsh AJ, Davis RJ. Transcription factor AP-1 regulation by mitogen-activated protein kinase signal transduction pathways. J Mol Med 1996; 74: 589–607.
99. Su B, Karin M. Mitogen-activated protein kinase cascades and regulation of gene expression. Curr Opin Immunol 1996; 8:402–411.
100. Woodgett JR, Avruch J, Kyriakis J. The stress activated protein kinase pathway. Cancer Surv 1996; 27:127–138.
101. Minden A, Karin M. Regulation and function of the JNK subgroup of MAP kinases. Biochim Biophys Acta Rev Cancer 1997; 1333:F85–F104.
102. Wilhelm D, Bender K, Knebel A, Angel P. The level of intracellular glutathione is a key regulator for the induction of stress-activated signal transduction pathways including Jun N-terminal protein kinases and p38 kinase by alkylating agents. Mol Cell Biol 1997; 17:4792–4800.

12

Clinical Trials of α-Lipoic Acid in Diabetic Polyneuropathy and Cardiac Autonomic Neuropathy

Dan Ziegler
Diabetes Research Institute, Heinrich-Heine-University, Düsseldorf, Germany

Polyneuropathy involving the somatic and autonomic nervous system is responsible for substantial morbidity and increased mortality among diabetic patients. Near normoglycemia is now generally accepted as the primary approach to prevention of diabetic neuropathy (1,2). However, in diabetic patients with advanced stages of peripheral neuropathy, relatively long periods of near-normal glycemic control for several months or even years may be needed to retard the progression of nerve dysfunction (3). Because normoglycemia is not achievable in most diabetic patients, the effects of several medical treatments derived from the pathogenetic concepts of diabetic neuropathy have been evaluated in numerous randomized clinical trials during the past two decades. However, due to various reasons, none of these compounds has been marketed as yet in the major European countries or in the United States. Nonetheless, in symptomatic diabetic neuropathy, additional pharmacological treatment of painful neuropathic symptoms is frequently required to maintain the patients' quality of life. Although treatment of pain with antidepressants is effective, it may be of limited value because of frequent adverse reactions (4). Other symptomatic approaches including anticonvulsants, mexiletine, and topical capsaicin either have not been unequivocally effective, have shown only partial effects, or caution has been expressed as to potential neurotoxic side effects in view of longer term treatment (4). Furthermore, these medications are designed to modulate symptoms without influencing the underlying neuropathy.

Cardiovascular autonomic neuropathy (CAN) is a serious complication of diabetes that is associated with a poor prognosis and may result in severe clinical symptoms (5). Although CAN is appreciated as a clinical entity since 1945, in the past it has received less attention than peripheral sensorimotor neuropathy, one reason being that noninvasive quantitative and reliable methods for assessment of cardiovascular autonomic function are available since only the last two decades. After the introduction of cardiovascular reflex tests based on changes in heart rate variability (HRV) and blood pressure regulation into clinical routine, it became evident that CAN may be frequently detected at early stages in asymptomatic diabetic patients (5).

The question of long-term primary prevention of CAN has been previously addressed only in trials that studied the role of near normoglycemia in Type 1 diabetic patients. These studies have shown that the development of abnormalities in HRV can be prevented or retarded by intensive insulin therapy (1,6). Secondary intervention trials in patients with advanced CAN have demonstrated that its progression can be delayed during long-term near normoglycemia, but periods of more than 2 years are needed (3,5).

I. ROLE OF OXIDATIVE STRESS IN DIABETIC NEUROPATHY: CLINICAL AND EXPERIMENTAL EVIDENCE

A growing body of evidence suggests that oxidative stress resulting from enhanced free radical formation and/or defects in antioxidant defense is implicated in the development of various disorders, including neurodegenerative diseases (7) and diabetic complications (8,9). Increased free radical formation and changes in hemostatic variables related to endothelial damage have been found in Type 2 diabetic patients with microalbuminuria (10). Impaired endothelium-dependent vasodilation is improved by administration of vitamin C, suggesting that nitric oxide inactivation by increased oxygen free radical activity contributes to abnormal vascular reactivity in diabetes (11). Furthermore, impaired cellular scavenging activity against oxidative stress (12) and elevated levels of plasma hydroperoxides in conjunction with a trend to lower vitamin E levels (13) have recently been demonstrated in patients with Type 2 diabetes.

In experimental diabetic neuropathy, oxygen free radical activity in the sciatic nerve is increased (9). Treatment with α-lipoic acid, a potent lipophilic free radical scavenger (14), results in prevention of neurovascular abnormalities associated with experimental diabetic neuropathy (15). It has been demonstrated that reduced digital nerve conduction velocity (NCV), nerve blood flow, and glutathione levels in diabetic rats are normalized and in vitro lipid peroxidation of neural tissue reduced by α-lipoic acid in a dose-dependent manner (15,16), suggesting that the improvement in neurovascular changes were induced by improving oxygen free radical scavenging activity. One mechanism of reduced nerve blood flow is the inhibitory effect of superoxide anion on nitric oxide synthase. Because nitric oxide synthase is reduced in experimental diabetic neuropathy (17), α-lipoic acid might prevent this inhibition by reducing oxidative stress (15). A recent study has also demonstrated that treatment with α-lipoic acid may correct neuropeptide deficits in diabetic rats, indicating that the compound may boost neurotrophic support (18). Administration of low doses of an α-lipoic acid–gamma-linolenic acid conjugate corrects the nerve conduction and nerve blood flow deficits (19) and sciatic nerve contents of nerve growth factor, substance P, and neuropeptide Y (20) in diabetic rats, suggesting a marked synergistic action of these compounds. These experimental findings provide the rationale for a potential therapeutic value of α-lipoic acid in diabetic patients with neuropathy.

II. MULTICENTER CONTROLLED CLINICAL TRIALS

Randomized clinical trials (RCTs) are a widely accepted means of applying experimental methods to a clinical setting and have been advocated as the gold standard for comparing and evaluating different treatments (21). However, the quality of the RCTs that evaluated the effects of medical treatment in diabetic polyneuropathy was poor. Cavaliere et al. (22) assessed the quality of scientific evidence for the efficacy of various pathogenetically oriented treatment approaches for diabetic polyneuropathy examined in RCTs published between 1981 and 1992. They used a quality system covering the internal (scientific) validity (the ability to demonstrate a treatment effect if it really exists) and external validity (the possibility of generalizing the study results to patients seen in clinical practice). The analysis based on 38 RCTs in total revealed a devastating picture: The methods of randomization were unspecified and a detailed a priori estimate of the sample size needed to detect a treatment difference was not reported in 95% of the RCTs, respectively. Only 11% of the RCTs had sufficient statistical power to detect a clinically meaningful difference (22). More generally spoken, a recent analysis by Freiman et al. (23) revealed that only 4 of 71 controlled clinical trials (5.6%) that reported nega-

Table 1 Multicenter, Randomized, Double-Blind, Placebo-Controlled Trials Using α-Lipoic Acid in Diabetic Peripheral and Cardiac Autonomic Neuropathy

	ALADIN Study[a]	DEKAN Study[b]	ALADIN 3 Study[c]
Number	328	73	509
Design	Four parallel groups	Two parallel groups	Three parallel groups
Dose	1,200/600/100 mg α/P I.V.	800 mg α/P PO	600 IV/1800 mg PO(α-α/α-P/P-P)
Duration of treatment	3 wk	4 mo	3 wk + 6 mo
Effect	Symptoms+, NDS+	HRV+, TSS	TSS, NIS+

α, α-Lipoic acid; P, placebo; +, improvement; IV, intravenous; PO, orally.
[a]Diabetologia, 38, 1995.
[b]Diabetes Care, 20, 1997.
[c]Diabetes Care, 22, 1999.

tive results ($p > 0.1$) in major medical journals between 1960 and 1977 included a sample size large enough to have a 90% chance of detecting a 25% difference in treatment effects. In another analysis, the situation did not improve as the number was 4 of 65 trials (6.2%) (23). Thus, as recently stated by Altman and Bland (24), absence of evidence is not evidence of absence. In other words, to interpret most published RCTs as providing evidence of an ineffectiveness of the respective treatment in diabetic neuropathy would be clearly misleading, because the likelihood to detect differences in the parameters of nerve function between the treatment groups was too low in view of the small sample sizes.

Adequate designs for RCTs in diabetic neuropathy have to consider the following aspects: type and stage of neuropathy, homogeneity of the study population, outcome measures (neurophysiological markers, intermediate clinical end points, ultimate clinical outcomes, quality of life), natural history, sample size, study duration, reproducibility of neurophysiological and intermediate end points, regression to the mean, true and perceived placebo effects, measures of treatment effect, and the generalizability of the overall trial result to individual patients (25). The results of three multicenter RCTs that evaluated the effects of α-lipoic acid in Type 2 diabetic patients with polyneuropathy are summarized and discussed below (Table 1).

A. ALADIN Study

The improvement in neuropathic symptoms during a 3-week period of intravenous treatment with 600 mg α-lipoic acid/day as compared with vitamin B_1

(26) in conjunction with the recent experimental evidence (15) formed the rationale for a large-scale, 3-week, multicenter, randomized, double-blind, placebo-controlled trial (*A*lpha-*L*ipoic *A*cid in *D*iabetic *N*europathy: ALADIN) (27). Assuming from previous studies a placebo response of about 30% and a drug response of about 60%, the a priori estimate of the required sample size yielded $n = 67$ patients per group, with $\alpha = 0.05$ and $\beta = 0.1$ for the two-tailed log-rank test.

The efficacy and safety of intravenous infusion of α-lipoic acid were evaluated in 328 NIDDM outpatients with symptomatic peripheral neuropathy who were randomly assigned to treatment using three doses (α-lipoic acid 1200 mg/day, 600 mg/day, 100 mg/day) or placebo. Neuropathic symptoms (pain, burning, paresthesias, and numbness) were assessed by the total symptom score (TSS) at baseline and each visit (days 2–5, 8–12, and 15–19) before infusion. In addition, the Hamburg Pain Adjective List (HPAL), a multidimensional specific pain questionnaire, and the Neuropathy Symptom and Disability Scores (NDS) were assessed at baseline and at day 19 (27).

According to the protocol, 260 patients ($n = 65$, 1200 mg/day; $n = 63$, 600 mg/day; $n = 66$, 100 mg/day; $n = 66$, placebo) completed the study. No significant differences were noted for the mean changes in HbA_1 and blood glucose levels between the four groups studied. TSS in the feet decreased from baseline to day 19 (mean ± SD) by −4.5 ± 3.7 (−58.6%) points in α-lipoic acid 1200, −5.0 ± 4.1 (−63.5%) points in α-lipoic acid 600, −3.3 ± 2.8 (−43.2%) points in α-lipoic acid 100, and −2.6 ± 3.2 (−38.4%) points in placebo (α-lipoic acid 1200 vs. placebo, $p = 0.003$; α-lipoic acid 600 vs. placebo, $p < 0.001$). The response rates after 19 days, defined as an improvement in the TSS of at least 30%, were 70.8% in α-lipoic acid 1200, 82.5% in α-lipoic acid 600, 65.2% in α-lipoic acid 100, and 57.6% in placebo (α-lipoic acid 600 vs. placebo, $p = 0.002$). The total scale of the HPAL was significantly reduced in α-lipoic acid 1200 and α-lipoic acid 600 as compared with placebo after 19 days (both $p < 0.01$). Detailed analysis of pain revealed that both the affective and sensory components of pain, representing pain experience and pain perception, could be improved. NDS decreased by −1.8 ± 0.3 points in α-lipoic acid 1200, by −1.5 ± 0.3 points in α-lipoic acid 600, by −0.9 ± 0.3 in α-lipoic acid 100, and by −1.0 ± 0.2 in placebo after 19 days ($p = 0.03$ for α-lipoic acid 1200 vs. placebo). The rates of adverse events were 32.6% in α-lipoic acid 1200, 18.2% in α-lipoic acid 600, 13.6% in α-lipoic acid 100, and 20.7% in placebo. These findings demonstrate that parenteral treatment with α-lipoic acid over 3 weeks using a dose of 600 mg/day in NIDDM patients is associated with a significant reduction of various symptoms of peripheral neuropathy including pain, paresthesias, and numbness as compared with placebo. Furthermore, it is evident that a dose of 100 mg/day does not exert an effect superior to that seen with placebo. An increase in the dosage to 1200 mg/day is associated with an enhanced rate of adverse events rather than with maximized efficacy. The increased risk of gastrointestinal side effects associated with 1200 mg/day precludes from using this dose (27).

It may be argued that nerve conduction studies have not been used in this study as objective measures of neuropathy. However, electrophysiological changes are not relevant in patients with pain. In addition, in a short-term study of this kind, a significant difference between the groups treated with α-lipoic acid and the placebo group regarding NCV would not appear likely to occur. Previous studies using drugs such as the aldose reductase inhibitors have shown that NCV was either unchanged (28) or only a minimal increase was seen within several weeks of treatment (29) that was subject to substantial criticism as to whether it represented a clinically meaningful degree of change or merely a physiological variation (30). By contrast, neuropathic symptoms have been shown susceptible to intervention within a few weeks. Painful symptoms but not motor and sensory NCV were improved after 4 weeks of treatment with sorbinil as compared with placebo (28), and withdrawal of tolrestat resulted in a rapid worsening of pain scores (31).

It may also be argued that the exclusion of 51 patients due to failures to adhere to the protocol potentially could have introduced bias. However, an additional analysis of the results of the ALADIN Study based on the intention to treat revealed no appreciable differences in the outcome of the parameters studied when compared with the per-protocol analysis, indicting that the adherence to the study protocol did not introduce bias. In summary, it has been demonstrated that in diabetic subjects a relief of neuropathic symptoms can be achieved by short-term intravenous with α-lipoic acid.

B. DEKAN Study

An effective treatment aimed at improving or retarding the progression of reduced HRV, the hallmark and earliest sign of CAN, might potentially favorably influence the poor prognosis among these patients.

The efficacy and safety of α-lipoic acid were studied in a randomized, double-blind, placebo-controlled, multicenter trial (*De*utsche *K*ardiale *A*utonome *N*europathie: DEKAN Study) in NIDDM patients with CAN (32). Inclusion criteria were age $\geq$ 18 and $\leq$70 years, NIDDM treated with diet, oral antidiabetic agents and/or insulin, spectral power of HRV in the low-frequency band (0.05–0.15 Hz) and/or high-frequency band (0.15–0.5 Hz) below the 2.5 centile of age-related normal ranges (33). Eligible patients were randomly assigned to treatment with an oral dose of 800 mg/day (200 mg four times daily) α-lipoic acid ($n = 39$) or placebo ($n = 34$) for 4 months. Parameters of HRV at rest, including the coefficient of variation (CV), root mean squared successive difference (RMSSD), and spectral power in the low-frequency (0.05–0.15 Hz) and high-frequency (0.15–0.5 Hz) bands, and the QTc interval were assessed at baseline, 2 weeks, and at the end of each month of study using a validated computer system (33). Seventeen patients (α-lipoic acid, $n = 10$; placebo, $n = 7$) dropped out of the study, but only 3 (α-lipoic acid, $n = 1$; placebo, $n = 2$) of these dropouts were due to adverse reactions.

Mean blood pressure, heart rate, and HbA_1 levels did not differ between the groups during the study. RMSSD increased from baseline to 4 months by 1.5 (−37.6–77.1) ms (median [min–max]) in the group treated with α-lipoic acid and decreased by −0.1 (−19.2–32.8) ms in the placebo group ($p < 0.05$ for α-lipoic acid vs. placebo). Power spectrum in the low-frequency band increased by 0.06 (−0.09–0.62) bpm^2 (beats per minute squared) in α-lipoic acid, whereas it declined by −0.01 (−0.48–1.86) bpm^2 in placebo ($p < 0.05$ for α-lipoic acid vs. placebo). Furthermore, there was a trend toward a favorable effect of α-lipoic acid versus placebo for the CV and for the high-frequency band power spectrum. QTc interval was shortened insignificantly by −8.8 (−87.9–46.5) ms in α-lipoic acid and remained unchanged in placebo (0.0 [−118–77.9]). No differences between the groups were noted regarding the rates of adverse events. These findings suggest that oral treatment with α-lipoic acid for 4 months using a well-tolerated dose of 800 mg/day in NIDDM patients is associated with a significant (two indices) or borderline (two indices) improvement in HRV but not QTc interval as compared with placebo (32).

Apart from the DEKAN study, the effects of antioxidants on CAN have not been previously examined in a controlled clinical trial. However, a recent study has demonstrated that glutathione, a physiological antioxidant, normalizes reduced HRV during the squatting test (baroreflex changes) induced by acute hyperglycemia in healthy nondiabetic subjects (34). Presumably, such an effect is mediated by a reduction in free radical activity. In the isolated perfused diabetic rat heart, treatment with vitamin E completely prevented a progressive loss of histofluorescent nerve fibers in the myocardium and intraneural catecholamines (35). There are no studies using α-lipoic acid in experimental diabetic cardiac neuropathy, but the compound normalizes reduced glucose uptake and glucose utilization and consequently oxygen uptake, myocardial ATP levels, and cardiac output in the isolated diabetic rat heart model

(36). However, it is not known whether and to which degree these experimental findings relate to the chronic process that characterizes human diabetic autonomic neuropathy.

C. ALADIN 3 Study

This was a randomized, double-blind, placebo-controlled, multicenter trial including type 2 diabetic outpatients with symptomatic distal symmetric polyneuropathy. Patients were allocated to three parallel groups receiving α-lipoic acid or placebo: group 1 (n = 167), α-lipoic acid 600 mg intravenously for 3 weeks, followed by α-lipoic acid 600 mg three times a day orally for 6 months; group 2 (n = 174), α-lipoic acid 600 mg intravenously for 3 weeks, followed by placebo orally for 6 months; group 3 (n = 168), placebo intravenously for 3 weeks, followed by placebo orally for 6 months. At baseline, there were no significant differences between the groups regarding the demographic variables such as age, sex, body mass index, duration of diabetes, and HbA_{1c}. After 3 weeks, the Neuropathy Impairment Score (NIS) decreased significantly from baseline by -4.34 ± 0.35 (± SEM) in the patients treated with α-lipoic acid and by -3.49 ± 0.58 points in the placebo group ($p = 0.016$ for α-lipoic acid vs. placebo). The NIS of the lower limbs (NIS[LL]) declined by -3.32 ± 0.26 on α-lipoic acid and -2.79 ± 0.42 points on placebo ($p = 0.055$). After completion of the 6-month oral phase, the reduction in the NIS was -5.82 ± 0.73 in group 1, -5.76 ± 0.69 in group 2, and -4.37 ± 0.83 points in group 3 ($p = 0.095$ for group 1 vs. 3), whereas the reduction in NIS[LL] was -4.39 ± 0.51 in group 1, -4.20 ± 0.52 in group 2, and -3.37 ± 0.54 points in group 3 ($p = 0.086$ for group 1 vs. 3). Regarding the TSS, no significant differences were noted between the groups at baseline and after 6 months. These results indicate a trend toward an improvement of neuropathic deficits but not symptoms after 6 months of oral treatment with α-lipoic acid (600 mg three times a day) after a 3-week intravenous phase in type 2 diabetic patients with polyneuropathy. The percentages of adverse events were comparable in the three groups throughout the study.

III. FUTURE ASPECTS

Dyck et al. (37) recently calculated the sample size needed in a clinical trial based on the 2-year follow-up of the Rochester Diabetic Neuropathy Study. The estimates were derived from the changes of a composite score including NIS of the lower limbs plus seven tests (NIS[LL]+7: VPT great toe; R-R variation to DB; peroneal CMAP, MNCV, and MNDL; tibial MNDL; and sural SNAP) that among other measures performed best at showing monotone worsening over time. Assuming that a treatment effect of two NIS points is clinically meaningful, a 2-year study would need 68 patients in each treatment arm to have a power of 0.90 at the two-sided 0.05 level. If the effect of treatment is to halt the progression of neuropathy without improving it, a study of 3.7 years would be required. A 4-year study would require 45 patients per arm to achieve power of 0.90 to detect a treatment effect that inhibits progression of neuropathy, and a clinically meaningful effect could be expected after approximately 2.4 years. Thus, a conservative estimate would yield 70–100 patients per arm for a period of at least 3 years to achieve a high probability of detecting a clinically meaningful effect (37). A 4-year RCT evaluating the effects of α-lipoic acid in diabetic polyneuropathy (Neurological Assessment of Thioctic Acid in Diabetic Neuropathy 1 Study) has been designed on the basis of these estimates. The design of this trial is summarized in Table 2.

In conclusion, it is conceivable that the initial diabetes-related changes in the nerve are mediated by oxidative stress that, on a long-term basis, could result in progressive neuronal damage and therefore would be of pathogenetic relevance. Studies in proof of the promising results reported herein are needed. An ongoing pivotal long-term trial of oral treatment with α-lipoic acid designed along the recent guidelines of the Peripheral Nerve Society (38) aimed at slowing the progression of clinical neuropathy using a reliable clinical end

Table 2 Outline of the NATHAN 1 (*N*eurological *A*ssessment of *Th*ioctic *A*cid in Diabetic *N*europathy) Study

Design: Randomized, double-blind, placebo-controlled, multicenter trial
Subjects: Two parallel groups of type 1 or type 2 diabetic patients ($n = 500$ enrolled)
Medication: Thioctic acid 600 mg or placebo tablets once daily orally
Duration: Screening, 2 wk; placebo run-in, 6 wk; treatment, 192 wk; follow-up, 4 wk (interim analysis, at 96 wk)
Inclusion criteria: Stage 1 or 2a polyneuropathy [NIS(LL) + 7 ≥ 97.5 centile; TSS ≤ 5]
Primary outcome measure: NIS(LL) + 7 tests score (VDT; HBDB; peroneal CMAP, MNCV, and MNDL; tibial MNDL; sural SNAP)
Secondary outcome measures: NSC, TSS, CDT, HP, other NIS and NC

VDT: vibration detection threshold; HBDB: heart beat to deep breathing; CMAP: compound muscle action potential; MNCV: motor nerve conduction velocity; MNDL: motor nerve distal latency; SNAP: sensory nerve action potential; NSC: neuropathy symptoms and changes; CDT: coding detection threshold; HP: heat as pain; NC: nerve conduction.

point addresses the question as to whether the observed improvement in neuropathic symptoms and autonomic dysfunction can be translated into long-term effects on objective neurophysiological parameters and neuropathic deficits.

ACKNOWLEDGMENTS

The ALADIN and DEKAN studies were supported by ASTA Medica AG, Frankfurt am Main, Germany.

REFERENCES

1. The Diabetes Control and Complications Trial Research Group. The effect of intensive diabetes therapy on the development and progression of neuropathy. Ann Intern Med 1995; 122:561–568.
2. Diabetes Control and Complications Trial (DCCT) Research Group. Effect of intensive diabetes treatment on nerve conduction in the Diabetes Control and Complications Trial. Ann Neurol 1995; 38:869–880.
3. Kennedy WR, Navarro X, Goetz FC, Sutherland DER, Najarian JS. Effects of pancreatic transplantation on diabetic neuropathy. N Engl J Med 1990; 322: 1031–1037.
4. Ziegler D. Diagnosis and management of diabetic peripheral neuropathy. Diabetic Med 1996; 13:S34–S38.
5. Ziegler D. Diabetic cardiovascular autonomic neuropathy: prognosis, diagnosis, and treatment. Diabetes Metab Rev 1994; 10:339–383.
6. Ziegler D, Piolot R, Gries FA. The natural history of diabetic neuropathy is governed by the degree of glycaemic control. A 10-year prospective study in IDDM. Diabetologia 1996; 39(suppl 1):A35.
7. Jenner P. Oxidative damage in neurodegenerative disease. Lancet 1994; 344: 796–798.
8. Baynes JW. Role of oxidative stress in development of complications in diabetes. Diabetes 1991; 40:405–412.
9. Cameron NE, Cotter MA. The relationship of vascular changes to metabolic factors in diabetes mellitus and their role in the development of peripheral nerve complications. Diabetes Metab Rev 1994; 10:189–224.
10. Collier A, Rumley A, Rumley AG, Paterson JR, Leach JP, Lowe GDO, Small M. Free radical activity and hemostatic factors in NIDDM patients with and without microalbuminuria. Diabetes 1992; 41:909–913.
11. Ting HH, Timimi FK, Boles KS, Creager SJ, Ganz P, Creager MA. Vitamin C improves endothelium-dependent vasodilation in patients with non-insulin-dependent diabetes mellitus. J Clin Invest 1996; 97:22–28.

12. Yoshida K, Hirokawa J, Tagami S, Kawakami Y, Urata Y, Kondo T. Weakened cellular scavenging activity against oxidative stress in diabetes mellitus: regulation of glutathione synthesis and efflux. Diabetologia 1995; 38:201–210.
13. Nourooz-Zadeh J, Tajaddini-Sarmadi J, McCarthy S, Betteridge DJ, Wolff SP. Elevated levels of authentic plasma hydroperoxides in NIDDM. Diabetes 1995; 44:1054–1058.
14. Suzuki YJ, Tsuchiya M, Packer L. Thioctic acid and dihydrolipoic acid are novel antioxidants which interact with reactive oxygen species. Free Rad Res Commun 1991; 15:255–263.
15. Nagamatsu M, Nickander KK, Schmelzer JD, Raya A, Wittrock DA, Tritschler H, Low PA. Lipoic acid improves nerve blood flow, reduces oxidative stress and improves distal nerve conduction in experimental diabetic neuropathy. Diabetes Care 1995; 18:1160–1167.
16. Nickander KK, McPhee BR, Low PA, Tritschler H. Alpha-lipoic acid: antioxidant potency against lipid peroxidation of neural tissues in vitro and implications for diabetic neuropathy. Free Rad Biol Med 1996; 21:631–639.
17. Kihara M, Low PA. Impaired vasoreactivity to nitric oxide in experimental diabetic neuropathy. Exp Neurol 1994; 132:180–185.
18. Garrett NE, Malcangio M, Dewhurst M, Tomlinson DR. α-Lipoic acid corrects neuropeptide deficits in diabetic rats via induction of trophic support. Neurosci Lett 1997; 222:191–194.
19. Cameron NE, Cotter MA, Horrobin DH, Tritschler HJ. Effects of α-lipoic acid on neurovascular function in diabetic rats: interaction with essential fatty acids. Diabetologia 1998; 41:390–399.
20. Hounsom L, Horrobin DF, Tritschler H, Corder R, Tomlinson DR. A lipoic acid-gamma linolenic acid conjugate is effective against multiple indices of experimental diabetic neuropathy. Diabetologia 1998; 41:839–843.
21. Pringle M, Churchill R. Randomized controlled trials in general practice. Br Med J 1995; 311:1382–1383.
22. Cavaliere D, Scorpiglione N, Belfiglio M, Carinci F, Cubasso D, Labbrozzi D, Mari E, Massi Benedetti M, Pontano C, Tognoni G, Nicolucci A. Quality assessment of randomised clinical trials on medical treatment of diabetic neuropathy. Diab Nutr Metab 1994; 7:287–294.
23. Freiman JA, Chalmers TC, Smith H, Kuebler RR. The importance of beta, the type II error, and sample size in the design and interpretation of the randomized controlled trial: survey of two sets of ''negative'' trials. In: Bailar JC, Mosteller F, eds. Medical Uses of Statistics. Boston: NEJM Books, 1992:357–373.
24. Altman DG, Bland JM. Absence of evidence is not evidence of absence. Br Med J 1995; 311:485.
25. Ziegler D. The design of clinical trials for treatment of diabetic neuropathy. Neurosci Res Commun 1997; 21:83–91.
26. Ziegler D, Mayer P, Mühlen H, Gries FA. Effekte einer Therapie mit α-Liponsäure gegenüber Vitamin B_1 bei der diabetischen Neuropathie. Diab Stoffw 1993; 2:443–448.

27. Ziegler D, Hanefeld M, Ruhnau KJ, Meißner HP, Lobisch M, Schütte K, Gries FA, The ALADIN Study Group. Treatment of symptomatic diabetic peripheral neuropathy with the antioxidant α-lipoic acid. A 3-week randomized controlled trial (ALADIN Study). Diabetologia 1995; 38:1425–1433.
28. Young RJ, Ewing DJ, Clarke BF. A controlled trial of sorbinil, an aldose reductase inhibitor, in chronic painful diabetic neuropathy. Diabetes 1983; 32:938–942.
29. Judzewitsch RG, Jaspan JB, Polonsky KS, Weinberg CR, Halter JB, Halar E, Pfeifer MA, Vukadinovic C, Bernstein L, Schneider M, Liang K-Y, Gabbay KH, Rubenstein AH, Porte D. Aldose reductase inhibition improves nerve conduction velocity in diabetic patients. N Engl J Med 1983; 308:119–125.
30. Young RR, Shahani BT. Nerve conduction velocity in diabetes. N Engl J Med 1983; 308:190–191.
31. Santiago JV, Sönksen PH, Boulton AJM, Macleod A, Beg M, Bochenek W, Graepel GJ, Gonen B, The Tolrestat Study Group. Withdrawal of the aldose reductase inhibitor tolrestat in patients with diabetic neuropathy: effect on nerve function. J Diab Comp 1993; 7:170–178.
32. Ziegler D, Conrad F, Ulrich H, Reichel G, Schatz H, Gries FA, the DEKAN Study Group. Effects of treatment with the antioxidant α-lipoic acid on cardiac autonomic neuropathy in NIDDM patients. A 4-month randomized controlled multicenter trial (DEKAN Study). Diabetes Care 1997; 20:369–373.
33. Ziegler D, Laux G, Dannehl K, Spüler M, Mühlen H, Mayer P, Gries FA. Assessment of cardiovascular autonomic function: age-related normal ranges and reproducibility of spectral analysis, vector analysis, and standard tests of heart rate variation and blood pressure responses. Diabetic Med 1992; 9:166–175.
34. Marfella R, Verrazzo G, Acampora R, La Marca C, Giunta R, Lucarelli C, Paolisso G, Ceriello A, Giugliano D. Glutathione reverses systemic hemodynamic changes induced by acute hyperglycemia in healthy subjects. Am J Physiol 1995; 268:E1167–E1173.
35. Rösen P, Ballhausen T, Bloch W, Addicks K. Endothelial relaxation is disturbed by oxidative stress in the diabetic rat heart: influence of tocopherol as antioxidant. Diabetologia 1995; 38:1157–1168.
36. Strödter D, Lehmann E, Lehmann U, Tritschler H-J, Bretzel RG, Federlin K. The influence of thioctic acid on metabolism and function of the diabetic heart. Diabetes Res Clin Pract 1995; 29:19–26.
37. Dyck PJ, Davies JL, Litchy WJ, O'Brien PC. Longitudinal assessment of diabetic polyneuropathy using a composite score in the Rochester Diabetic Neuropathy Study cohort. Neurology 1997; 49:229–239.
38. Peripheral Nerve Society. Diabetic polyneuropathy in controlled clinical trials: consensus report of the Peripheral Nerve Society. Ann Neurol 1995; 38:478–482.

13
Oxidative Stress, NF-κB Activation, and Late Diabetic Complications

Peter P. Nawroth, Valentin Borcea, Angelika Bierhaus, Martina Joswig, and Stephan Schiekofer
University of Heidelberg, Heidelberg, Germany

Hans J. Tritschler
ASTA Medica AWD GmbH, Frankfurt, Germany

Oxidative stress is widely believed to play a central role in the pathogenesis of late diabetic complications. Recently, the understanding of oxidative stress in diabetes has been improved by the availability of assays exactly determining defined products of reactive oxygen species. These studies have revealed oxidative stress to occur before diabetic complications are present, further supporting the concept that oxidative stress is pivotal for the development of diabetic complications. Studies looking at the oxidative stress-activated transcription factor NF-κB help to understand the cellular consequences of oxidative stress at the molecular level. However, the occurrence of oxidative stress and oxygen species-mediated secondary end products are not sufficient proof for the hypothesis of oxidative stress-dependent diabetic complications. It has to be demonstrated that antioxidant therapy does not only reduce plasmatic markers of oxidative stress and subsequent NF-κB activation but also late diabetic complications.

I. OXIDATIVE STRESS IN PATIENTS WITH DIABETES MELLITUS

Several studies have shown that increased production of reactive oxygen species and antioxidant depletion occurs in patients with diabetes mellitus (1–11). Oxidative stress may lead to endothelial cell damage and vascular dysfunction through various mechanisms (12–32).

Lately, considerable effort has been devoted to gain insights into the role of oxidative stress in the development and progression of late micro- and macrovascular complications in diabetes (17,23,27,28,31–34). Although hyperglycemia is an acknowledged pathogenic factor in diabetic complications, it is not known through which mechanism an excess of glucose results in tissue damage. Accumulating data support the hypothesis that oxidative stress might play an important role in the pathogenesis of late diabetic complications. Several pathways are leading to oxidative stress associated with acute or chronic hyperglycemia, such as the polyol pathway, prostanoid synthesis, glucose autoxidation, and protein glycation by increasing the production of free radicals (35–39). A close relationship of oxidative stress with glycemic control has been described, showing a significant positive correlation between malondialdehyde (MDA) and both fasting blood sugar and glycosilated hemoglobin (40). Moreover, many injurious effects of hyperglycemia on endothelial functions, such as delayed cell replication, impaired endothelial cell-dependent relaxation, and the activation of NF-κB, are reversed by antioxidants (38,41).

Several studies indicate that not only increased production of free radicals but also the depletion of antioxidative capacities may play an important role in the pathogenesis of late diabetic complications (42,43). In this regard, a prospective study has described an association between low lipid-standardized α-tocopherol levels and the incidence of type 2 diabetes, suggesting a link between hyperglycemia-induced depletion of antioxidants and the pathology of diabetes (44). Recently, it has been shown that oxidative stress appears to be primarily related to the underlying metabolic disorder, occurring before manifestation of late diabetic complications, consistent with the idea that oxidative stress is an early event in the pathology of diabetes and its complications (45). The imbalance between lipid peroxidation products and antioxidant capacities in diabetic patients has been demonstrated using a precise technique for measurement of plasma lipid hydroperoxides. A significantly higher ratio of hydroperoxides to cholesterol-standardized α-tocopherol has been found in diabetics compared with control subjects (45). Further, it has been described that endothelial dysfunction is associated with oxidant injury and tubular damage and may precede microalbuminuria in development of diabetic nephropathy (46). Free radicals produced by the system myeloperoxidase/hydrogen peroxide/halogen derivatives activate proteinases, which break down collagen and other components of the extracellular matrix present in the basal membrane of the glomeruli and in the mesangium. It has been shown that hydroxyl radicals may depolarize glomerular heparan sulfate in vitro and in experimental nephrotic syndrome, leading to loss of glomerular basement membrane integrity and albuminuria (47). Thus, oxygen radicals and proteinases can cause and amplify glomerular damage.

II. HYPOTHESIS OF ADVANCED GLYCATION END PRODUCTS AND ITS RECEPTOR

A. Advanced Glycation End Products

Advanced glycation end products (AGEs) are a heterogeneous group of irreversible adducts resulting from nonenzymatic glycation and oxidation of proteins, lipids, and nucleic acids. Glucose and other reducing sugars react in a nonenzymatic reaction (Maillard reaction) with the N-terminal residues and/or ϵ-amino groups of proteins initially forming a Schiff base. Rearrangement of this aldimine leads after a short time to the formation of more stable but still reversible Amadori adducts. The open chain of the resulting ketoamin can react with other amino groups. Oxidation, dehydration, and condensation reactions finally lead to the production of irreversible crosslinks, which are proteinase resistant.

The formation of AGEs in vitro and in vivo depends on the turnover rate of the modified substrate, sugar concentration, and time. Recent studies have shown that AGEs can be formed not only at long-living proteins but occur also on short-living proteins (48), peptides (48), lipids (49), and nucleic acids (50–52).

AGE formation and protein crosslinking alter the structural and functional properties of proteins, lipid components, and nucleic acids. AGEs have also been shown to induce cellular signaling, activation of transcription factors, and consequently gene expression in vitro and in vivo (32). They have been suggested to represent general markers of oxidative stress and long-term damage to proteins and to induce pathogenic changes in endothelial cells. Thus, AGEs are not only markers but also mediators of chronic vasuclar diseases and late diabetic complications.

B. Formation of AGEs in Diabetes

AGE formation proceeds slowly under normal glycemic conditions but is enhanced in the presence of hyperglycemia, oxidative stress, and/or conditions in which protein and lipid turnover are prolonged. For example, *N*-epsilon-(carboxymethyl)lysine (CML), one of the various AGE structures postulated to date, has been found to be a product of both glycoxidation (combined nonenzymatic glycation and oxidation) and lipid peroxidation reactions (53). CML and pentosidine have been shown to accumulate in diabetic kidneys in colocalization with a marker of lipid peroxidation (MDA), suggesting an association of local oxidative stress with the etiology of diabetic glomerular lesions (54). Evidence for an age-dependent increase in CML accumulation in distinct localizations and acceleration of this process in diabetes has been provided by immunolocalization of CML in skin, lung, heart, kidney, intestine, intervertebral discs, and particularly in arteries (55). In diabetic kidneys, AGEs were preferentially localized in vascular lesions (56), renal cortex (57), expanded mesangial areas (58), and the glomerular basement membrane (56–59). An increased CML content in serum proteins of diabetic patients (55) and a correlation of serum AGE levels with the progressive loss of kidney function was found (60). The increased formation of tissue AGEs has been described to precede and to correlate with early manifestations of renal and retinal complications in patients with diabetes (61).

Increased levels of AGE-modified low-density lipoprotein (LDL) with a markedly impaired clearance have been found in the plasma of diabetic patients, suggesting a pathway for pathogenic modification of LDL (62). The mediating role of AGEs in development of late diabetic complications (Table 1) (49,63–70) has been studied in animal models by short- and long-term administration of AGEs. Short-term administration of AGEs led to increased vascular permeability and leakage, impaired endothelial relaxation, subendothelial mononuclear recruitment, activation of NF-κB, and subsequent VCAM-1 gene expression (71–73). Long-term administration of AGEs resulted in arteriolar basement thickening and complex vascular dysfunction (74) and in glomerular basement thickening, mesangial expansion, glomerulosclerosis, and proteinuria (68).

C. AGE–RAGE Interactions

The principal means through which AGEs exert their cellular effects is via specific cellular receptors (Table 2). One of them, the receptor for AGE (RAGE), a 35-kDa protein, is also expressed by endothelial cells (23,75,76).

Table 1 The Role of AGEs in Diabetic Complications

Formation of HbA_{1c} as a marker of production of AGEs: poor glycemic control increases formation of AGEs and AGE-dependent cell activation (37,41,63)
Toxic effects of AGEs on retinal endothelial cells (64) and positive correlation between accumulation of AGEs, expression of vascular endothelial growth factor, and nonproliferative and proliferative diabetic retinopathy (65)
Inhibition of development of experimental diabetic retinopathy by aminoguanidine treatment (49).
Excessive deposition of intra- and extracellular AGEs in human diabetic peripheral nerve (66)
Inhibition of AGE formation prevents diabetic peripheral nerve dysfunction (67)
Accumulation of AGEs in the kidney of diabetic patients (56,60)
Injection of AGE-albumin in normal rats induces symptoms of diabetic nephropathy (68)
Blocking of AGE binding to RAGE reduces albuminuria (69)
Inhibitor AGEs reduces urinary ablumin excretion, mesangial expansion, and glomerular basement membrane thickening (70)

Table 2 AGE Binding Proteins and Their Localization

AGE binding proteins	Localization
AGE-R_1 (OST-48)	Monocytes/macrophages, endothelial cells, T lymphocytes, mesangial cells, neurons
AGE-R_2 (80KH)	Monocytes/macrophages, endothelial cells, T lymphocytes, fibroblasts, mesangial cells, neurons
AGE-R_3 (Galectin-3 or GBP-35)	Monocytes/macrophages, endothelial cells, T lymphocytes,
RAGE	Endothelial cells, monocytes/ macrophages, smooth muscle cells, mesangial cells, neurons, T lymphocytes, erythrocytes
Lactoferrin, lysozyme	Endothelial cells
Fructosylline-specific binding protein	Monocytes
Macrophage scavenger receptor	Macrophages

An induction of endothelial RAGE expression has been shown on vessels from patients with arteriosclerosis, diabetes, uremia, and vasculitis (77–79). Binding of AGEs to their cellular binding sites results in generation of oxygen free radicals and depletion of antioxidants such as glutathione and ascorbate (32,80). The consequently enhanced cellular oxidative stress leads to activation of the redox-sensitive transcription factor NF-κB in endothelial cells, smooth muscle cells, mesangial cells, and monocytes/macrophages (23,25,32,78–81).

III. ACTIVATION OF NF-κB

The multiprotein complex NF-κB resides as an inactive form in the cytoplasm associated with its inhibitor, IκB (Table 3). NF-κB translocates to the nucleus after phosphorylation and proteolitic degradation of IκB. NF-κB activation is modulated by redox reactions that increase the cytosolic phosphorylation, and degradation of IκB and requires a thioredoxin-dependent status in the nucleus (82–85). NF-κB-dependent genes and their products [include] IκBα, RAGE, cytokines (tumor necrosis factor-α, interleukin-6 and -8), adhesion molecules (VCAM-1, ICAM-1, ELAM), receptors for coagulation factors such as the procoagulant tissue factor endothelin-1, inducible nitric oxide synthase, inducible cyclooxygenase, heme oxygenase type 1, and 5-lipoxygenase (23,77,86). Because transcription of IκBα is autoregulated by NF-κB (87), activation of NF-κB terminates itself (86,88), leading to a short-living acute cellular response. Recent studies showed that IκBβ mediates a more sustained activation of NF-κB that lasts up to 48 h (89,90).

Activation of NF-κB and induction of increased binding activity of NF-κB are believed to have a pivotal role in the pathogenesis and progression of chronic diseases, such as diabetes and atherosclerosis (39,86,91,92). Accumu-

Table 3 Proteins of the NF-κB and IκB Families

Proteins of the NF-κB family	Proteins of the IκB family
P50 (p150)	IκBα
P52/p49 (p100)	IκBβ
P65 (relA)	IκNγ
c-rel	IκBε
relB	IκB-R

lating data indicate a close link between hyperglycemia, oxidative stress, formation of AGEs, and induction of NF-κB to the etiology of late diabetic complications. Increased glucose concentration has been shown to induce NF-κB activation in endothelial cells (38) and to increase NF-κB binding activity in peripheral blood mononuclear cells isolated from diabetic patients with poor glycemic control (37), suggesting that NF-κB activation is an early event in response to elevations in glucose contributing to diabetes-induced endothelial cell injury.

AGEs interacting with endothelial cell RAGE have been identified as relevant mediators of NF-κB activation by generating intracellular oxidative stress (39,41,76,80). Recently, it has been shown that the binding of AGEs or amyloid-β peptides to RAGE leads to perpetuated NF-κB activation in vitro and in vivo resulting in a 1-week translocation of NF-κB (p50/p65) from the cytoplasm into the nucleus (39). The AGE–RAGE-mediated NF-κB activation was initiated by the degradation of both IκBα and IκBβ. The key event in maintaining the activation of NF-κB is the induction of de novo synthesis of p65-mRNA, leading to a constantly growing pool of free NF-κBp65. Thus, AGEs are capable of activating NF-κB in vitro and in vivo, pointing to a central role of AGE-mediated NF-κB activation in late diabetic complications.

IV. INHIBITION OF DIABETIC COMPLICATIONS BY ANTIOXIDANT TREATMENT

In patients with diabetes mellitus, oxidative stress is increased by enhanced production of free radicals and by antioxidant depletion, resulting in an increased susceptibility to oxidative damage and possibly development of late diabetic complications. Endogenous antioxidant proteins such as superoxide dismutase, glutathione peroxidase, and metal-binding proteins may protect the body against the effect of prooxidant reactions. Multiple antioxidants, including α-lipoic acid, vitamins C and E, urate, carotenoids, flavonoids, the amino acid methionine, and protein-bound zinc and selenium, are interacting additively in these biological systems. In vitro and in vivo studies using antioxidants support the concept of radical-mediated diabetic complications.

A. Vitamin E

Vitamin E is the most abundant antioxidant in LDL. In vitro it scavenges peroxyl radicals 10,000-fold avidly, and then these react with fatty acids. But in LDL, vitamin E is located in the more rigid outer layer of the particle, whereas the free radicals seem to accumulate in the more fluid core and might therefore not be scavenged effectively by the antioxidant. However, vitamin E has been shown to inhibit lipid peroxidation and to reduce protein glycation in diabetic patients (93–95).

Intervention studies have shown that vitamin E treatment could prevent early changes of diabetic glomerular dysfunction in diabetic rats through activation of diacylglyceral kinase, decreasing diacylglycerol and protein kinase C levels (96,97). Further, vitamin E has been demonstrated to improve significantly diabetes-induced abnormal contractility and endothelial dysfunction (98) and to exhibit cardiovascular protection in diabetes (99). Thus, these studies support the concept of oxidative stress-mediated diabetic complications.

B. Vitamin C

Vitamin C is the most effective water-soluble antioxidant in the organism. It acts as a potent electron donor, which is then reduced back to ascorbic acid primarily by glutathione. Ascorbate is the first antioxidant consumed in plasma exposed in vitro to aqueous peroxyl radicals, followed by sulfhydryl groups, urate, and vitamin E. Vitamin C supplementation has been shown to regenerate vitamin E and to increase glutathione levels (94).

Treatment with vitamin C improved endothelium-dependent vasodilatation in patients with insulin-dependent diabetes mellitus (100) and decreased albuminuria, glomerular transforming growth factor-β, and glomerular size in diabetic rats (101). These data are in support for a role of water-soluble antioxidants in diabetic complications.

C. α-Lipoic Acid

α-Lipoic acid occurs naturally in physiological systems as a cofactor for enzymatically catalyzed acyl transfer reactions. It has powerful antioxidant actions in vitro and in vivo (102,103). α-Lipoic acid exists in oxidized and reduced forms and regenerates NAD^+ from NADH (104–106). It acts as a universal antioxidant both in the membrane and the aqueous phase by reducing peroxyl, ascorbyl, and chromanoxyl radicals (107) and by decreasing microsomal lipid peroxidation (108). α-Lipoic acid participates in establishing a cellular antioxidant network, raising intracellular glutathione levels, reducing the oxidized amino acid cysteine to cystine and regenerating other important antioxidants such as the vitamins C and E. On the cellular level, α-lipoic acid has also been shown to prevent single oxygen-induced DNA damage (104,109). Also of interest, and related to diabetic complications, are the findings regarding the effects of α-lipoic acid with respect to the glucose homeostasis and the production of AGEs (110). α-Lipoic acid has been found to reduce glycemia and to stimulate glucose uptake and transport activity in skeletal muscle both human and experimental diabetes (111,112).

One of the earliest events in atherogenesis is the adhesion of monocytes to the endothelium and its migration into the arterial intima. Endothelin-1, which is increased in diabetes and is believed to be relevant for the progression of nephropathy (113), has been shown to increase monocyte chemotaxis in a dose-dependent manner (97). α-Lipoic acid inhibits migration (114). α-Lipoic acid has also been shown to be an effective inhibitor of aldose reductase (115). Aldose reductase inhibitors have been suggested to prevent or reduce the different components of vascular dysfunction, cataract, neuropathy, and nephropathy in animal models of diabetes.

Several intervention studies have been performed to establish the role of α-lipoic acid as a powerful antioxidant in diabetes. Therapeutic effects of α-lipoic acid in the prevention of diabetic retinopathy and cataract have been described (116). The neuroprotective effect of α-lipoic acid in the treatment of symptomatic diabetic peripheral neuropathy by reducing oxidative stress and improving nerve blood flow and distal nerve conduction is well documented (117–119). The increased blood flow is consistent with the vascular protective effect of α-lipoic acid.

Recently, it has been reported that α-lipoic acid completely prevented the AGE-dependent depletion of glutathione and ascorbate in vitro and reduced in a time- and dose-dependent manner the AGE albumin-mediated activation of NF-κB in endothelial cells as long as α-lipoic acid was added at least 30 min before AGE albumin stimulation (Fig. 1) (41). It was shown that the inhibition of NF-κB activation was not due to physical interactions with protein DNA binding, because α-lipoic acid did not prevent binding activity of recombinant NF-κB when it was included directly into the binding reaction. Furthermore, it was demonstrated by Western blots that α-lipoic acid inhibited the release and translocation of NF-κB from the cytoplasm into the nucleus. In addition, α-lipoic acid reduced the NF-κB-mediated transcription of tissue factor and endothelin-1, both of them being relevant for endothelial cell dysfunction in diabetes (41). Ongoing studies demonstrated that α-lipoic acid-dependent downregulation of NF-κB is also evident in monocytes of diabetic patients under α-lipoic acid therapy (Fig. 1) (37,41). Thus, α-lipoic acid reduces oxidative stress-dependent NF-κB activation in vitro and in vivo. It is of interest that these effects are present even in patients with poor glycemic control.

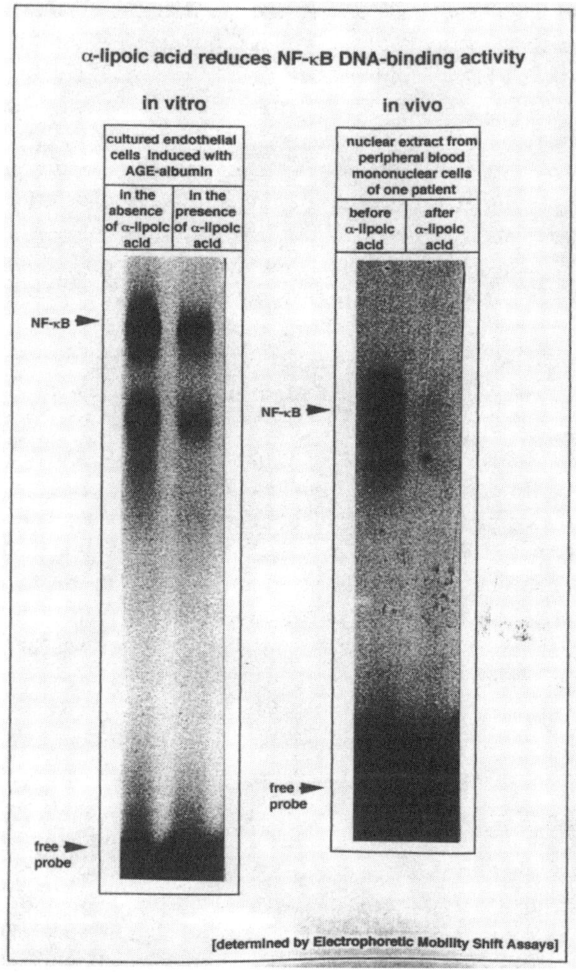

Figure 1 Inhibition of NF-κB DNA binding activity by α-lipoic acid in vitro (left) and in vivo (right).

The effects of α-lipoic acid on the development of late diabetic complications have been studied with respect to the progressive endothelial cell damage and albuminuria in patients with diabetes mellitus (120). The progression of endothelial cell damage has been evaluated in a pilot study over 18 months that assessed the course of plasma thrombomodulin as a marker of endothelial

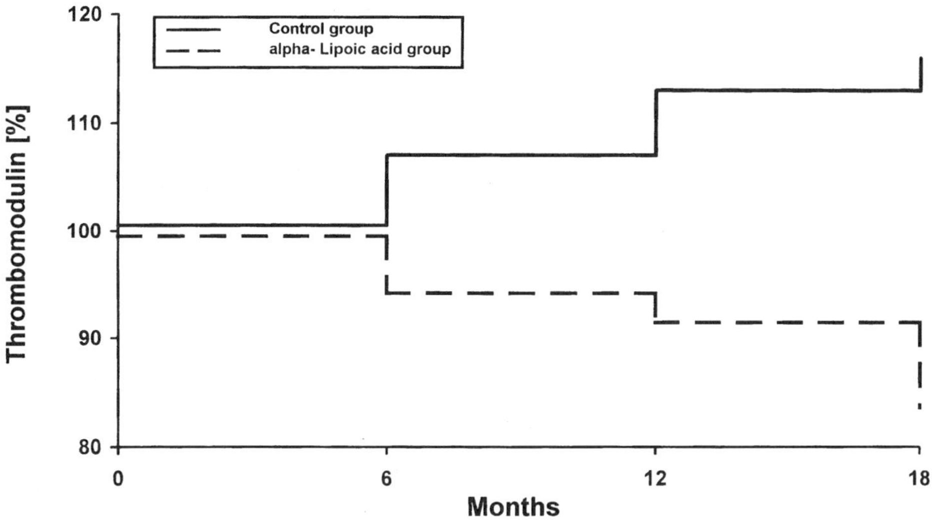

Figure 2 Progression of thrombomodulin in 205 patients with diabetes mellitus studied over 18 months according to the use of α-lipoic acid expressed as relative values (% of study entry values). ——, $n = 151$ patients without α-lipoic acid treatment; ---, $n = 54$ patients treated with 600 mg/day α-lipoic acid.

injury. It has been shown that α-lipoic acid significantly reduced the time-dependent increase of plasma thrombomodulin that was seen in the control patients (Fig. 2). Treatment with α-lipoic acid was found to be the only factor significantly predicting a decrease of the urinary albumin concentration and a decrease of plasma thrombomodulin in multiple regression analysis (120).

V. SUMMARY

There is increasing evidence that oxidative stess plays a major role in the development of late diabetic complications. Oxidative stress generated by hyperglycemia, AGEs, or other factors of cellular activation results in activation of NF-κB activation correlates in diabetic patients with glucose control and can be reduced by treatment with α-lipoic acid. The vasculoprotective action of α-lipoic acid supports the hypothesis shown in Figure 3.

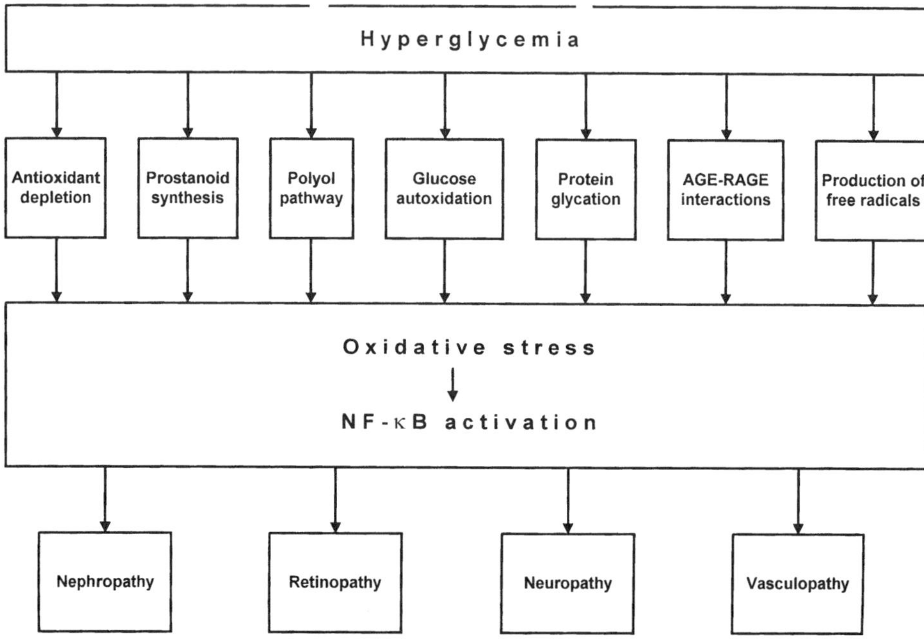

Figure 3 Possible linkage between hyperglycemia-induced oxidative stress, subsequent activation of NF-κB, and development of secondary complications in patients with diabetes mellitus.

REFERENCES

1. Nourooz Zadeh J, Tajaddini Sarmadi J, McCarthy S, Betteridge DJ, Wolff SP. Elevated levels of authentic plasma hydroperoxides in NIDDM. Diabetes 1995; 44:1054–1058.
2. Rabini RA, Fumelli P, Galassi R, et al. Increased susceptibility to lipid oxidation of low-density lipoproteins and erythrocyte membranes from diabetic patients. Metabolism 1994; 43:1470–1474.
3. Ghiselli A, Laurenti O, De-Mattia G, Maiani G, Ferro-Luzzi A. Salicylate hydroxylation as an early marker of in vivo oxidative stress in diabetic patients. Free Radic Biol Med 1992; 13:621–626.
4. Karpen CW, Cataland S, O'Dorisio TM, Panganamala RV. Production of 12-hydroxyeicosatetraenoic acid and vitamin E status in platelets from type I human diabetic subjects. Diabetes 1985; 34:526–531.
5. Griesmacher A, Kinderhauser M, Andert S, Schreiner W, Toma C, Knoebl P,

Pietschmann P, Prager R. Enhanced serum levels of TBARS in diabetes mellitus. Am J Med 1995; 98:469–475.

6. Srivastava S, Joshi CS, Sethi PP, Agrawal AK, Srivastava SK, Seth PK. Altered platelet functions in non-insulin-dependent diabetes mellitus (NIDDM). Thromb Res 1994; 76:451–461.
7. Gopaul NK, Anggard EE, Mallet AI, Betteridge DJ, Wolff SP, Nourooz-Zadeh J. Plasma 8-epi-PGF_2 alpha levels are elevated in individuals with non-insulin-dependent diabetes mellitus. FEBS Lett 1995; 368:225–229.
8. Asayama K, Uchida N, Nakane T, et al. Antioxidants in the serum of children with insulin-dependent diabetes mellitus. Free Radic Biol Med 1993; 15:597–602.
9. De-Mattia G, Laurenti O, Bravi C, Ghiselli A, Iuliano L, Balsano F. Effect of aldose reductase inhibition on glutathione redox status in erythrocytes of diabetic patients. Metabolism 1994; 43:965–968.
10. Sinclair AJ, Taylor PB, Lunec J, Girling AJ, Barnett AH. Low plasma ascorbate levels in patients with type 2 diabetes mellitus consuming adequate dietary vitamin C. Diabet Med 1994; 11:893–898.
11. Nourooz-Zadeh J, Halliwell B, Tritschler H, Betteridge DJ. Decreased lipid standardised α-tocopherol in non-insulin dependent diabetes mellitus. Diab Stoffw 1997; 6(suppl 2):20–23.
12. Zhao B, Zhang Y, Liu B, Nawroth P, Dierichs R. Endothelial cells injured by oxidized low density lipoprotein. Am J Hematol 1995; 49:250–252.
13. Zhang W, Khanna P, Chan LL, Campbell G, Ansari NH. Diabetes-induced apoptosis in rat kidney. Biochem Mol Med 1997; 61:58–62.
14. Messent M, Sinclair DG, Quinlan GJ, Mumby SE, Gutteridge JM, Evans TW. Pulmonary vascular permeability after cardiopulmonary bypass and its relationship to oxidative stress. Crit Care Med 1997; 25:425–429.
15. Holman RG, Maier RV. Oxidant-induced endothelial leak correlates with decreased cellular energy levels. Am Rev Respir Dis 1990; 141:134–140.
16. Rösen P, Ballhausen T, Bloch W, Addicks K. Endothelial relaxation is disturbed by oxidative stress in the diabetic rat heart: influence of tocopherol as antioxidant. Diabetologia 1995; 38:1157–1168.
17. Giugliano D, Ceriello A, Paolisso G. Diabetes mellitus, hypertension, and cardiovascular disease: which role for oxidative stress? Metabolism 1995; 44:363–368.
18. Mertsch K, Grune T, Siems WG, Ladhoff A, Saupe N, Blasig IE. Hypoxia and reoxygenation of brain endothelial cells in vitro: a comparison of biochemical and morphological response. Cell Mol Biol (Noisy-le-grand) 1995; 41:243–253.
19. Ciolino HP, Levine RL. Modification of proteins in endothelial cell death during oxidative stress. Free Radic Biol Med 1997; 22:1277–1282.
20. Halliwell B. Free radicals, proteins and DNA: oxidative damage versus redox regulation. Biochem Soc Trans 1996; 24:1023–1027.
21. Pieper GM, Siebeneich W, Roza AM, Jordan M, Adams MB. Chronic treatment

in vivo with dimethylthiourea, a hydroxyl radical scavenger, prevents diabetes-induced endothelial dysfunction. J Cardiovasc Pharmacol 1996; 28:741–745.
22. Shi MM, Godleski JJ, Paulauskis JD. Regulation of macrophage inflammatory protein-1alpha mRNA by oxidative stress. J Biol Chem 1996; 271:5878–5883.
23. Hori O, Yan SD, Ogawa S, et al. The receptor for advanced glycation end-products has a central role in mediating the effects of advanced glycation end-products on the development of vascular disease in diabetes mellitus. Nephrol Dial Transplant 1996; 11(suppl 5):13–16.
24. Lewis MS, Whatley RE, Cain P, McIntyre TM, Prescott SM, Zimmerman GA. Hydrogen peroxide stimulates the synthesis of platelet-activating factor by endothelium and induces endothelial cell-dependent neutrophil adhesion. J Clin Invest 1988; 82:2045–2055.
25. Aghajanian AA, Oguogho A, Sinzinger H. Isoprostanes, a new substance group in angiology—of future significance? Vasa 1997; 26:65–69.
26. Rattan V, Shen Y, Sultana C, Kumar D, Kalra VK. Diabetic RBC-induced oxidant stress leads to transendothelial migration of monocyte-like HL-60 cells. Am J Physiol 1997; 273(2 Pt 1):E369–375.
27. Chappey O, Dosquet C, Wautier MP, Wautier JL. Advanced glycation end products, oxidant stress and vascular lesions. Eur J Clin Invest 1997; 27:97–108.
28. Tesfamariam B. Free radicals in diabetic endothelial cell dysfunction. Free Radic Biol Med 1994; 16:383–391.
29. Ceriello A, Giacomello R, Stel G, et al. Hyperglycemia-induced thrombin formation in diabetes. The possible role of oxidative stress. Diabetes 1995; 44: 924–928.
30. Ceriello A, Curcio F, dello-Russo P, et al. The defence against free radicals protects endothelial cells from hyperglycaemia-induced plasminogen activator inhibitor 1 over-production. Blood Coagul Fibrinolysis 1995; 6:133–137.
31. Brownlee M. Advanced glycation end products in diabetic complications. Curr Opin Endocrinol Diabetes 1996; 3:291–297.
32. Schmidt AM, Hori O, Brett J, Yan SD, Wautier JL, Stern D. Cellular receptors for advanced glycation end products. Implications for induction of oxidant stress and cellular dysfunction in the pathogenesis of vascular lesions. Arterioscleros Thrombus 1994; 14:1521–1528.
33. Baynes JW, Thorpe SR. The role of oxidative stress in diabetic complications. Curr Opin Endocrinol 1996; 3:277–284.
34. Giugliano D, Ceriello A, Paolisso G. Oxidative stress and diabetic vascular complications. Diabetes Care 1996; 19:257–267.
35. Ceriello A. Acute hyperglycaemia and oxidative stress generation. Diabet Med 1997; 14(suppl 3):S45–49.
36. Reddi AS, Bollineni JS. Renal cortical expression of mRNAs for antioxidant enzymes in normal and diabetic rats. Biochem Biophys Res Commun 1997; 235:598–601.
37. Hofmann AM, Schiekofer S, Kanitz M, et al. Insufficient glycemic control in-

creases NF-B binding activity in peripheral blood mononuclear cells isolated from patients with diabetes mellitus. Diabetes Care (in press).
38. Pieper GM, Riaz-ul-Haq. Activation of nuclear factor-kappaB in cultured endothelial cells by increased glucose concentration: prevention by calphostin C. J Cardiovasc Pharmacol 1997; 30:528–532.
39. Bierhaus A, Klevesath M, Schwanninger M. et al. Perpetuated NF-κB activation: A receptor mediated, transcription dependent pathway. Exp Med (in press).
40. Noberasco G, Odetti P, Boeri D, Maiello M, Adezati L. Malondialdehyde (MDA) level in diabetic subjects. Relationship with blood glucose and glycosylated hemoglobin. Biomed Pharmacother 1991; 45:193–196.
41. Bierhaus A, Chevion S, Chevion M, et al. Advanced glycation end product-induced activation of NF-κB is suppressed by α-lipoic acid in cultured endothelial cells. Diabetes 1997; 46:1481–1490.
42. Sundaram RK, Bhaskar A, Vijayalingam S, Viswanattham M, Mohan R, Shanmugasundaram KR. Antioxidant status and lipid peroxidation in type II diabetes with and without complications. Clin Sci (Colch) 1996; 90:255–260.
43. Maxwell SR, Thomason H, Sandler D, et al. Antioxidant status in patients with uncomplicated insulin-dependent and non-insulin-dependent diabetes mellitus. Eur J Clin Invest 1997; 27:484–490.
44. Salonen JT, Nyyssonen K, Tuomainen TP, et al. Increased risk of non-insulin dependent diabetes mellitus at low plasma vitamin E concentrations: a four year follow up study in men. BMJ 1995; 311:1124–1127.
45. Nourooz-Zadeh J, Rahimi A, Tajaddini-Sarmadi J, et al. Relationships between plasma measures of oxidative stress and metabolic control in NIDDM. Diabetologia 1997; 40:647–653.
46. Yaqoob M, Patrick AW, McClelland P, et al. Relationship between markers of endothelial dysfunction, oxidant injury and tubular damage in patients with insulin-dependent diabetes mellitus. Clin Sci (Colch) 1993; 85:557–562.
47. Raats CJI, Bakker MAH, van den Born J, Berden JHM. Hydroxyl radicals depolimerize heparan sulfate in vitro and in experimental nephrotic syndrome. J Biol Chem 1997; 42:26734–26741.
48. Vlassara H. Advanced glycation end-products and atherosclerosis. Ann Med 1996; 28:419–426.
49. Hammes HP, Martin S, Federlin K, Geisen K, Brownlee M. Aminoguanidine treatment inhibits the development of experimental diabetic retinopathy. Proc Natl Acad Sci USA 1991; 88:11555–11558.
50. Bucala R, Model P, Cerami A. Modification of DNA by reducing sugars: a possible mechanism for nucleic acid aging and age-related dysfunction in gene expression. Proc Natl Acad Sci USA 1984; 81:105–109.
51. Gugliucci A, Bendayan M. Histones from diabetic rats contain increased levels of advanced glycation end products. Biochem Biophys Res Commun 1995; 212:56–62.
52. Papoulis A, Youssef A, Bucala R. Identification of *N*2-(1-carboxyethyl) gua-

nine (CEG) as a guanine advanced glycosylation end product. Biochemistry 1995; 34:684–655.

53. Fu MX, Requena JR, Jenkins AJ, Lyons TJ, Baynes JW, Thorpe SR. The advanced glycation end product, *N* epsilon-(carboxymethyl)lysine, is a product of both lipid peroxidation and glycoxidation reactions. J Biol Chem 1996; 271: 9982–9986.
54. Horie K, Miyata T, Maeda K, et al. Immunohistochemical colocalization of glycoxidation products and lipid peroxidation products in diabetic renal glomerular lesions. Implication for glycoxidative stress in the pathogenesis of diabetic nephropathy. J Clin Invest 1997; 100:2995–3004.
55. Schleicher ED, Wagner E, Nerlich AG. Increased accumulation of the glycoxidation product *N*(epsilon)-(carboxymethyl)lysine in human tissues in diabetes and aging. J Clin Invest 1997; 99:457–468.
56. Nishino T, Horii Y, Shiiki H, et al. Immunohistochemical detection of advanced glycosylation end products within the vascular lesions and glomeruli in diabetic nephropathy. Hum Pathol 1995; 26:308–313.
57. Mitsuhashi T, Nakayama H, Itoh T, et al. Immunochemical detection of advanced glycation end products in renal cortex from STZ-induced diabetic rat. Diabetes 1993; 42:826–832.
58. Shikata K, Makino H, Sugimoto H, et al. Localization of advanced glycation endproducts in the kidney of experimental diabetic rats. J Diabetes Complications 1995; 9:269–271.
59. Gugliucci A, Bendayan M. Reaction of advanced glycation endproducts with renal tissue from normal and streptozotocin-induced diabetic rats: an ultrastructural study using colloidal gold cytochemistry. J Histochem Cytochem 1995; 43:591–600.
60. Makita Z, Radoff S, Rayfield EJ, et al. Advanced glycosylation end products in patients with diabetic nephropathy N Engl J Med 1991; 325:836–842.
61. Beisswenger PJ, Makita Z, Curphey TJ, et al. Formation of immunochemical advanced glycosylation end products precedes and correlates with early manifestations of renal and retinal disease in diabetes. Diabetes 1995; 44:824–829.
62. Bucala R, Makita Z, Vega G, et al. Modification of low density lipoprotein by advanced glycation end products contributes to the dyslipidemia of diabetes and renal insufficiency. Proc Natl Acad Sci USA 1994; 91:9441–9445.
63. Makita Z, Vlassara H, Rayfield E. Hemoglobin-AGE: a circulating marker of advanced glycosylation. Science 1992; 258:651–653.
64. Chibber R, Molinatti PA, Rosatto N, Lambourne B, Kohner EM. Toxic action of advanced glycation end products on cultured retinal capillary pericytes and endothelial cells: relevance to diabetic retinopathy. Diabetologia 1997; 40:156–164.
65. Murata T, Nagai R, Ishibashi T, Inomuta H, Ikeda K, Horiuchi S. The relationship between accumulation of advanced glycation end products and expression of vascular endothelial growth factor in human diabetic retinas. Diabetologia 1997; 40:764–769.

66. Sugimoto K, Nishizawa Y, Horiuchi S, Yagihashi S. Localization in human diabetic peripheral nerve of *N*(epsilon)-carboxymethyllysine-protein adducts, an advanced glycation endproduct. Diabetologia 1997; 40:1380–1387.
67. Cameron NE, Cotter MA, Dines K, Love A. Effects of aminoguanidine on peripheral nerve function and polyol pathway metabolites in streptozotocin-diabetic rats. Diabetologia 1992; 35:946–950.
68. Vlassara H, Striker LJ, Teichberg S, Fuh H, Li YM, Steffes M. Advanced glycation end products induce glomerular sclerosis and albuminuria in normal rats. Proc Natl Acad Sci USA 1994; 91:11704–11708.
69. Wautier JL, Zoukourian C, Chappey O, et al. Receptor-mediated endothelial cell dysfunction in diabetic vasculopathy. Soluble receptor for advanced glycation end products blocks hyperpermeability in diabetic rats. J Clin Invest 1996; 97:238–243.
70. Yamauchi A, Takei I, Makita Z, et al. Effects of aminoguanidine on serum advanced glycation endproducts, urinary albumin excretion, mesangial expansion, and glomerular basement membrane thickening in Otsuka Long-Evans Tokushima fatty rats. Diabetes Res Clin Pract 1997; 34:127–133.
71. Esposito C, Gerlach H, Brett J, Stern D, Vlassara H. Endothelial receptor-mediated binding of glucose-modified albumin is associated with increased monolayer permeability and modulation of cell surface coagulant properties. J Exp Med 1989; 170:1387–1407.
72. Schmidt AM, Hori O, Chen JX, et al. Advanced glycation endproducts interacting with their endothelial receptor induce expression of vascular cell adhesion molecule-1 (VCAM-1) in cultured human endothelial cells and in mice. A potential mechanism for the accelerated vasculopathy of diabetes. J Clin Invest 1995; 96:1395–1403.
73. Vlassara H, Fuh H, Donnelly T, Cybulsky M. Advanced glycation endproducts promote adhesion molecule (VCAM-1, ICAM-1) expression and atheroma formation in normal rabbits. Mol Med 1995; 1:447–456.
74. Vlassara H, Fuh H, Makita Z, Krungkrai S, Cerami A, Bucala R. Exogenous advanced glycosylation end products induce complex vascular dysfunction in normal animals: a model for diabetic and aging complications. Proc Natl Acad Sci USA 1992; 89:12043–12047.
75. Yan SD, Stern D, Schmidt AM. What's the RAGE? The receptor for advanced glycation end products (RAGE) and the dark side of glucose. Eur J Clin Invest 1997; 27:179–181.
76. Bierhaus A, Hofmann MA, Ziegler R, Nawroth PP. AGE's and their interaction with AGE-receptors in vascular disease and diabetes mellitus. Cardiovasc Res 1998; 37:586–600.
77. Bierhaus A, Illmer T, Kasper M. Advanced glycation end product (AGE)-mediated induction of tissue factor in cultured endothelial cells is dependent on RAGE. Circulation 1997; 96:2262–2271.
78. Bierhaus A, Ritz E, Nawroth PP. Expression of receptors for advanced glycation end-products in occlusive vascular and renal disease. Nephrol Dial Transplant 1996; 11(suppl 5):87–90.

79. Abel M, Ritthaler U, Zhang Y. Expression of receptors for advanced glycosylated end-products in renal disease. Nephrol Dial Transplant 1995; 10:1662–1667.
80. Yan SD, Schmidt AM, Anderson GM. Enhanced cellular oxidant stress by the interaction of advanced glycation end products with their receptors/binding proteins. J Biol Chem 1994; 269:9889–9897.
81. Yan SD, Yan SF, Chen X, et al. Non-enzymatically glycated tau in Alzheimer's disease induces neuronal oxidant stress resulting in cytokine gene expression and release of amyloid beta-peptide. Nat Med 1995; 1:693–699.
82. Flohe L, Brigelius-Flohe R, Saliou C, Traber MG, Packer L. Redox regulation of NF-kappa B activation. Free Radic Biol Med 1997; 22:1115–1126.
83. Jin DY, Chae HZ, Rhee SG, Jeang KT. Regulatory role for a novel human thioredoxin peroxidase in NF-kappa B activation. J Biol Chem 1997; 272: 30952–30961.
84. Piette J, Piret B, Bonizzi G. Multiple redox regulation in NF-kappa B transcription factor activation. Biol Chem 1997; 378:1237–1245.
85. Alkalay I, Yaron A, Hatzubai A, Orian A, Ciechanover A, Ben-Beriah Y. Stimulation-dependent I kappa B alpha phosphorylation marks the NF-kappa B inhibitor for degradation via the ubiquitin-proteasome pathway. Proc Natl Acad Sci USA 1995; 92:10599–10603.
86. Baeuerle PA, Baltimore D. NF-κB: ten years after. Cell 1996; 87:13–20.
87. de-Martin R, Vanhove B, Cheng Q, Hofer E, Csizmadia V, Winkler H, Bach FH. Cytokine-inducible expression in endothelial cells of an I kappa B alpha-like gene is regulated by NF kappa B. EMBO J 1993; 12:2773–2779.
88. Read MA, Whitley MZ, Williams AJ, Collins T. NF-kappa-B and I-kappa-B-alpha: an inducible regulatory system in endothelial activation. J Exp Med 1994; 179:503–512.
89. Thompson JE, Phillips RJ, Erdjument-Bromage H, Tempst P, Ghosh S. I kappa B-beta regulates the persistent response in a biphasic activation of NF-kappa B. Cell 1995; 80:573–582.
90. Johnson DR, Douglas I, Jahnke A, Ghosh S, Pober JS. A sustained reduction in IkappaB-beta may contribute to persistent NF-kappa B activation in human endothelial cells. J Biol Chem 1996; 271:16317–16322.
91. Collins T. Endothelial nuclear factor-kappa B and the initiation of the atherosclerotic lesion. Lab Invest 1993; 68:499–508.
92. Hofmann AM, Schiekofer S, Klevesath MS, et al. Peripheral blood mononuclear cells isolated from patients with diabetic nephropathy demonstrate increased activation of the oxidative-stress sensitive transcription factor NF-κB Diabetologia (in press).
93. Jain SK, McVie R, Jaramillo JJ, et al. The effect of modest vitamin E supplementation on lipid peroxidation products and other cardiovascular risk factors in diabetic patients. Lipids 1996; 31(suppl):S87–90.
94. Stall W, Sies H. Antioxidant defense: vitamins E and C and carotenoids. Diabetes. 1997; 46(suppl 2):S14–18.

95. Ceriello A, Giugliano D, Quatraro A, Donzella C, Dipalo G, Lefebvre PJ. Vitamin E reduction of protein glycosylation in diabetes. New prospect for prevention of diabetic complications? Diabetes Care 1991; 14:68–72.
96. Ishii H, Koya D, King GL. Protein kinase C activation and its role in the development of vascular complications in diabetes mellitus. J Mol Med 1998; 76: 21–31.
97. Koya D, Lee IK, Ishii H, Kanoh H, King GL. Prevention of glomerular dysfunction in diabetic rats by treatment with D-alpha-tocopherol. J Am Soc Nephrol 1997; 8:426–435.
98. Karasu C, Ozansoy G, Bozkurt O, Erdogan D, Omeroglu S. Antioxidant and triglyceride-lowering effects of vitamin E associated with the prevention of abnormalities in the reactivity and morphology of aorta from streptozotocin-diabetic rats. Antioxidants in Diabetes-Induced Complications (ADIC) study group. Metabolism 1997; 46:872–879.
99. Gazis A, Page S, Cockcroft J. Vitamin E and cardiovascular protection in diabetes. BMJ 1997; 314:1845–1846.
100. Timimi FK, Ting HH, Haley EA, Roddy MA, Ganz P, Creager MA. Vitamin C improves endothelium-dependent vasodilation in patients with insulin-dependent diabetes mellitus. J Am Coll Cardiol 1998; 31:552–557.
101. Craven PA, DeRubertis FR, Kagan VE, Melhem M, Studer RK. Effects of supplementation with vitamin C or E on albuminuria, glomerular TGF-beta, and glomerular size in diabetes. J Am Soc Nephrol 1997; 8:1405–1414.
102. Chevion S, Hofman M, Ziegler R, Chevion M, Nawroth PP. The antioxidant properties of thioctic acid: characterization by cyclic voltammetry. Biochem Mol Biol Int 1997; 41:317–327.
103. Packer L, Witt EH, Tritschler HJ. Alpha-lipoic acid as a biological antioxidant. Free Radic Biol Med 1995; 19:227–250.
104. Scott BC, Aroma EI, Evans PJ, et al. Lipoic and dihydrolipoic acids as antioxidants. A critical evaluation. Free Radic Res 1994; 20:119–133.
105. Roy S, Sen CK, Tritschler HJ, Packer L. Modulation of cellular reducing equivalent homeostasis by alpha-lipoic acid. Mechanisms and implications for diabetes and ischemic injury. Biochem Pharmacol 1997; 53:393–399.
106. Suzuki YJ, Tsuchiya M, Packer L. Thioctic acid and dihydrolipoic acid are novel antioxidants which interact with reactive oxygen species. Free Radic Res Commun 1991; 15:225–236.
107. Kagan VE, Shvedova A, Serbinova E, et al. Dihydrolipoic acid—a universal antioxidant in the membrane and the aqueous phase. Reduction of peroxyl, ascorbyl and chromanoxyl radicals. Biochem Pharmacol 1992; 44:1637–1649.
108. Scholich H, Murphy ME, Sies H. Antioxidant activity of dihydrolipoate against microsomal lipid peroxidation and its dependence on alpha-tocopherol. Biochim Biophys Acta 1989; 1001:256–261.
109. Devasagayam TP, Subramanian M, Pradhan DS, Sies H. Prevention of singlet oxygen-induced DNA damage by lipoate. Chem Biol Interact 1993; 86: 79–92.

110. Suzuki YJ, Tsuchiya M, Packer L. Lipoate prevents glucose-induced protein modifications. Free Radic Res Commun 1992; 17:211–217.
111. Khamaisi M, Potashnik R, Tirosh A, et al. Lipoic acid reduces glycemia and increases muscle GLUT4 content in streptozotocin-diabetic rats. Metabolism 1997; 46:763–768.
112. Estrada DE, Ewart HS, Tsakiridis T, et al. Stimulation of glucose uptake by the natural coenzyme alpha-lipoic acid/thioctic acid: participation of elements of the insulin signaling pathway. Diabetes 1996; 45:1798–1804.
113. Bruzzi I, Remuzzi G, Benigni A. Endothelin: a mediator of renal disease progression. J Nephrol 1997; 10:179–183.
114. Achmad TH, Rao GS. Chemotaxis of human blood monocytes toward endothelin-1 and the influence of calcium channel blockers. Biochem Biophys Res Commun 1992; 189:994–1000.
115. Ou P, Nourooz-Zadeh J, Tritschler HJ, Wolff S. Activation of aldose reductase in rat lens and metal-ion chelation by aldose reductase inhibitors and lipoic acid. Free Radic Res 1996; 25:337–346.
116. Packer L. Antioxidant properties of lipoic acid and its therapeutic effects in prevention of diabetes complications and cataracts. Ann NY Acad Sci 1994; 738:257–264.
117. Ziegler D, Hanefeld M, Ruhnau KJ, et al. Treatment of symptomatic diabetic peripheral neuropathy with the anti-oxidant α-lipoic acid. A 3-week multicentre randomized controlled trial (ALADIN Study). Diabetologia 1995; 38:1425–1433.
118. Nagamatsu M, Nickander KK, Schmelzer JD, et al. Lipoic acid improves blood flow, reduces oxidative stress, and improves distal nerve conduction in experimental diabetic neuropathy. Diabetes Care 1995; 18:1160–1167.
119. Packer L, Tritschler HJ, Wessel K. Neuroprotection by the metabolic antioxidant alpha-lipoic acid. Free Radic Biol Med 1997; 22:359–378.
120. Borcea V, Isermann B, Henkels M, et al. Effect of the antioxidant alpha-lipoic acid on the progression of endothelial cell damage and albuminuria in patients with diabetes mellitus. Submitted.

14

Role of Oxidative Stress and Antioxidants on Adhesion Molecules and Diabetic Microangiopathy

Klaus Kusterer, Jörg Bojunga, Gerald Bayer, Thomas Konrad, Eva Haak, Thomas Haak, and Klaus H. Usadel
University of Frankfurt, Frankfurt, Germany

Hans J. Tritschler
ASTA Medica AWD GmbH, Frankfurt, Germany

Each cell can mobilize an armory of antioxidant defense systems. Under normal metabolic conditions, the production of free radicals and the antioxidant capacity are balanced. Hyperglycemia in diabetes mellitus is associated with an increased production of free radicals. Furthermore, observational studies indicate lower levels of antioxidants like vitamin E, vitamin C, carotene, ascorbate, and thiols in patients with diabetes mellitus (1,2). Imbalance between free radical production and the antioxidant defense system leads to oxidative stress. In diabetic patients, oxidative stress can be demonstrated by increased levels of lipid peroxidation products (3–8). There is a body of evidence that vascular and neurological complications in patients with diabetes mellitus are a consequence of oxidative stress (9–12).

I. FREE RADICALS AND DIABETES MELLITUS

Various sources of free radicals are considered in patients with diabetes mellitus. Free radicals are produced during autooxidation (10). Furthermore, glu-

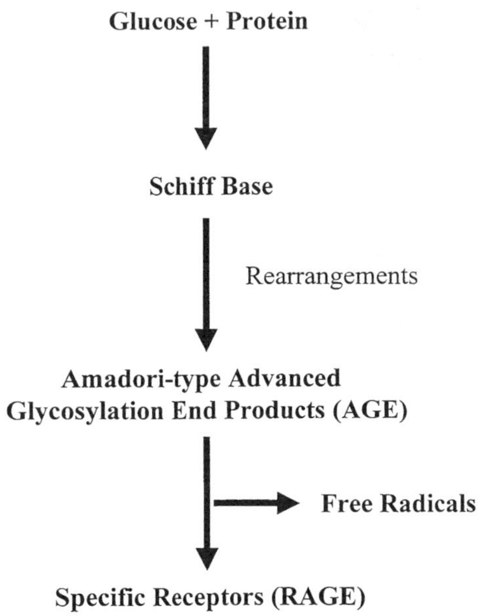

Figure 1 The production of AGEs. The interaction of AGEs with their specific receptors (RAGEs) generates free radicals.

cose is known to form glycosylation products with protein (Fig. 1). These Schiff bases rearrange and form more stable Amadori-type glycosylation end products (13). Some of these early glycosylation end products on collagen or proteins of the vessel wall undergo a complex series of chemical rearrangements to form irreversible advanced glycosylation end products (AGE). Receptors specific for AGEs (RAGE) have been identified on endothelial cells, monocytes, neurons, and smooth muscle cells (14–20). AGE–RAGE interaction induces free radicals (18).

The sorbitol pathway is another mechanism involved in glucotoxicity (21) (Fig. 2). Glucose is reduced to sorbitol by aldose reductase. Then sorbitol is oxidized by sorbitol dehydrogenase to fructose. The second reaction is coupled with the reduction of NAD^+ to NADH (Fig. 1). The pathophysiological consequences are similar to changes during ischemia, and the increased $NADH/NAD^+$ ratio has been termed pseudohypoxia (11). During hyperglycemia, the sorbitol pathway activity is increased. The increased ratio of NADH/

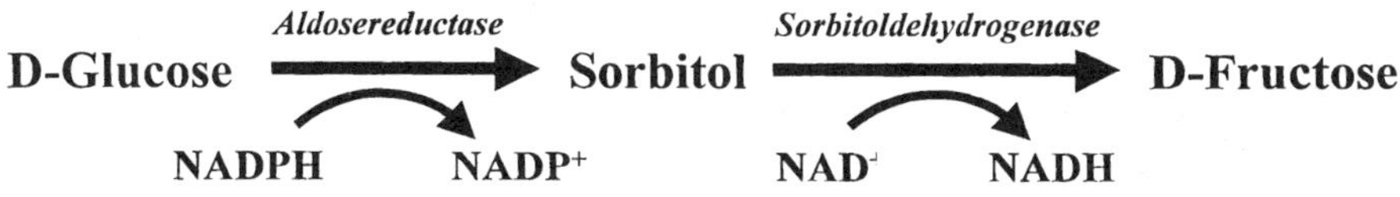

Figure 2 Sorbitol oxidation increases cytosolic NADH/NAD$^+$, which is linked to hyperglycemic pseudohypoxia (11).

NAD$^+$ enhances the synthesis of prostaglandins, which leads to free radical production. Further, the oxidation of NADH to NAD$^+$ in the electron transport chain in the mitochondria involves increased production of superoxide radical (Fig. 3).

The superoxide radical is normally catalyzed by superoxide dismutase to hydrogen peroxide. The iron-dependent Fenton reaction leads to the aggressive hydrogen peroxide radical that further attacks the side chains of lipids,

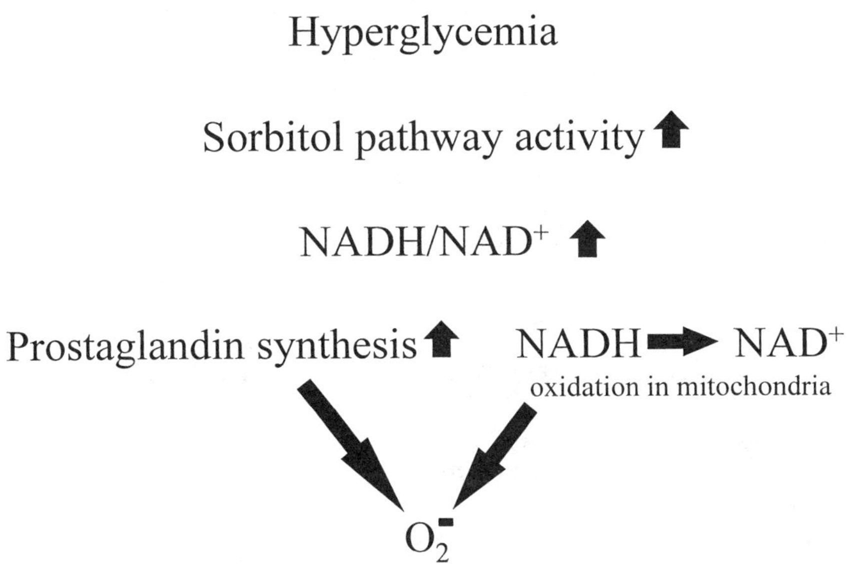

Figure 3 Hyperglycemia activates the sorbitol pathway. Sorbitol oxidation increases cytosolic NADH/NAD$^+$. Increased NADH/NAD$^+$ ratios increase prostaglandin synthesis, leading to free radical production. In the mitochondria, the superoxide radical is generated by oxidation of NADH in the electron transport chain.

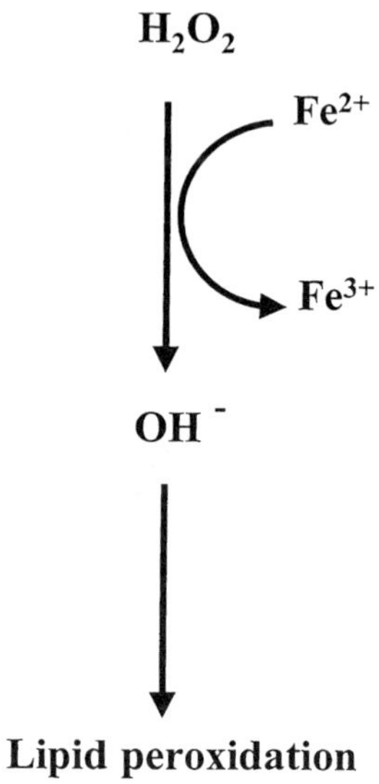

Figure 4 The superoxide radical is rapidly dismutized to H_2O_2 by superoxide dismutase. The iron-dependent Fenton reaction produces a hydrogen peroxide radical, which induces lipid peroxidation.

resulting in lipid peroxidation products (22) (Fig. 4). Patients with diabetes mellitus have increased lipid peroxidation products (3–8).

II. ENDOTHELIUM-DEPENDENT VASODILATION

In physiological terms, hyperglycemia increases blood pressure and leads to endothelial dysfunction with impaired vascular reactivity (23). Hypoxia is accompanied with an influx of calcium, which might activate nitric oxide (NO) synthase followed by vasodilation and hyperemia (11) (Fig. 5). In diabetes, increased free radicals might quench NO, leading to ischemia (11,24). In vitro acetylcholine-induced vasodilation of vasculature from diabetic animals is impaired (25,26). The rate of NO synthesis in vivo compared with the rate of NO quenching is unclear. We measured the blood flow of the arteria iliaca in diabetic and nondiabetic rats. The NO-mediated stimulation by acetylcholine was impaired in diabetic rats, but in contrast to in vitro experiments, treatment

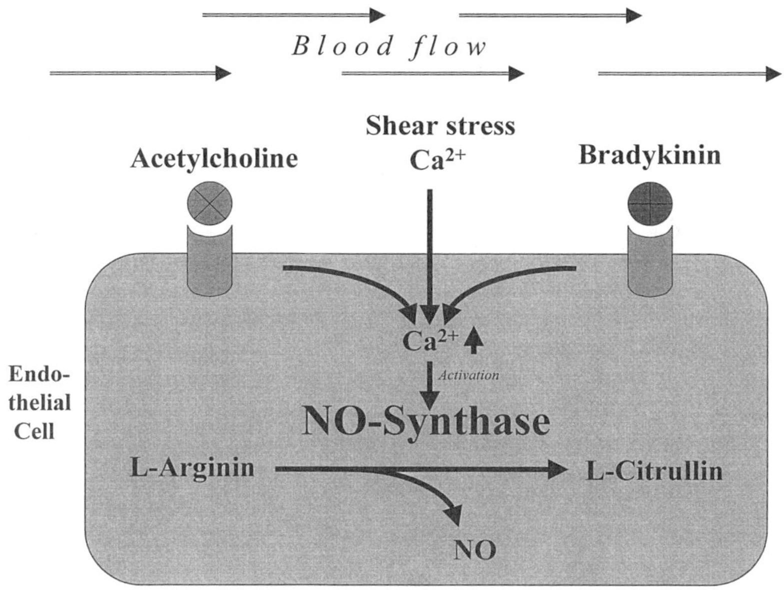

Figure 5 The increase of cytosolic calcium activates nitric oxide synthase.

with antioxidants did not restore the impaired endothelium-dependent vasodilation (unpublished results).

III. ISCHEMIA–REPERFUSION IN DIABETES MELLITUS

Microvascular dysfunction has been studied extensively in animal models. One of the most widely used models is streptozotocin-induced diabetes in the rat. In this model, rats are treated with a single toxic dose of streptozotocin, which destroys the islets of Langerhans (27). The effect of hyperglycemia on the microvasculature is then evaluated after 4–12 weeks (21,28–37). Glycemic control by insulin treatment can prevent the microvascular dysfunction. In diabetic humans, metabolic status is not stable, and episodes of normoglycemia are followed by phases of hyper- and hypoglycemia. Thus, blood sugar levels vary considerably, and in consequence to the pathophysiological changes presented above, the status of oxidative stress changes and blood flow will go up and down. Therefore, it is reasonable to assume that under realistic conditions, a diabetic patient undergoes episodes of ischemia and reperfusion during the time until manifestation of microangiopathy. The time intervals of the increased blood sugar levels are sufficient to induce leukocyte adherence to the vascular endothelium.

We therefore propose an additional pathophysiological approach to the understanding of microangiopathy (Fig. 6). A patient with diabetes mellitus has frequent episodes of ischemia followed by reperfusion. During ischemia, there is a loss of energy-rich phosphates leading to an accumulation of hypoxanthine (38). In the endothelial cell, xanthine dehydrogenase is converted to xanthine oxidase. During reperfusion, superoxide radical and hydrogen perox-

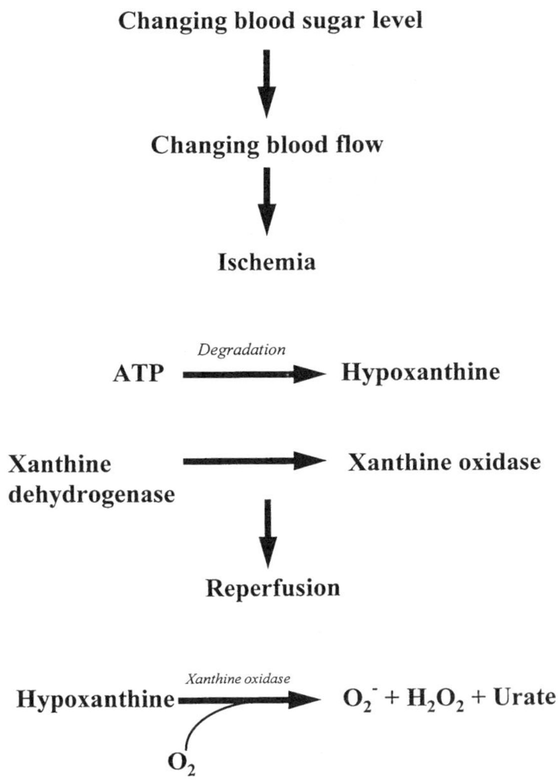

Figure 6 Changes in blood sugar are associated with changes in blood flow. Frequent episodes of hyperglycemia in a diabetic patient will induce frequent episodes of ischemia–reperfusion. Ischemia–reperfusion generates free radicals and induces leukocyte adherence to vascular endothelium followed by tissue injury.

ide are produced by the oxidation of hypoxanthine. In addition, ischemia–reperfusion induces the adherence of leukocytes to the endothelium. The adherent leukocytes migrate to the tissue of the vessel wall and release their inflammatory mediators, including free radicals. Free radicals are produced by leukocytes by the following reaction:

$$2O_2 + NADPH \xrightarrow[\text{oxidase}]{} 2O_2^- + NADP^+ + H^+$$

To test this hypothesis, we first evaluated the effect of lipoic acid on leukocyte adherence induced by ischemia–reperfusion. Lipoic acid was chosen because its beneficial effect in diabetic neuropathy has been demonstrated in animals and multicenter trials of clinically manifested polyneuropathy. Lipoic acid is an effective radical scavenger (39). Nerve conductance and blood flow of the nerves improved by the treatment with lipoic acid (37). In multicenter clinical trials, symptoms in diabetic patients with polyneuropathy improved (40). Ischemia–reperfusion experiments were performed in groups of rats receiving either solvent propylenglycol or 25, 50, or 100 mg/kg intravenous (IV) lipoic acid, respectively, 30 min before the beginning of the ischemia. Ischemia of 30 min was produced by means of a plastic ring in mesentery vessels. With in vivo microscopy, leukocyte adherence was measured during 10, 20, and 30 min of reperfusion. Leukocyte adherence was reduced dose dependently by lipoic acid. Diabetic animals were treated either with propylenglycol or lipoic acid at 100 mg/kg intraperitoneally (IP) 5 days a week for 1 month. After 1 month of treatment with propylenglycol IP, the acute pretreatment with lipoic acid 100 mg/kg IV did not prevent the increased leukocyte adhesion in diabetic rats. Treatment with lipoic acid (100 mg/kg/day IP) from the induction of diabetes combined with an IV bolus 10 min before the experiment reduced ischemia–reperfusion-induced leukocyte adhesion from $7550 \pm 1073/\text{mm}^2$ vein cross-section to 1774 ± 840 ($p < 0.001$).

In conclusion, the therapeutic agent for polyneuropathy, lipoic acid, reduces reperfusion injury. Thus, ischemia–reperfusion caused by changing blood sugar levels might contribute to the pathogenesis of diabetic polyneuropathy, and the benefical effects of lipoic acid in diabetic polyneuropathy might be partially explained by the inhibition of leukocyte adherence.

IV. ADHESION MOLECULES

The migration of leukocytes from the bloodstream into inflamed tissue requires a cascade of events in the microcirculation (41). The sequence of bind-

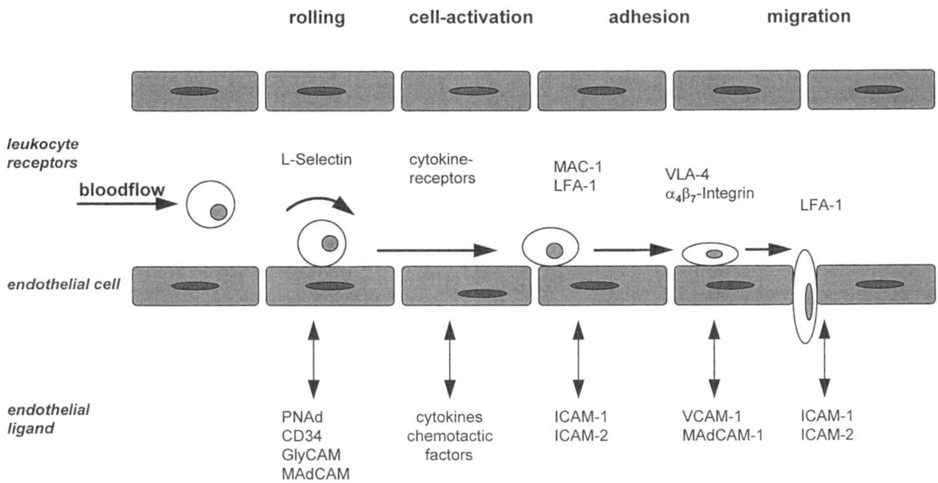

Figure 7 The migration of leukocytes from the bloodstream to the tissue starts with rolling of the leukocytes, which is mediated by selectins. Chemoattractants or cytokines increase the expression of adhesion molecules on the endothelium or increase the avidity of the integrins on the leukocytes, leading to adhesion of leukocytes to the endothelium and finally to emigration from the bloodstream.

ing events starts with leukocytes rolling along the endothelium (Fig. 7). This first step is mediated by selectins (42–47). Upon activation by inflammatory signals such as chemoattractants, rolling progresses to firmer adhesion, due to interaction of the integrins on leukocytes with adhesion molecules of the immunoglobulin family, such as ICAM-1 or VCAM-1, on the endothelium. Monoclonal antibodies that interfere with different steps of the cell-binding cascade have shown a beneficial effect on ischemia–reperfusion injury (48).

Enhanced expression of ICAM-1 and P-selectin has been demonstrated in the diabetic human retina and choroid (49). This increased expression of cell adhesion molecules may contribute to the retinal and choroidal microangiopathy in diabetic patients. A potential mechanism for the accelerated vasculopathy has been proposed recently (14). The interaction of AGEs with their endothelial receptor induced the expression of VCAM-1 in cultured human endothelial cells and in mice (14). AGE–RAGE interaction generates free radicals that activate NF-κB. NF-κB regulates in addition to other genes the expression of VCAM-1. The incubation of human umbilical vein endothelial cells with AGE increased the endothelial expression of VCAM-1. Preincubation of the cells with lipoic acid suppressed VCAM-1 expression to baseline levels (50). The AGE-induced endothelial binding of monocytes was also reduced by lipoic acid (50).

Soluble adhesion molecules are detectable only in small quantities in the serum of healthy individuals (51,52). However, increased serum levels of soluble adhesion molecules have been described in different pathologic situations, including ischemia–reperfusion injuries (53,54), insulin-dependent (IDDM) (55), and non–insulin-dependent diabetes mellitis (NIDDM) (56). In IDDM, circulating ICAM-1 and VCAM-1 but not ELAM-1 was elevated. The increased levels were found in IDDM patients with and without microangiopathy. In first-degree relatives of NIDDM, the levels of E-selectin relates to vascular risk in contrast to soluble VCAM-1, which showed no difference compared with control subjects (56). Thus, elevated levels of circulating adhesion molecules can be used as a risk marker for developing microangiopathy. The pathophysiological role of the circulating adhesion molecules is unclear. It might be that they just indicate endothelial cell stimulation by oxidative stress or that they are a reaction to protect the endothelium from further leukocyte attack. The second hypothesis might be reasonable because we could recently demonstrate that leukocyte adhesion during ischemia–reperfusion can be reduced by the application of naturally occurring soluble recombinat ICAM-1 (57).

V. CONCLUSION

In line with many other investigators, oxidative stress is an important pathogenic factor for the development of microangiopathy in diabetic patients. In addition to the well-characterized soruces of free radicals, we propose a new concept for free radical production: Changes of metabolic control are coupled to episodes of ischemia–reperfusion with subsequent free radical production and leukocytes adherence. Lipoic acid prevents increased leukocyte adherence in diabetic and nondiabetic rats, which might contribute to its beneficial effect in diabetic neuropathy.

REFERENCES

1. Godin TV, Wohaieb SA, Garnett ME, Goumeniouk AD. Antioxidant enzyme alterations in experimental and clinical diabetes. Mol Cell Biochem 1988; 84: 223–231.

2. Packer L, Witt EH, Tritschler HJ. α-Lipoic acid as a biological antioxidant. Free Radic Biol Med 1995; 19:227–250.
3. Jennings PE, Jones AF, Florkowski CM, Lunec J, Barnett AH. Increased diene conjugates in diabetic subjects with microangiopathy. Diabetic Med 1987; 4: 452–456.
4. Valazques E, Winocour HP, Kesteven P, Alberti KGMM, Laker MF. Relation of lipid peroxides to macrovascular disease in type 2 diabetes. Diabetic Med 1991; 8:752–758.
5. MacRury SM, Gordon D, Wilson R, Bradley H, Gemmell CG, Paterson JR, et al. A comparison of different methods of assessing free radical activity in type 2 diabetes and peripheral vascular disease. Diabetic Med 1993; 10:331–335.
6. Griesmacher A, Kinder-Hauser M, Andert S, Schreiner W, Toma C, Knoebel P, et al. Enhanced serum level of TBARS in diabetes mellitus. Am J Med 1995; 98:469–475.
7. Sundaram RK, Bhaskar A, Vijayalingam S, Viswanatthan M, Mohan R, Shanmugasundaram KR. Antioxidant status and lipid peroxidation in type II diabetes with and without complications. Clin Sci 1996; 90:255–260.
8. Nourooz-Zadeh J, Tajaddini-Samadi J, McCarthy S, Betteridge DJ. Elevated levels of authentic plasma hydroperoxides in NIDDM. Diabetes 1995; 44:1054–1058.
9. Giugliano D, Ceriello A, Paolisso G. Oxidative stress in diabetic vascular complications. Diabetes Care 1996; 19:257–267.
10. Baynes JW. Perspectives in diabetes. Role of oxidative stress in development of complications in diabetes. Diabetes 1991; 40:405–412.
11. Williamson JR, Chang K, Frangos M, Hasan KS, Ido Y, Kawamura T, et al. Perspectives in diabetes hyperglycemic pseudohypoxia and diabetic complications. Diabetes 1993; 42:801–813.
12. Nourooz-Zadeh J, Rahimi A, Tajaddini-Sarmadi J, Tritschler H, Rosen P, Halliwell B, et al. Relationships between plasma measures of oxidative stress and metabolic control in NIDDM. Diabetologia 1997; 40:647–653.
13. Brownlee M, Cerami A, Vlassara H. Advanced glycosylation end products in tissue and the biochemical basis of diabetic complications. N Engl J Med 1988; 318:1315–1321.
14. Schmidt AM, Hori O, Chen JX, Li JF, Crandall J, Zhang J, et al. Advanced glycation endproducts interacting with their endothelial receptor induce expression of vascular cell adhesion molecule-1 (VCAM-1) in cultured human endothelial cells and in mice. A potential mechanism for the accelerated vasculopathy of diabetes. J Clin Invest 1995; 96:1395–1403.
15. Ritthaler U, Deng Y, Zhang Y, Greten J, Abel M, Sido B, et al. Expression of receptors for advanced glycation end products in peripheral occlusive vascular disease. Am J Pathol 1995; 146:688–694.
16. Schmidt AM, Mora R, Cao R, Yan SD, Brett J, Ramakrishnan R, et al. The endothelial cell binding site for advanced glycation end products consist of a

complex: an integral membrane protein and a lactoferrin-like polypeptide. J Biol Chem 1994; 269:9882–9888.
17. Wu VY, Cohen MP. Identification of aortic endothelial cell binding proteins for Amadori adducts in glycated albumin. Biochem Biophys Res Commun 1993; 193:1131–1136.
18. Stitt AW, Li YM, Gardiner TA, Bucala R, Archer DB, Vlassara H. Advanced glycation end products (AGEs) co-localize with AGE receptors in the retinal vasculature of diabetic and of AGE-infused rats. Am J Pathol 1997; 150:523–531.
19. Yang Z, Makita Z, Hori Y, Brunelle S, Cerami A, Sehajpal P, et al. Two novel rat liver membrane proteins that bind advanced glycosylation end products: relation to macrophage receptor for glucose-modified proteins. J Exp Med 1991; 174:515–524.
20. Yan SD, Stern D, Schmidt AM. What's the RAGE? The receptor for advanced glycation end products (RAGE) and the dark side of glucose. Eur J Clin Invest 1997; 27:179–181.
21. Tilton RG, Chang K, Neyengaard JR, Van den Enden M, Ido Y, Williamson JR. Inhibition of sorbitol dehydrogenase. Effects on vascular and neural dysfunction in streptozotocin-induced diabetic rats. Diabetes 1995; 44:234–242.
22. Farber JL, Kyle ME, Coleman JB. Biology of disease: mechanisms of cell injury by activated oxygen species. Lab Invest 1990; 62:670–679.
23. Tooke JE. Perspectives in Diabetes Microvascular function in human diabetes. A physiological perspective. Diabetes 1995; 44:721–726.
24. Stevens MJ, Dananberg J, Feldman EL, Lattimer SA, Kamijo M, Thomas TP, et al. The linked roles of nitric oxide, aldose reductase and (Na^+, K^+)-ATPase in the slowing of nerve conduction in the streptozotocin diabetic rat. J Clin Invest 1994; 94:853–859.
25. Rösen P, Ballhausen T, Bloch W, Addicks K. Endothelial relaxation is disturbed by oxidative stress in the diabetic rat heart: influence of tocopherol as antioxidant. Diabetologia 1995; 38:1157–1168.
26. Cameron NE, Cotter MA. Impaired contraction and relaxation in aorta from streptozotocin-diabetic rats: role of polyol pathway. Diabetologia 1992; 35: 1011–1019.
27. Brosky G, Logothetopoulos J. Streptozotocin diabetes in the mouse and guinea pig. Diabetes 1969; 18:606–611.
28. Cameron NE, Cotter MA, Dines KC, Maxfield EK. Pharmacological manipulation of vascular endothelium function in non-diabetic and streptozotocin-diabetic rats: effects on nerve conduction, hypoxic resistance and endoneurial capillarization. Diabetologia 1993; 36:516–522.
29. Low PA, Nickander KK. Oxygen free radical effects in sciatic nerve in experimental diabetes. Diabetes 1991; 40:873–877.
30. Low PA, Ward K, Schmelzer JD, Brimijoin S. Ischemic conduction failure and energy metabolism in experimental diabetic neuropathy. Am J Physiol 1985; 248:E457–E462.

31. Cotter MA, Love A, Watt MJ, Cameron NE, Dines KC. Effects of natural free radical scavangers on peripheral nerve and neurovascular function in diabetic rats. Diabetologia 1995; 38:1285–1294.
32. Cameron NE, Cotter MA, Dines KC, Maxfield EK. Anti-oxidant and pro-oxidant effects on nerve conduction velocity, endoneurial blood flow and oxygen tension in non-diabetic and streptozotocin-diabetic rats. Diabetologia 1994; 37:449–459.
33. Cameron NE, Cotter MA. Neurovascular dysfunction in diabetic rats. Potential contribution of autoxidation and free radicals examined using transition metal chelating agents. J Clin Invest 1995; 96:1159–1163.
34. Cameron NE, Cotter MA, Maxfield EK. Anti-oxidant treatment prevents the development of peripheral nerve dysfunction in streptozotocin-diabetic rats. Diabetologia 1993; 36:299–304.
35. Cameron NE, Cotter MA, Hohman TC. Interactions between essential fatty acid, prostanoid, polyol pathway and nitric oxide mechanisms in the neurovascular deficit of diabetic rats. Diabetologia 1996; 39:172–182.
36. Bravenboer B, Kappelle AC, Hamers FPT, van Buren T, Erkelens DW, Gispen WH. Potential use of glutathione for the prevention and treatment of diabetic neuropathy in the streptozotocin-induced diabetic rat. Diabetologia 1992; 35: 813–817.
37. Nagamatsu M, Nickander KK, Schmelzer JD, Raya A, Wittrock DA, Tritschler H, et al. Lipoic acid improves nerve blood flow, reduces oxidative stress, and improves distal nerve conduction in experimental diabetic neuropathy. Diabetes Care 1995; 18:1160–1167.
38. McCord JM. Oxygen-derived free radicals in postischemic tissue injury. N Engl J Med 1985; 312:159–163.
39. Matsugo S, Yan L-J, Han D, Tritschler HJ, Packer L. Elucidation of antioxidant activity of α-lipoic acid toward hydroxyl radical. Biochem Biophys Res Commun 1995; 208:161–167.
40. Ziegler D, Hanefeld M, Ruhnau KJ, Meiner HP, Lobisch M, Schütte K, et al. Treatment of symptomatic diabetic perpheral neuropathy with the anti-oxidant α-lipoic acid. A 3-week multicentre randomized controlled trial (ALADIN study). Diabetologia 1995; 38:1425–1433.
41. Springer TA. Traffic signals for lymphocyte recirculation and leukocyte emigration: the multistep paradigm. Cell 1994; 76:301–314.
42. Lawrence MB, Springer TA. Leukocytes roll on a selectin at physiologic flow rates: distinction from and prerequisite for adhesion through integrins. Cell 1991; 65:859–873.
43. Ley K, Tedder TF. Leukocyte interactions with vascular endothelium. New insights into selectin-mediated attachment and rolling. J Immunol 1995; 155:525–528.
44. Ley K, Bullard DC, Arbones ML, Bosse R, Vestweber D, Tedder TF, et al. Sequential contribution of L- and P-selectin to leukocyte rolling in vivo. J Exp Med 1995; 181:669–675.
45. Morita Y, Clemens MG, Miller LS, Rangan U, Kondo S, Miyasaka M, et al.

Reactive oxidants mediate TNF-α-induced leukocyte adhesion to rat mesenteric venular endothelium. Am J Physiol 1995; 269:H1833–H1842.

46. Tedder TF, Steeber DA, Chen A, Engel P. The selectins: vascular adhesion molecules. FASEB J 1995; 9:866–873.
47. McEver RP, Moore KL, Cummings RD. Leukocyte trafficking mediated by selectin-carbohydrate interactions. J Biol Chem 1995; 270:11025–11028.
48. Kubes P, Jutila M, Payne D. Therapeutic potential of inhibiting leukocyte rolling in ischemia/reperfusion. J Clin Invest 1995; 95:2510–2519.
49. McLeod, Lefer DJ, Merges C, Lutty GA. Enhanced expression of intracellular adhesion molecule-1 and P-selectin in the diabetic human retina and choroid. Am J Pathol 1995; 147:642–653.
50. Kunt T, Forst T, Wilhelm A, Tritschler H, Pfuetzner A, Harzer O, et al. Alpha lipoic acid reduces expression of vascular cell adhesion molecule-1 and endothelial adhesion of human monocytes after stimulation with advanced glycation endproducts. Clin Sci 1999; 96:75–82.
51. Rothlein R, Mainolfi EA, Czajkowski M, Marlin SD. A form of circulating ICAM-1 in human serum. J Immunol 1991; 147:3788–3793.
52. Seth R, Raymond FD, Makgoba MW. Circulating ICAM-1 isoforms: diagnostic prospects for inflammatory and immune disorders. Lancet 1991; 338:83–84.
53. Haught WH, Mansour M, Rothlein R, Kishimoto TK, Mainolfi EA, Hendricks JB, et al. Alterations in circulating intercellular adhesion molecule-1 and L-selectin: further evidence for chronic inflammation in ischemic heart disease. Am Heart J 1996; 132:1–8.
54. Gearing AJH, Newman W. Circulating adhesion molecules in disease. Immunol Today 1993; 14:506–512.
55. Fasching P, Veitl M, Rohac M, Streli C, Schneider B, Waldhäusl W, et al. Elevated concentrations of circulating adhesion molecules and their association with microvascular complications in insulin-dependent diabetes mellitus. J Clin Endocrinol Metab 1996; 81:4313–4317.
56. Bannan S, Mansfield MW, Grant PJ. Soluble vascular cell adhesion molecule-1 and E-selectin levels in relation to vascular risk factors and to E-selectin genotype in the first degree relatives of NIDDM patients and in NIDDM patients. Diabetologia 1998; 41:460–466.
57. Kusterer K, Bojunga J, Enghofer M, Heidenthal E, Usadel KH, Kolb H, et al. Soluble intercellular adhesion molecule 1 reduces leukocyte adhesion to vascular endothelium in ischemia-reperfusion injury in mice. Am J Physiol 1998; 275: G377–G380

15

Molecular Basis of α-Tocopherol Action and Its Protective Role Against Diabetic Complications

Angelo Azzi, Roberta Ricciarelli, and Sophie Clément
University of Bern, Bern, Switzerland

Nesrin Özer
Marmara University, Istanbul, Turkey

Atherosclerosis is a pathology frequently associated with diabetes (1–4). Migration and proliferation of smooth muscle cells (smc) from the media to the intima of the arterial wall take place early at the beginning of the atherosclerotic process (5).

Proliferation of smc is accompanied by an increased expression of extracellular matrix protein, which contributes to the development of diabetic vascular complications (6–8). Several studies have shown beneficial effects of antioxidant vitamins, in particular vitamin E, in protection against the vascular complications seen in diabetic patients (9–12).

In recent years, the mechanism of action of vitamin E has been discussed (13,14) because its simple role as an antioxidant and protective component of the cell membrane (15) is becoming insufficient to explain the action of this compound.

Vitamin E deficiency leads to premature cell aging and to the binding of immunoglobulin G to erythrocytes (16), and it has been shown to play an important role in porphyrin metabolism (17). Moreover, reports suggest an effect of vitamin E on the arachidonic acid cascade, related to the biosynthesis of prostaglandins (18). A specific neuropathology ataxia with vitamin E deficiency (AVED) has also been found to be due to familiar vitamin E deficiency (19–21).

In our laboratory we found that α-tocopherol (the most active form of vitamin E) inhibits vascular smooth muscle cell proliferation (22–25). smc are under the control of several growth factors that activate a cascade of kinases and phosphatases ending with the activation of transcription factors (such as AP-1 and NF-κB) and those proteins involved in the cell cycle progression, in particular protein kinase C (PKC) (26).

First described 20 years ago as a proteolytically activated serine/threonine kinase, PKC still justifies the attention of researchers, providing new surprises. The enormous number of weekly publications requires a continuous effort to summarize and simplify the knowledge on the field. Since its original discovery, PKC has expanded into a family of closely related proteins, which can be subdivided on the basis of certain structural and biochemical properties. The original members of the PKC family are the Ca^{2+}-dependent or conventional (c) α, β_I, β_{II}, and γ isoforms. Later, with the discovery of Ca^{2+}-independent PKC isoenzymes, the group of a new or novel (n) isoforms has been classified, including ε, η, and θ PKCs. Finally, there are the so-called atypical (a) ζ, τ, λ, and μ isoforms, which take an intermediate position between the nPKC and aPKC isoforms. For a complete description of the structures, there are several recent reviews (27–29).

PKC has played an important role in the field of cancer research since the discovery that the tumor-promoting phorbol ester class of compounds caused PKC activation. For the first time, a connection between the process of signal transduction and tumor promotion could be made. Since then, PKC isoforms have been implicated in several pathways not always related to carcinogenesis. Today, the observation that individual isoenzymes are located in different subcellular compartments and undergo different regulation strongly suggests that each isoform has a unique individual role. For example, PKCμ has been found to be associated with the B-cell antigen receptor complex (30), PKCη is thought to mediate transcriptional activation of the human transglutaminase 1 gene (31), and PKCθ has been described to stimulate the transcription factor complex AP-1 in T lymphocytes (32). Implication of specific PKC isoenzymes has also been shown in pathological conditions such as Alzheimer's (33–36), atherosclerosis (37–39), and diabetes (40–42).

In our laboratory we observed the inhibition of PKC activity and smc proliferation by physiological concentrations of α-tocopherol. By using isoform-specific inhibitors and activators, we found that PKCα is the selective target of α-tocopherol action. β-Tocopherol, an antioxidant almost as potent as α-tocopherol, did not show any effect on cell proliferation of PKC activity, suggesting that the mechanism of action of α-tocopherol is not related to its antioxidant properties. Our results could offer a model to explain the beneficial effects of vitamin E on diabetic vascular complication.

I. METHODS

Rat A7r5 aortic vascular smc were obtained from American Type Culture Collection. Purified PKCα and protein phosphatase type 2A were from UBI (New York). Tissue culture media and polyclonal antibodies to PKCα, δ, and ε isoforms were from Life Technologies, Inc. (Grand Island, NY). Fetal calf serum (FCS) was from PAA (Linz, Austria). Anti-rat PKC ζ polyclonal antibody, purified PKCα, and trimeric PP2A were from Upstate Biotechnology (Lake Placid, NY). Polyclonal anti-PKCμ antibody, caliculin A, okadaic acid, phorbol 12-myristate 13-acetate, and Gö 6976 were from LC Laboratories (Woburn, MA). Ly379196 was a gift of Eli Lilly (Indianapolis, IN). (γ-^{32}P) ATP (3000 Ci/mmol), $^{32}P_i$, monoclonal anti-PKCα (clone MC5), ECL detection system, and ECL Hyperfilm were from Amersham International (Buckinghamshire, UK). Anti-protein kinase Cα rabbit polyclonal used for the kinase reactions of the immunoprecipitated protein was from Oxford Biomedical Research, Inc. (Oxford, MI). Phosphorylase-β, phosphorylase kinase, streptolysin-O, Histone III-SS, and phorbol dibutyrate were from Sigma (St. Louis, MO). C_2-ceramide was from BioMol (Hamburg, Germany). Phenylmethylsulfonylfluoride (PMSF), leupeptin, pepstatin, and aprotinin were from Böhringer (Mannheim, Germany). Protein A-Sepharose 4B was from Pharmacia Biotech Inc. PKCζ antisense oligodeoxynucleotide was from MWG Biotech (Ebersberg, Germany). The peptide PLSRTLSVAAKK used as substrate for assay PKC activity was synthesized by Dr. Servis (Epalinges, Switzerland). Myelin basic protein (4-14 fragment) was produced by Bachem (Switzerland). RRR-α-tocopherol and RRR-β-tocopherol are obtained from Henkel (LaGrange, IL). Tocopherols are adsorbed to FCS before the addition to the cells, as described (43). Protein concentration was determined using a Pierce kit according to the manufacturer's procedures.

A. Cell Cultures

Rat A7r5 cells are maintained in Dulbecco's modified Eagle's medium (DMEM) containing 1.0 g/L glucose, 60 U/mL penicillin, 60 mg/mL streptomycin, and supplemented with 10% (v/v) FCS. Cells in a subconfluent state were made quiescent by incubation in DMEM containing 0.2% FCS for 48

h. Cells were then washed with phosphate-buffered saline (PBS) and treated as indicated in the figure legends. Cell viability, determined by Trypan blue exclusion method, was 90–95% in all experiments. Cells are used between passages 7 and 15.

B. Animals

Thirty male albino rabbits aged 2–4 months were assigned randomly to one of the following four groups. All rabbits were fed 100 g/day vitamin E-free diet as described (44,45). One group of rabbits was only fed the diet without addition of treatments. The second group received daily injections of 50 mg/kg vitamin E. The diet of the third group contained 2% cholesterol, and the fourth received the same diet with daily injections of 50 mg/kg vitamin E. After 4 weeks, the thoracic aortas were removed, and media strips were minced, homogenized, and cytosolic and membrane extracts were prepared for analysis of PKC activity (46).

C. Cell Proliferation

Quiescent A7r5 cells were restimulated to grow by addition of 10% FCS. α-Tocopherol was added to cells at the indicated concentrations. Cell number was determined 30 h later by using a hemocytometer. To measure DNA synthesis, cells were pulsed for 1 h with [^{3}H]thymidine (1 μCi/well) during the S phase (11 h after entry into the cycle). After labeling, cells were processed as described (22), and radioactivity was determined.

D. PKC Activity in Permeabilized Cells

Quiescent A7r5 cells were subjected to different treatments as indicated in the figure legends. During the last hour of the preincubation period, cells were treated with 100 nM phorbol 12-myristate 13-acetate. Aliquots of cells were resuspended in a reaction buffer containing 5.2 mM $MgCl_2$, 94 mM KC1, 12.5 mM HEPES pH 7.4, 12.5 mM EGTA, and 8.2 mM $CaCl_2$, and assays were started by adding [γ-^{32}P]ATP (9 cpm/pmol, final concentration 250 μM), peptide substrate (final concentration 70 μM), and streptolysin-O (0.3 IU). Samples were incubated at 37 °C for 10 min, quenched, and analyzed as described previously (22,47).

E. Immunoprecipitation of PKC Isoforms

After treatment, cells were harvested in 1 mL lysis buffer (50 mM Tris pH 7.5, 150 mM NaCl, 1% [v/v] Triton X-100, 1 mM EGTA, 2 mM EDTA, chymostatin, leupeptin, antipain, pepstatin [5 mg/L each], 1 mg/L E64, and 1 mM PMSF. Cell lysates were forced through a 25-gauge syringe (15 times) and cleared by centrifugation at 15,800 × g for 10 min. Immunoprecipitation was carried out on equal amounts of protein with the indicated anti-PKC antibody (3 μg) incubated for 1–3 h at 4 °C followed by adsorption to protein A-Sepharose beads (10 mg) for 1 h at 4 °C. Precipitated samples were recovered by centrifugation and proteins were either resolved by SDS-PAGE or used in autophosphorylation and kinase reactions.

F. Western Blot Analyses

Immunocomplexes were dissolved in Laemmli's sample buffer and separated by electrophoresis on a 10% polyacrylamide gel followed by electrotransfer to poly (vinylidene difluoride) (PVDF) membranes (DuPont, NEN Research Products). Membranes were incubated at room temperature with 0.1 mg/mL anti-PKC isoforms. Proteins were detected with the ECL system (Amersham).

G. Autophosphorylation of PKC Isoforms

Immunoprecipitated PKCs bound to protein A-Sepharose beads were washed three times with lysis buffer and once with the same buffer containing 0.4 M NaCl and without EDTA/EGTA. Samples were incubated in 40 mL of a mixture containing 5 μCi of [γ-^{32}P]ATP, 10 mM ATP, 400 μM $MgCl_2$, 5 mM $CaCl_2$, 400 μM phosphatidylserine, 100 nM phorbol 12,1-dibutyrate, 1 mM sodium orthovanadate, and 20 mM Tris, pH 7.4 at 37 °C for 10 min. The reactions were terminated by addition of 10 μL of boiling SDS sample buffer and electrophoresed on a 10% polyacrylamide gel. Gels were stained using the SYPRO protein gel stain kit (Molecular Probes), blotted, and radioactivity in the membranes was detected by using a BioRad GS-250 Molecular Imager. Alternatively, gels were dried down for autoradiography on Kodak X-Omat S films. Quantification was done by using a BioRad GS-700 imaging densitometer.

H. Activity of Immunoprecipitated PKCα

Confluent A7r5 cells, after the treatment described in the figure legends, were lysed in a buffer containing 150 mM NaCl, 50 mM Tris-HCl pH 8.0, 1%

Nonidet P-40, 0.5% deoxycholate, 0.1% SDS, 10 mM NaF, protease inhibitor cocktail (Böhringer), 1 mM Na_3VO_4, and 1 mM PMSF. Extracts were prepared by passing the lysates through a 25-gauge needle (15 times) and cleared by centrifugation at 15,800 × g for 10 min. Anti-protein kinase Cα antibody (3 μg) was added to the supernatants for 1 h at 4 °C, and afterward protein A-Sepharose was added for an additional hour. The resulting immunocomplexes were collected by centrifugation, washed in lysis buffer, and finally in kinase buffer (50 mM Tris-HCl pH 7.4, 10 mM NaF, 0.5 mM EDTA, 0.5 mM EGTA, 2 mM $MgCl_2$, 1 mM PMSF, and protease inhibitor cocktail). Kinase reactions with the immunocomplexes were carried out in a 40-μL final volume of an activation buffer containing 20 mM Tris-HCl pH 7.4, 10 mM $MgCl_2$, 10 mM ATP, 2.5 μCi (γ-^{32}P) ATP (600 Ci/mmol), 0.4 mg/mL histone III-S, 1.2 mM $CaCl_2$, 40 mg/mL phosphatidylserine, and 3.3 mM dioleylglycerol. Reactions were terminated by adding 20 μL boiling SDS sample buffer and frozen until use. Samples were loaded in a 10% SDS-PAGE and blotted on a PVDF membrane for 1 h at 100 mA. Histone phosphorylation was detected by using a phosphorimager, and the signals were quantified by densitometric scanning and normalized in respect to the amount of immunoprecipitated PKCα, which was detected by immunoblots using the MC5 anti-PKC antibody.

I. In Vivo Labeling of Cells

Quiescent A7r5 cells (6 × 10^5) were incubated in phosphate-free DMEM (Amimed) with 0.25 mCi/mL $^{32}P_j$ during 14 h at 37 °C. Then cells were stimulated with 10% dialyzed FCS (Sigma) in the presence of the indicated agents and further incubated for 7 h. During the last hour, cells received 100 nM phorbol 12-myristate 13-acetate (PMA). Cells were then washed exhaustively with PBS, lysed in SDS buffer, and subjected to immunoprecipitation for PKCα. PKCα was resolved on SDS-PAGE, and its phosphorylation was analyzed on a BioRad Molecular Imager GS-250. Staining with the SYPRO kit has been used to control protein loading of the gels.

J. Protein Phosphatase Activity Assay

Purified PP_2A (25 ng) resuspended in 10 μL assay buffer (Tris 50 mM, EDTA 1 mM pH 7.6) was preincubated with a solution of either α-tocopherol (50 μM) or β-tocopherol (50 μM) for 10 min at 30 °C. Control reactions contained vehicle (ethanol 0.1%) alone. Assays were started by addition to the mixtures of [^{32}P]phosphorylase-α solution (8.5 mg protein, 9 × 10^4 dpm) and further incubated for 10 min at 30 °C. Reactions were stopped by adding 120 μL ice-cold trichloroacetic acid 10% and 150 mg albumin in 20 μL H_2O. Samples were left on ice and centrifuged 2 min at 12,000 × g. The clear supernatant was counted in a liquid scintillation counter.

K. PKCα/Protein Phosphatase Assay

PKCα (16 nM) was incubated for 10 min at 30°C with PP_2A or PP_1 at the indicated concentrations, in 40 μL activation buffer containing 10 mM MOPS (3-[N-morpholino]propanesulfonic acid), pH 7.2, 0.5 mM DTT (1,4-dithio-DL-threitol), 100 μM $MBP_{4\text{-}14}$ (myelin basic protein peptide fragment 4-14), 0.25 mM ATP, 20 mM $MgCl_2$, 5 μg phosphatidylserine, 5 μg diacylglicerides, and 5 μCi [^{32}P]-ATP. Reaction was stopped with 20 μL 25% TCA (trichloroacetic acid). Aliquots of 50 μL were spotted onto 3 × 3 cm P81 Whatman filters, washed twice with 0.75% phosphoric acid, and then washed once with acetone. Radioactivity was counted in a liquid scintillation analyzer.

II. α-TOCOPHEROL IS A SPECIFIC INHIBITOR OF CELL PROLIFERATION

α-Tocopherol, at concentrations between 10 and 50 μM, was shown to inhibit rat A7r5 smc proliferation (Fig. 1), whereas β-tocopherol appeared ineffective (48). When α-tocopherol and β-tocopherol were added together, no inhibition of cell proliferation was seen. Both compounds were transported equally in

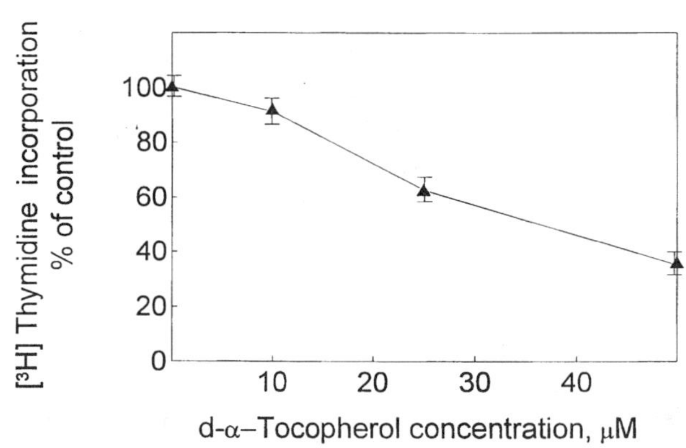

Figure 1 Inhibition of SMC proliferation. Quiescent cells were restimulated with FCS in the presence of the indicated concentrations of α-tocopherol. For DNA synthesis determination, [^{3}H]thimydine was given to the cells in the S-phase. The control represents 84,332 ± 5150 cpm.

cells and did not compete with each other for uptake (48). The oxidized product of α-tocopherol, α-tocopheryl quinone, and several other water- and lipid-soluble antioxidants were not inhibitory, indicating that the effects of α-tocopherol were not related to its antioxidant properties (48).

Inhibitory effects of α-tocopherol were also observed in primary human aortic smc, Balb/3T3 mouse fibroblasts, and NB-2a mouse neuroblastoma but not in Chinese hamster ovary (CHO), Saos-2 human osteosarcoma cells, or P388 mouse macrophages.

III. α-TOCOPHEROL IS A SPECIFIC INDIRECT INHIBITOR OF PKC

A. α-Tocopherol Inhibits PKC Activity

During the transition $G_0 \rightarrow G_1$ phase of the cell cycle, an α-tocopherol-sensitive increase in PKC activity not paralleled by changes in the mRNA levels of the PKCα, β, δ, ε, and ζ isoforms was observed (Fig. 2) (Ricciarelli R., et al., 1997, unpublished results). Similarly, no changes in the protein levels of the major isoform (PKCα), expressed during the transition were observed in the presence or absence of α-tocopherol (Fig. 2).

Maximal PKC inhibition by α-tocopherol was found 6–7 h after the entry of cells into the G_1 phase (Fig. 2, inset), and this inhibition was only observed when α-tocopherol was added at the time of restimulation (22).

PKC activity has been also measured in homogenates of aortas from rabbits fed different dietary supplements. As shown in Table 1, an approximate 50% reduction in PKC activity is observed in vitamin E-treated animals compared with controls (vitamin E-poor diet). With cholesterol supplementation, PKC activity increases to 10.2 Δ-absorbency units/min/mg protein, which is significantly reduced by vitamin E treatment.

B. PKC Isoforms in A7r5 smc

The finding that PKC is involved in the α-tocopherol inhibition of smc proliferation (22) prompted the question of which isoform(s) is(are) affected by α-tocopherol. In A7r5 cells the presence of PKCα, δ, ε, ζ, and μ was documented (Fig. 3, lane A). To determine the specificity of the reaction, the corresponding competitor peptides were used (lane B). The PKCβ isoform was determined in a separate experiment as well and shown to be present in smc. It was also

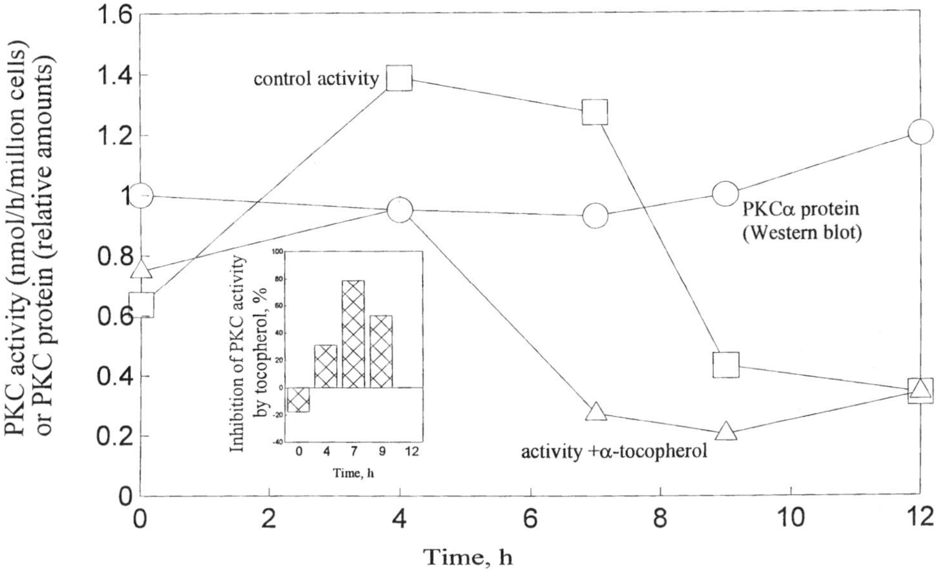

Figure 2 Inhibition of PKC activity by α-tocopherol is a function of the cell cycle. Quiescent A7r5 cells were stimulated for different times with FCS in the absence or presence of 50 μM α-tocopherol. At the indicated points, PMA-stimulated PKC activity in permeabilized cells was measured. PKCα levels were analyzed by Western analysis and the signals scanned by densitometry. Data are expressed as arbitrary units of absorbency. The inset shows the percentage of PKC inhibition by α-tocopherol at different incubation times. Data are representative of four independent experiments.

found that long PMA treatment downregulated the PKCα, δ, ε (lane C) and β and μ isoforms (not shown).

C. α-Tocopherol Selectively Inhibits PKCα

Nanomolar concentrations of Gö 6976 have been shown to inhibit PKCα and β, whereas even micromolar concentrations have no effect on the activity of PKCδ, ε, or ζ (49).

As can be seen in Figure 4, when PKCα and β isoforms were inhibited by Gö 6976, the residual activity was not sensitive to α-tocopherol, indicating that the PKCδ, ε, ζ, and μ isoforms were not involved in the α-tocopherol-induced PKC inhibition. Differently, after PKCβ activity was inhibited by the specific inhibitor Ly379196 (42), the effect of α-tocopherol was still present,

Table 1 PKC Activity from smc Homogenates Obtained from Differently Treated Rabbits

Treatment	PKC activity
Control	8.4 ± 1.1
Vitamin E	4.5 ± 2.5*
Cholesterol	10.2 ± 2.4
Cholesterol + vitamin E	4.5 ± 1.0†

* $p < 0.01$ compared with control group.
† $p < 0.02$ with respect to cholesterol group.
Aortic media are minced and homogenized, and nuclei are sedimented by centrifugation. Supernatants are centrifuged again at 100,000 × g to obtain cytosolic fractions. Pellets are used for preparation of membrane fractions. Protein kinase C activity is measured in both fractions. Since the homogenates did not show significant membrane/cytosol distribution changes, only the values of total PKC activity are reported. Results are expressed as mean ± SD (n = 5). Statistical analysis was performed by one-way analysis of variance (ANOVA).

indicating that this isoform of PKC is not involved in α-tocopherol inhibition (Table 2).

Further evidence was obtained by the experiments reported in Figures 5 and 6. Figure 5 shows that after the inhibition of PKCα and β by Gö 6976 and ζ by PKCζ specific antisense oligonucleotide, the remaining PKC isoforms (δ, ε, and μ) were not affected by α-tocopherol. Finally, when PKCα, β, δ, ε, and μ isoforms were downregulated, the residual PKCζ was not sensitive to α-tocopherol either in the absence or presence of the activator C_2-ceramide (50) (Fig. 6).

Taken together, the above experiments suggested that PKCα is the specific target for α-tocopherol. To further substantiate this finding, immunoprecipitation of the different PKC isoforms and the determination of the kinase and autophosphorylating activity were carried out.

D. Effect of α-Tocopherol on PKC Isoforms Autophosphorylation

PKC autophosphorylation in immunoprecipitates has been found to correlate with its enzymatic activity and has been taken as a reliable indication of PKC activity (28).

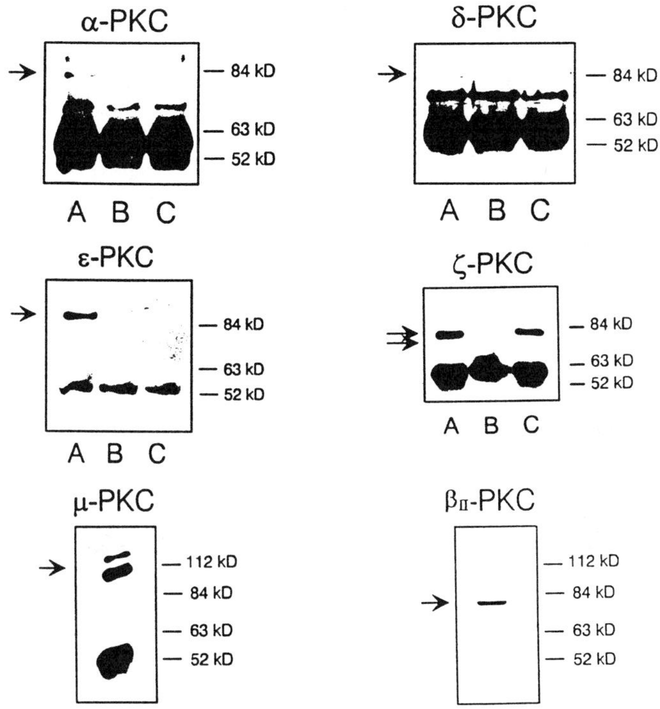

Figure 3 Characterization of PKC isoforms in A7r5 cells. Cells (1×10^6) at 90% confluence were harvested. PKC isoforms were immunoprecipitated with the corresponding antibodies and subjected to SDS-PAGE and immunoblotting as described in Methods. A, control; B, plus competitor peptide; C, cells treated for 24 h with 1 μM PMA.

Cells were incubated in the absence or presence of α-tocopherol or β-tocopherol for 7 h during the G_1 phase. Then extracts were prepared, and immunoprecipitation of the individual PKC isoforms was performed. Autophosphorylation activity and protein amounts were determined for each isoform. In Figure 7, the effects on PKCα and PKCζ are shown. The bar graphs correspond to the PKC activity, and values are normalized with respect to the protein content. As can be seen, only PKCα from α-tocopherol-treated cells was less active relative to its control. The activity of all other PKC isoforms was not affected by the treatment of cells with α-tocopherol (data not shown).

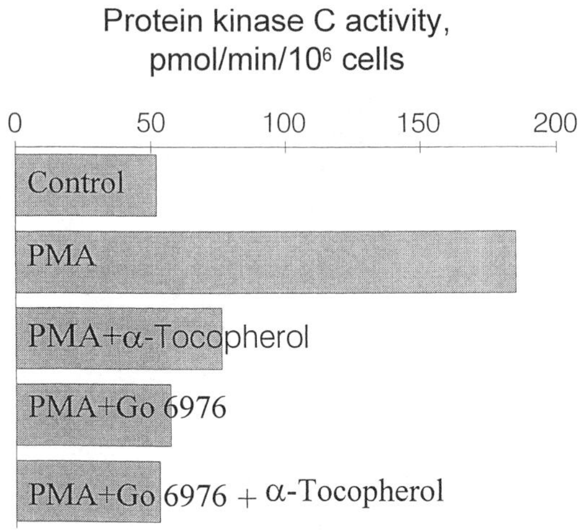

Figure 4 Selective inhibition of PKCα by α-tocopherol. Quiescent A7r5 cells were restimulated for 7 h with FCS in the absence or presence of 50 μM α-tocopherol. Gö 6976 (20 nM) was added to the permeabilized cells where indicated, and PMA-stimulated PKC activity was measured as described in Methods.

E. α-Tocopherol Selectively Inhibits PKCα Activity and Phosphorylation State

To establish whether the incubation of cells with α-tocopherol resulted in a change in the phosphorylation state of PKCα, an in vivo labeling reaction was carried out. Cells were labeled with $^{32}P_i$ overnight, and after stimulation with

Table 2 Effect of the PKC β-Specific Inhibitor Ly379196 on the α-Tocopherol-Induced Inhibition of PKC

Treatment	cpm	% Change	Inhibition
PMA	13,428	100	0
α-tocopherol	8,928	67	33%
Ly379196	15,280	113	−13
Ly379196 + α-tocopherol	9,228	69	31%

Quiescent A7r5 cells were restimulated for 7 h with FCS in the absence or presence of 50 μM α-tocopherol. Ly379196 (20 nM) was added to the permeabilized cells where indicated, and PMA-stimulated PKC activity was measured as described in Method. PMA, phorbol 12-myristate 13-acetate.

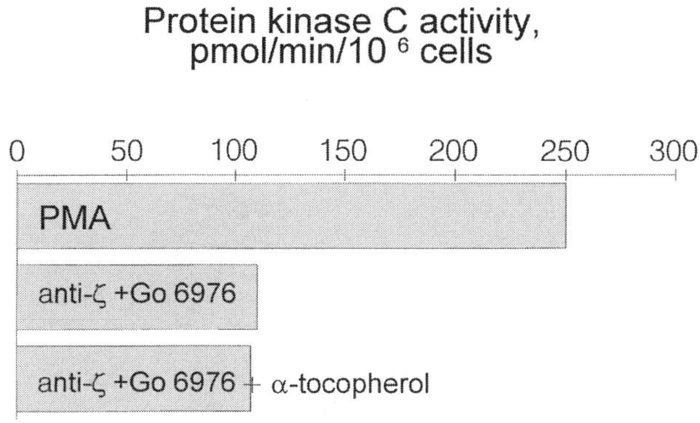

Figure 5 Selective inhibition of PKCα by α-tocopherol. Quiescent cells were treated for 24 h with 1 mM phosphorothioate antisense oligodeoxynucleotide designed to hybridize PKCζ mRNA (anti-ζ). Then cells were restimulated with FCS for 7 h in the absence or presence of 50 μM α-tocopherol. Gö 6976 was added to the PKC assay as described above.

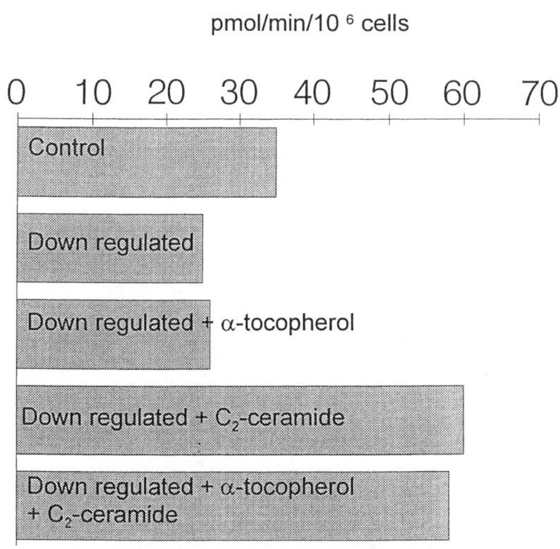

Figure 6 Effect of α-tocopherol on PKCζ. Quiescent cells were treated for 24 h with 1 μM PMA (downregulation, DR) and afterward treated for 7 h with 50 μM α-tocopherol. C_2-ceramide (20 μM) was added to the PKC assay in permeabilized cells as described.

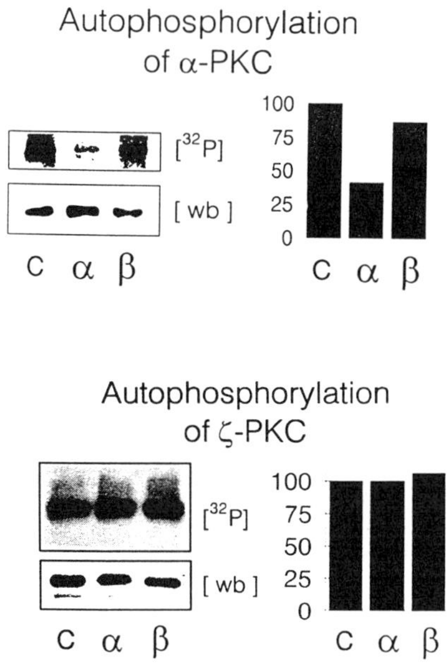

Figure 7 Autophosphorylation activity of different PKC isoforms. Quiescent cells were restimulated for 7 h with FCS in the absence (C) or presence of either 50 μM α-tocopherol (α) or β-tocopherol (β). PMA (100 nM) was added for the last hour of the preincubation period. Then, cell extracts were prepared, and PKC isoforms were immunoprecipitated with the indicated antibodies. Autophosphorylation reaction of the individual isoforms was performed as described in Methods. Samples were electrophoresed and blotted, and the calculated ratio between incorporated radioactivity [^{32}P] and the protein levels (Western blot) is represented in the bar graphs for each condition. Data are representative of three independent experiments.

FCS for 7 h in the presence or absence of α-tocopherol, PKCα was immunoprecipitated, blotted, and the ^{32}P incorporation measured. Figure 8 shows a bar graph presentation of the radioactivity intensities integrated and normalized with respect to the protein levels of each sample. Relative to the control (N), the PMA-treated cells (P) showed a significant increase in ^{32}P incorporation into PKCα. Cells pretreated with α-tocopherol (column α) showed a large inhibition of PKCα phosphorylation, whereas cells preincubated with β-tocopherol (column β) showed much less inhibition. The inhibitory effect of α-tocopherol was reversed by two potent protein phosphatase inhibitors, okadaic acid 2 nM (not shown) or calyculin A 2 nM (column α + C). Figure 9 shows the PKCα activity measured after immunoprecipitation of the enzyme

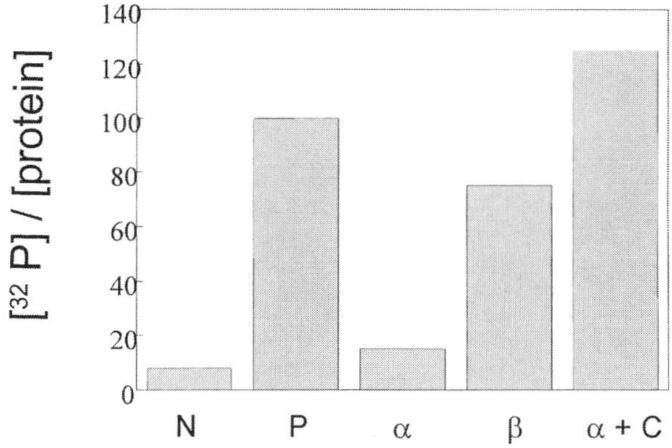

Figure 8 Effect of α-tocopherol and β-tocopherol on PKCα phosphorylation state. Quiescent A7r5 cells were incubated in phosphate-free DMEM medium (ICN) for 48 h. They received 0.25 mCi/ml P_i for the last 14 h. Cells were restimulated for 7 h with FCS in the absence (P) or presence of either 50 μM α-tocopherol (α) or β-tocopherol (β). PMA (100 nM) was added for the last hour to all samples except N. Caliculin A (2 nM) was added to cells for 1 h where indicated (α + C). Cell extracts were prepared and immunoprecipitated with anti-PKCα. Proteins were resolved by SDS-PAGE and radioactivity [^{32}P] and protein levels were quantified as described in Methods. The bar graph represents the ratio between cpm incorporated to PKCα and the protein levels. Data are representative of three independent experiments.

from cells preincubated with α-tocopherol or β-tocopherol at the late G_1 phase of the cell cycle. As can be seen, α-tocopherol inhibited PKCα activity more strongly compared with β-tocopherol.

In the case of PKCβ, no significant PKC activity changes were observed if the cells were preincubated with either α-tocopherol or β-tocopherol.

F. Protein Phosphatase PP2A Is Activated by α-Tocopherol and Can Dephosphorylate PKCα

The role of a phosphatase PP2A on the deactivation of PKCα has been postulated on the basis of previous experiments (22). To establish if a direct effect of PP2A on PKC took place, the following experiment was carried out (Fig. 10). The two enzymes were preincubated together and then the activity of PKCα was measured. It was observed that PP2A produced a deactivation of PKCα. The inhibition of approximately 50% in PKCα activity obtained at a ratio 1 PP2A/16 PKC molecules indicates a catalytic role of PP2A on PKC inactivation.

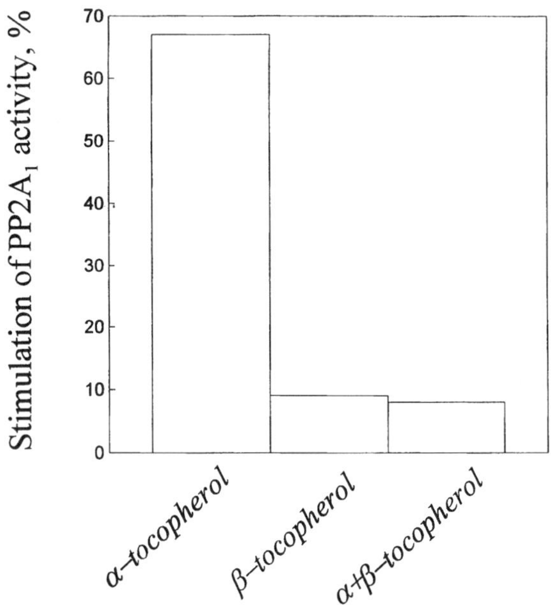

Figure 9 Determination of PKCα activity after its immunoprecipitation from cells treated with α-tocopherol or β-tocopherol. Cells were stimulated for 7 h with FCS in the absence (Control) or presence of either 50 μM α-tocopherol or β-tocopherol as indicated. During the last hour of preincubation, they received 100 nM PMA. Then extracts were prepared, PKCα was immunoprecipitated, and a kinase reaction using Histone III-SS was performed as described in Methods. Proteins were resolved by electrophoresis, and radioactive bands were quantified with a BioRad Molecular Analyst software. Protein levels were estimated by staining the gel with the SYPRO kit or by immunoblots with the MC5 monoclonal antibody. The ratio between radioactivity incorporated into the substrate and the amount of PKCα precipitated was expressed as arbitrary units of the densitometric scanning of the bands. Data are representative of three independent experiments.

The inhibition by α-tocopherol of PKCα at a cellular level may thus be related to a possible activation of PP2A by α-tocopherol. This hypothesis was investigated in the experiment outlined in Figure 11. Purified PP2A was incubated with [^{32}P]phosphorylase-α as a substrate; its activation by α-tocopherol, β-tocopherol, and a mixture of the two was analyzed. α-Tocopherol produced almost a twofold activation. β-Tocopherol was slightly inhibitory, and the mixture of both tocopherols was without significant effect. It thus appears that one of the cellular targets of α-tocopherol may be PP2A.

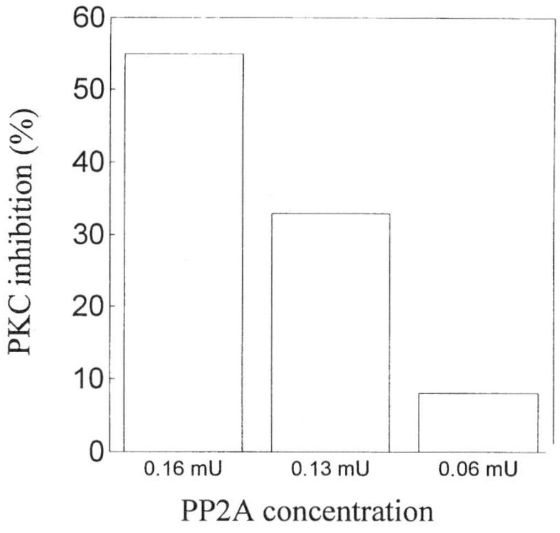

Figure 10 Inhibition of PKCα activity by PP2A. Purified PKCα (16 nM) was incubated for 10 min at 30°C with PP2A in 40 μL activation buffer as described in Methods. PKCα activity was determined using a peptide substrate as described previously. Data are representative of three independent experiments.

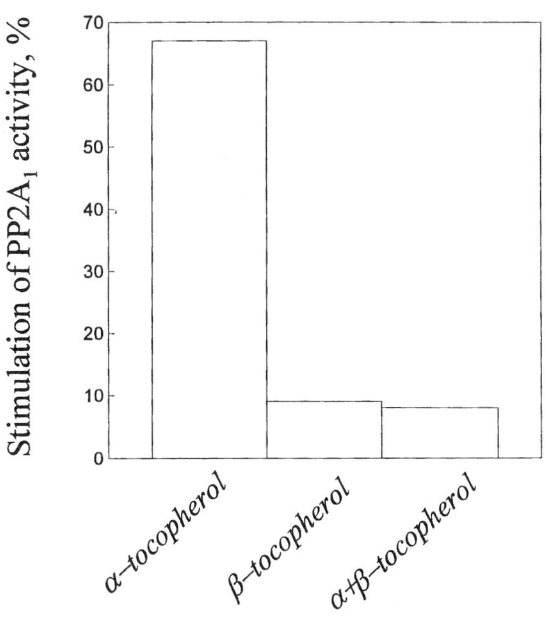

Figure 11 Effect of α-tocopherol and β-tocopherol on PP2A activity. Phosphatase activity, using pure PP2A, was assayed in the presence of different α-tocopherol or β-tocopherol concentrations as indicated. PP2A activity stimulation was calculated with respect to control samples. The background in the absence of the enzyme represented less than 3.5% of the initial total counts. Data are representative of three separate experiments.

IV. CONCLUSIONS

Cell proliferation, especially of smc and mesangial cells, plays an important role in the pathogenesis of diabetic complications. Increase in smc proliferation rate is of primary importance in the progression of atherosclerosis. Increased growth of mesangial cells, a cell type similar to smc, takes place during nephrosclerosis. PKC has been shown to be involved in both diseases. Smooth muscle cells from aortas of rabbits fed a high cholesterol diet show increased PKC activity. α-Tocopherol treatment of the animals has been shown to diminish such activity.

In vitro smooth muscle cells are subject to a fine control by α-tocopherol. Their proliferation is strongly diminished by α-tocopherol in a specific way. Many other cell types are, in fact, insensitive to α-tocopherol. α-Tocopherol is also unique in its action in smooth muscle cells, because other tocopherols, tocotrienols, and general antioxidants are not as potent as α-tocopherol. Some of them, such as probucol, are not effective at all. It is thus conceivable that the action of α-tocopherol is not mediated by its radical scavenging function.

Data on the competition of α-tocopherol and β-tocopherol suggest the existence of a receptor with the capacity of recognizing α-tocopherol as an agonist and β-tocopherol as an antagonist. The finding that a phosphatase PP2A is modulated in an opposite way to proliferation by several tocopherols may indicate a role of this enzyme in the cascade of events at the basis of α-tocopherol inhibition of cell proliferation. In the studies reported above, it has also been clarified that PKC, in smooth muscle cells, is inhibited by α-tocopherol. Also, such an event is α-tocopherol specific, with a specificity pattern similar to that of cell proliferation. PKC inhibition takes place only at cellular level and is associated with a diminution of PKC phosphorylation. This finding parallels the observed activation pattern of a phosphatase. Consequently, the entire picture relative to the understanding of smc inhibition may be understood in the following way. In the hypothesis that a receptor for α-tocopherol exists, this may produce PP2A increase expression. Alternatively, the latter enzyme could be by itself the receptor, distinguishing between α-tocopherol and β-tocopherol. In either case, the increased PP2A activity results in a dephosphorylation of PKC and in a reversible diminution of its activity. The role of α-tocopherol has also been described in terms of inhibition, in mesangial cells, of PKC activity via diminution of diacylglycerol, the physiological activator of PKC. Such a decrease would be the consequence of the specific activation by α-tocopherol of the enzyme diacylglycerol kinase.

The two described mechanisms of cell proliferation control by α-tocopherol are both centered on PKC regulation. In one (22,48), emphasis is given to the postranslational modifications of PKC mediated by an α-tocopherol-sensitive protein phosphatase. In the other (42), the role of α-tocopherol would be to subtract PKC major activator by biochemical conversion. Both mechanisms may coexist or acquire a major role in one or the other cell type.

ACKNOWLEDGMENTS

Supported by the Swiss National Science Foundation and by F. Hoffmann-La Roche, AG. We thank Mrs. Maria Feher for her expert help with cellular cultures.

REFERENCES

1. Ybarra J, Lopez-Talavera JC. Non insulin dependent diabetes mellitus, lipid metabolism and atherosclerosis [editorial]. Med Clin (Barc) 1998; 110:19–21.
2. Valek J. Prevention of atherosclerosis in diabetics. Cas Lek Cesk 1997; 136: 523–526.
3. Steiner G. Diabetes mellitus, dyslipoproteinaemias and atherosclerosis. Diabetologia 1997; 40:S147–S148.
4. Visseren FL, Bouter KP, Pon MJ, Hoekstra JB, Erkelens DW, Diepersloot RJ. Patients with diabetes mellitus and atherosclerosis: a role for cytomegalovirus? Diabetes Res Clin Pract 1997; 36:49–55.
5. Bornfeldt KE, Raines EW, Nakano T, Graves LM, Krebs EG, Ross R. Insulin-like growth factor-I and platelet-derived growth factor-BB induce directed migration of human arterial smooth muscle cells via signaling pathways that are distinct from those of proliferation. J Clin Invest 1994; 93:1266–1274.
6. Gilbert RE, Cox A, Wu LL, Allen TJ, Hulthen UL, Jerums G, Cooper ME. Expression of transforming growth factor-beta1 and type IV collagen in the renal tubulointerstitium in experimental diabetes: effects of ACE inhibition. Diabetes 1998; 47:414–422.
7. Park IS, Kiyomoto H, Abboud SL, Abboud HE. Expression of transforming growth factor-beta and type IV collagen in early streptozotocin-induced diabetes. Diabetes 1997; 46:473–480.
8. Sumida Y, Ura H, Yano Y, Misaki M, Shima T. Abnormal metabolism of type-IV collagen in normotensive non-insulin-dependent diabetes mellitus patients. Horm Res 1997; 48:23–28.

9. Karasu C, Ozansoy G, Bozkurt O, Erdogan D, Omeroglu S. Antioxidant and triglyceride-lowering effects of vitamin E associated with the prevention of abnormalities in the reactivity and morphology of aorta from streptozotocin-diabetic rats. Antioxidants in Diabetes-Induced Complications (ADIC) Study Group. Metabolism 1997; 46:872–879.
10. Gazis A, Page S, Cockcroft J. Vitamin E and cardiovascular protection in diabetes [editorial]. Br Med J 1997; 314:1845–1846.
11. Siman CM, Eriksson UJ. Vitamin E decreases the occurrence of malformations in the offspring of diabetic rats. Diabetes 1997; 46:1054–1061.
12. Viana M, Herrera E, Bonet B. Teratogenic effects of diabetes mellitus in the rat. Prevention by vitamin E. Diabetologia 1996; 39:1041–1046.
13. Shklar G, Schwartz JL. Vitamin E inhibits experimental carcinogenesis and tumour angiogenesis. Eur J Cancer B Oral Oncol 1996; 32B:114–119.
14. Pentland AP, Morrison AR, Jacobs SC, Hruza LL, Hebert JS, Packer L. Tocopherol analogs suppress arachidonic acid metabolism via phospholipase inhibition. J Biol Chem 1992; 267:15578–15584.
15. Lucy JA. Functional and structural aspects of biological membranes: a suggested structural role for vitamin E in the control of membrane permeability and stability. Ann NY Acad Sci 1972; 203:4–11.
16. Gillilan RE, Mondell B, Warbasse JR. Quantitative evaluation of vitamin E in the treatment of angina pectoris. Am Heart J 1977; 93:444–449.
17. Briggs M. Are vitamin E supplements beneficial? Med J Aust 1974; 1:434–437.
18. Diplock AT, Xu GL, Yeow CL, Okikiola M. Relationship of tocopherol structure to biological activity, tissue uptake, and prostaglandin biosynthesis. Ann NY Acad Sci 1989; 570:72–84.
19. Hentati A, Deng HX, Hung WY, Nayer M, Ahmed MS, He X, Tim R, Stumpf DA, Siddique T, Ahmed. Human alpha-tocopherol transfer protein: gene structure and mutations in familial vitamin E deficiency. Ann Neurol 1996; 39:295–300.
20. Doerflinger N, Linder C, Ouahchi K, Gyapay G, Weissenbach J, Le Paslier D, Rigault P, Belal S, Ben Hamida C, Hentati F, et al. Ataxia with vitamin E deficiency: refinement of genetic localization and analysis of linkage disequilibrium by using new markers in 14 families. Am J Hum Genet 1995; 56:1116–1124.
21. Ouahchi K, Arita M, Kayden H, Hentati F, Ben Hamida M, Sokol R, Arai H, Inove K, Mandel JL, Koenig M. Ataxia with isolated vitamin E deficiency is caused by mutations in the alpha-tocopherol transfer protein. Nat Genet 1995; 9:141–145.
22. Tasinato A, Boscoboinik D, Bartoli GM, Maroni P, Azzi A. *d*-Alpha-tocopherol inhibition of vascular smooth muscle cell proliferation occurs at physiological concentrations, correlates with protein kinase C inhibition, and is independent of its antioxidant properties. Proc Natl Acad Sci USA 1995; 92:12190–12194.
23. Boscoboinik D, Ozer NK, Moser U, Azzi A. Tocopherols and 6-hydroxy-chro-

man-2-carbonitrile derivatives inhibit vascular smooth muscle cell proliferation by a nonantioxidant mechanism. Arch Biochem Biophys 1995; 318:241–246.
24. Boscoboinik DO, Chatelain E, Bartoli GM, Stauble B, Azzi A. Inhibition of protein kinase C activity and vascular smooth muscle cell growth by *d*-alpha-tocopherol. Biochim Biophys Acta 1994; 1224:418–426.
25. Chatelain E, Boscoboinik DO, Bartoli GM, Stauble B, Azzi A. Inhibition of smooth muscle cell proliferation and protein kinase C activity by tocopherols and tocotrienols. Biochim Biophys Acta 1993; 1176:83–89.
26. Muller R, Mumberg D, Lucibello FC. Signals and genes in the control of cell-cycle progression. Biochim Biophys Acta 1993; 1155:151–179.
27. Azzi A, Boscoboinik D, Hensey C. The protein kinase C family. Eur J Biochem 1992; 208:547–557.
28. Newton AC. Protein kinase C: structure, function, and regulation. J Biol Chem 1995; 270:28495–28498.
29. Mellor H, Parker PJ. The extended protein kinase C superfamily [In Process Citation]. Biochem J 1998; 332:281–292.
30. Korinek V, Barker N, Morin PJ, van Wichen D, de Weger R, Kinzler KW, Vogelstein B, Clevers H. Constitutive transcriptional activation by a beta-catenin-Tcf complex in APC-/- colon carcinoma. Science 1997; 275:1784–1787.
31. Morin PJ, Sparks AB, Korinek V, Barker N, Clevers H, Vogelstein B, Kinzler KW. Activation of beta-catenin-Tcf signaling in colon cancer by mutations in beta-catenin or APC. Science 1997; 275:1787–1790.
32. Rubinfeld B, Robbins P, El-Gamil M, Albert I, Porfiri E, Polakis P. Stabilization of beta-catenin by genetic defects in melanoma cell lines. Science 1997; 275: 1790–1792.
33. Matsushima H, Shimohama S, Tanaka S, Taniguchi T, Hagiwara M, Hidaka H, Kimura J. Platelet protein kinase C levels in Alzheimer's disease. Neurobiol Aging 1994; 15:671–674.
34. Kinouchi T, Sorimachi H, Maruyama K, Mizumo K, Ohno S, Ishiura S, Suzuki K. Conventional protein kinase C (PKC)-alpha and novel PKC epsilon, but not delta, increase the secretion of an N-terminal fragment of Alzheimer's disease amyloid precursor protein from PKC cDNA transfected 3Y1 fibroblasts. FEBS Lett 1995; 364:203–206.
35. Boyce JJ, Shea TB. Phosphorylation events mediated by protein kinase C alpha and epsilon participate in regulation of tau steady-state levels and generation of certain ''Alzheimer-like'' phospho-epitopes. Int J Dev Neurosci 1997; 15:295–307.
36. Govoni S, Racchi M, Bergamaschi S, Trabucchi M, Battaini F, Bianchetti A, Binetti AG. Defective protein kinase C alpha leads to impaired secretion of soluble beta-amyloid precursor protein from Alzheimer's disease fibroblasts. Ann NY Acad Sci 1996; 777:332–337.
37. Haller H, Lindschau C, Quass P, Distler A, Luft FC. Differentiation of vascular smooth muscle cells and the regulation of protein kinase C-alpha. Circ Res 1995; 76:21–29.

38. Wang S, Desai D, Wright G, Niles RM, Wright GL. Effects of protein kinase C alpha overexpression on A7r5 smooth muscle cell proliferation and differentiation. Exp Cell Res 1997; 236:117–126.
39. Leng L, Du B, Consigli S, McCaffrey TA. Translocation of protein kinase C-delta by PDGF in cultured vascular smooth muscle cells: inhibition by TGF-beta 1. Artery 1996; 22:140–154.
40. Schaffer SW, Ballard C, Mozaffari MS. Is there a link between impaired glucose metabolism and protein kinase C activity in the diabetic heart? Mol Cell Biochem 1997; 176:219–225.
41. Malhotra A, Reich D, Reich D, Nakouzi A, Sanghi V, Geenen DL, Buttrick PM. Experimental diabetes is associated with functional activation of protein kinase C epsilon and phosphorylation of troponin I in the heart, which are prevented by angiotensin II receptor blockade. Circ Res 1997; 81:1027–1033.
42. Ishii H, Jirousek MR, Koya D, et al. Amelioration of vascular dysfunctions in diabetic rats by an oral PKC beta inhibitor. Science 1996; 272:728–731.
43. Chan AC, Tran K. The uptake of (R, R, R)alpha-tocopherol by human endothelial cells in culture. Lipids 1990; 25:17–21.
44. Konneh MK, Rutherford C, Li SR, Anggard EE, Ferns GA. Vitamin E inhibits the intimal response to balloon catheter injury in the carotid artery of the cholesterol-fed rat. Atherosclerosis 1995; 113:29–39.
45. Sirikci O, Ozer NK, Azzi A. Dietary cholesterol-induced changes of protein kinase C and the effect of vitamin E in rabbit aortic smooth muscle cells. Atherosclerosis 1996; 126:253–263.
46. Porreca E, Ciccarelli R, Di Febbo C, Cuccurullo F. Protein kinase C pathway and proliferative responses of aged and young rat vascular smooth muscle cells. Atherosclerosis 1993; 104:137–145.
47. Alexander DR, Graves JD, Lucas SC, Cantrell DA, Crumpton MJ. A method for measuring protein kinase C activity in permeabilized T lymphocytes by using peptide substrates. Evidence for multiple pathways of kinase activation. Biochem J 1990; 268:303–308.
48. Azzi A, Boscoboinik D, Marilley D, Ozer NK, Stauble B, Tasinato A. Vitamin E: a sensor and an information transducer of the cell oxidation state. Am J Clin Nutr 1995; 62:1337S–1346S.
49. Martiny-Baron G, Kazanietz MG, Mischak H, Blumberg PM, Kochs G, Hug H, Marme D, Schachtele C. Selective inhibition of protein kinase C isozymes by the indolocarbazole Go 6976. J Biol Chem 1993; 268:9194–9197.
50. Muller G, Ayoub M, Storz P, Rennecke J, Fabbro D, Pfizenmaier K. PKC zeta is a molecular switch in signal transduction of TNF-alpha, bifunctionally regulated by ceramide and arachidonic acid. EMBO J 1995; 14:1961–1969.

16

Protein Kinase C Activation, Development of Diabetic Vascular Complications, and Role of Vitamin E in Preventing These Abnormalities

Sven-Erik Bursell
Harvard Medical School, Beetham Eye Institute Eye Research, Boston, Massachusetts

George L. King
Joslin Diabetes Center, Harvard Medical School, Boston, Massachusetts

Hyperglycemia induces multiple changes in vasculature or in neuronal cells in animal models of diabetes or in diabetic patients. The multifactorial nature of the changes is not surprising because the flux of glucose and its metabolites are known to affect many cellular pathways. The main challenge in this area has been to identify hyperglycemia-induced biochemical changes that can have a significant impact on vascular dysfunction and subsequent development of pathologies. Multiple theories have been proposed to explain the pathogenesis of the various complications involving retina, glomeruli, peripheral nerves, cardiovascular tissues, wound healing, and pregnancy. No one single theory, however, has emerged to account for all these changes.

Extracellularly, glucose can react nonenzymatically with the primary amines of proteins, forming glycated compounds or oxidants (1). These products can secondarily act on inflammatory cells or vascular cells directly via receptor- or nonreceptor-mediated processes to cause vascular dysfunction (2,3). Excessive glucose can also be transported intracellularly, mainly by the glucose transporter GLUT-1, and the resulting metabolism can cause changes in the redox potential, increase sorbitol production via aldose reductase, or alter signal transduction pathways such as the activation of diacylglycerol (DAG) and protein kinase C (PKC) pathway activation (4–10). It is probable that all hyperglycemia-induced intra- and extracellular changes and their adverse effects are being mediated through the alteration of some of these signal transduction pathways.

The effect of hyperglycemia on signal transduction pathways has not been extensively studied except for the activation of the DAG–PKC pathway. This pathway is known to be important in vascular cells because it is associated with the regulation of vascular permeability, contractility, extrcellular matrix, cell growth, angiogenesis, cytokine actions, and leukocyte adhesions, all of which are abnormal in diabetes (11,12).

I. PROTEIN KINASE C

PKC includes at least 11 isoforms (α, $\beta 1$, $\beta 2$, γ, δ, ε, ζ, η, θ, λ, μ), representing the major downstream targets for lipid second messengers or phorbol esters (11–13). The conventional PKC isoforms (α, $\beta 1$, $\beta 2$, γ) are Ca^{2+}-dependent, containing two cysteine-rich, zinc finger-like motifs (C1 region), which are the binding sites of DAG or phorbol ester, and a Ca^{2+}/phospholipid (C2 region). New PKCs (δ, ε, η, θ, μ) are DAG sensitive but Ca^{2+} independent due to the absence of the C2 region. The two atypical PKCs, ζ, and λ, are insensitive to DAG and lack one of the cysteine-rich motifs in the C1 region, but they can be activated by phosphatidylserine.

The source of DAG resulting in PKC activation can be derived from the hydrolysis of phosphatidylinositides (PI) or from the metabolism of phosphatidylcholine (PC) by phospholipase C (PLC) or D (PLD). Recent data, however, have shown that each isoform can be regulated by more than one lipid second messenger (9) such as the activation of PKC ζ by PIP3 (12–14). Multiple isoforms can be expressed in different cell types, but despite extensive study, the attribution of a specific function to a specific isoform cannot be consistently established, suggesting that several isoforms can possibly mediate a similar range of functions and that their actions may be cell specific (12,15).

II. MECHANISMS OF HYPERGLYCEMIA-INDUCED PKC ACTIVATION

In association with the diabetic vascular complications, increased total DAG content has been demonstrated in a variety of tissues, including retina (16), aorta, heart (17), and renal glomeruli (18,19), in both diabetic animal models and patients (Table 1). This has also been observed in classically termed ''insulin-sensitive'' tissues such as the liver and skeletal muscle (20,21). In all vascular cells studied, increasing glucose levels from 5 to 22 mM in the media elevated the cellular DAG contents (17). Increased DAG levels in response to elevated glucose may not occur immediately and can take as long as 3–5 days to reach a maximum after elevating glucose levels (18,22). Xia et al. (22) also showed that increased DAG content was chronically maintained in the aorta of diabetic dogs even after 5 years of disease. In fact, Inoguchi et al. (17) reported that euglycemic control by islet cell transplant after 3 weeks was not able to completely reverse the increases in DAG level or PKC activation in the aorta of diabetic rats. These results clearly indicate that the activation of the DAG–PKC pathway can be chronically sustained.

Cellular DAG content can also be increased by agonist-stimulated hydrolysis of PI or PC such as PLC or PLD (11–13). Because inositol phosphate products are not increased by hyperglycemia in aortic cells and glomerular

Table 1 Summary of DAG Level and PKC Activity in Cultured Cells Exposed to High Glucose and Tissues Isolated from Diabetic Animals

	Diacylglycerol	Protein kinase C
Cultured cells		
Retinal endothelial cells	↑	↑
Aortic endothelial cells	↑	↑
Aortic smooth muscle cells	↑	↑
Renal mesangial cells	↑	↑
Pericytes	→	↑
Tissues		
Retina (diabetic rats and dogs)	↑	↑
Heart (diabetic rats)	↑	↑
Aorta (diabetic rats and dogs)	↑	↑
Renal glomeruli (diabetic rats)	↑	↑
Brain (diabetic rats)	ND	Not changed
Peripheral nerve	→↑	→↓

ND, not determined.

mesangial cells, increases in PI hydrolysis are most likely not involved in diabetes (22,23). Increases in DAG content could also arise from PC metabolism since Yasunare et al. (24) reported that PLD activity was increased by elevated glucose levels in aortic smooth muscle cells. They did not, however, quantitate the amount of total DAG. Most studies, however, have shown that the source of glucose-induced DAG increases were through the de novo synthesis pathway. In this case, labeling studies using [6-^{3}H]- or [U-^{14}C]-glucose demonstrated that elevated glucose levels increased the incorporation of labeled glucose into the glycerol backbone of DAG in aortic endothelial cells (25), aortic smooth muscle cells (22), and glomeruli (18). These studies clearly established that the increased DAG content was partially derived from glycolytic intermediates (26–28). Palmitic acid and oleic acid are the predominate fatty acids incorporated into DAG through the de novo pathway and from the metabolism of PC, which is consistent with the findings in vascular tissues from diabetic animals (25). In contrast, DAG derived from PLC activation consists mainly of 1-stearolyl, 2-arachidonyl fatty acid, which was not altered by glucose (25,29).

The activation of PKC by hyperglycemia may be tissue specific because it was noted in the retina (16), aorta, heart (17), and glomeruli (8,18) but not clearly demonstrated in the brain (16) and peripheral nerves (30) (Table 1). Similar increases in DAG levels and PKC activation have also been shown in multiple types of cultured vascular cells in response to increased glucose levels (Table 1) (8,16,22,31). Thus, it is likely that the DAG–PKC pathway is activated by the hyperglycemic-diabetic state in all vascular cells. Among the various PKC isoforms in vascular cells, PKC β and δ isoforms appear to be preferentially activated as shown by immunoblotting studies in aorta and heart of diabetic rats (17) and in cultured aortic smooth muscle cells exposed to high levels of glucose (32). However, increases in other isoforms such as PKC α, β2, and ε in the retina (18) and PKC α, β1, and δ in the glomerular cells from diabetic rats have also been noted (33,34). These results demonstrate that diabetes and hyperglycemia will activate the DAG–PKC pathways in many tissue types, including vascular tissues, and thus glucose and its metabolites can cause many cellular abnormalities. However, for a hyperglycemia-induced change to be credible as a causal factor of diabetic complications, it has to be shown to be able to be chronically altered, difficult to reverse, to cause similar vascular changes when activated without diabetes, and to be able to prevent complications when it is inhibited. Thus far, based on the evidence presented, DAG–PKC pathway activation appears to fulfill the first two criteria. In the following sections, data are presented to support a fulfillment of the final two criteria with respect to the DAG–PKC pathway.

III. FUNCTIONAL ALTERATIONS IN VASCULAR CELLS MEDIATED BY DAG–PKC ACTIVATION

Multiple cellular and functional abnormalities in the diabetic vascular tissues have been attributed to the activation of DAG–PKC pathways, including vascular blood flow, vascular permeability, Na^+-K^+ ATPase, and extracellular matrix components.

A. Vascular Blood Flow

Abnormalities in vascular blood flow and contractility have been found in many organs of diabetic animals or patients, including the kidney, retina, peripheral arteries, and microvessels of peripheral nerves. In the retina of diabetic patients without clinical retinopathy (35–38) and animals with short durations of disease (39–43), retinal blood flows have been shown to be decreased. However, retinal blood flow may be normal or increased with longer duration of retinopathy (37,38,44). Multiple lines of evidence have supported the hypothesis that the decreases in retinal blood flow are due to PKC activation. For example, introduction of a PKC agonist such as a phorbol ester into the retina will decrease retinal blood flow (16). On the other hand, decreases in retinal blood flow in diabetic rats have been reported to be normalized by PKC inhibitors (16,19). In nondiabetic animals, the intravitreal injection of a DAG kinase inhibitor resulted in increased retinal DAG levels, activation of PKC, and a concomitant reduction in retinal blood flow (1,31). DAG kinase metabolizes DAG to phosphatidic acid, so DAG kinase inhibition will result in an increase in the available DAG pool. The results from this study showed that increased retinal DAG levels resulted in retinal blood flow decreases comparable with those measured in the diabetic rats. In addition to the retina, decreases in blood flow have also been reported in the peripheral nerves of diabetic animals, which were normalized by PKC inhibition (45,46), although some reports have noted increases in neuronal blood flow in diabetic rats (6).

One of the potential mechanisms by which PKC activation could be causing vasoconstriction in the retina is by increasing the expression of endothelin-1 (ET-1) (47). We reported that the expression of ET-1, a potent vasoconstrictor, plays a primary role in the regulation of retinal hemodynamics (48) and is increased in the retina of diabetic rats. Additionally, intravitreous injection of an ET-A receptor antagonist BQ123 prevented the decrease in retinal blood flow in these diabetic rats (47). The decrease in blood flow to the retina could lead to local hypoxia. Hypoxia is known to be a potent inducer of vascular endothelial growth factor (VEGF), causing increases in permeability and microaneurysm formation (49,50).

Abnormalities in hemodynamics have been clearly documented to precede diabetic nephropathy (51,52). Elevated renal glomerular filtration rate (GFR) and modest increases in renal blood flow are characteristic findings in insulin-dependent diabetes mellitus (IDDM) patients (51,52) and experimental diabetic animals (53). Diabetic glomerular hyperfiltration is likely to be the result of hyperglycemia-induced decreases in arteriolar resistance, especially at the level of afferent arterioles (54,55), resulting in an elevation of glomerular filtration pressure. Multiple mechanisms have been proposed to explain the increases in GFR and glomerular filtration pressure, including an enhanced activity of angiotensin (56) and culturation in prostinoid productions (57–59). It is possible that the activation of DAG–PKC may also play a role in the enhancement of angiotensin actions because angiotensin mediates some of its activity by the activation of the DAG–PKC pathway (57). In addition, increases in vasodilatory prostanoids such as prostaglandin E_2 (PGE_2) and prastafandin I_2 could also be involved in causing glomerular hyperfiltration in diabetes (58,59). The enhanced production of PGE_2 induced by diabetes and hyperglycemia could be the result of sequential activation of PKC and cytosolic phospholipase A_2 ($cPLA_2$), a key regulator of arachidonic acid synthesis (60–63).

In the microvessels, increases in nitric oxide (NO) activities, a potent vasodilator, may also enhance glomerular filtration (64). Urinary excretions of NO2/NO3, stable metabolites of NO, have been reported to be increased in diabetes of short duration (64–66), possibly due to enhanced expression of inducible NO synthase (iNOS) gene and increased production of NO in mesangial cells (67). In addition, both increases in iNOS gene expression and NO production can be mimicked by PKC agonist and inhibited by PKC inhibitors when induced by hyperglycemia (67), suggesting that NO production might be increased in diabetes through PKC-induced iNOS overexpression. In addition, Graier et al. (68) suggested that NO production was enhanced by the elevation of glucose levels, possibly by the increased flux of Ca^{2+} and its activation of eNOS. However, Craven et al. (69) reported that the production of glomerular NO and its second messenger, cGMP, in diabetic rats in response to cholinergic agents were decreased and that PKC inhibitors restored the glomerular cGMP production. Several authors also reported that elevated levels of glucose decreased NOS expression in vascular smooth muscle cells and that these effects of glucose were reversed by PKCβ inhibitors (70,71). Thus, PKC can regulate renal hemodynamics by increasing or decreasing NO production dependent on the cell type and tissue location.

In the macrovessels, increases in contractility found in diabetes are due to a delay in the relaxation response after contraction induced by cholinergic agents (72–75). These abnormal responses can also be prevented by PKC inhibitors (76), suggesting that PKC activation plays a general role in causing abnormal peripheral hemodynamics in diabetes.

B. Vascular Permeability and Neovascularization

Increased vascular permeability is another characteristic systemic vascular abnormality in diabetic animals, in which increased permeability to albumin can occur as early as after 4–6 weeks of diabetes (77), suggesting endothelial cell dysfunctions. PKC activation can directly increase the permeability of albumin and other macromolecules through barriers formed by endothelial cells (78,79) and skin chamber granulation tissues (80), probably by phosphorylating cytoskeletal proteins forming the intracellular junctions (81,82). Interestingly, phorbol ester-induced increases in endothelial permeability may be regulated by PKC β1 activation (83), which is consistent with the preferential activation of PKC β isoforms in diabetes.

PKC activation could also regulate vascular permeability and neovascularization via the expression of growth factors, such as the VEGF/vascular permeability factor (VPF), which is increased in ocular fluids from diabetic patients and has been implicated in the neovascularization process of proliferative retinopathy (49). We reported that both the mitogenic and the permeability-inducing actions of VEGF/VPF are due in part to the activation of the PKC β isoform via tyrosine phosphorylation of PLC (84). Further, in vivo studies in the rat have shown that VEGF-associated increases in retinal vascular permeability are mediated through the PKC pathway (85). Inhibition by the PKC β isoform selective inhibitor LY333531 resulted in the decrease of both endothelial cell proliferation and angiogenesis (84) and permeability increases induced by VEGF (85). In addition, Williams et al. (50) showed that the expression of VEGF was increased in aortic smooth muscle cells by elevating glucose concentration and was inhibited by PKC inhibitors.

In the kidney, the expression of transforming growth factor-β (TGF-β) has been shown to be increased in the glomeruli of diabetic patients and experimental animals. Similar increases of TGF-β have also been reported in cultured mesangial cells exposed to high glucose levels (9). Because TGF-β can directly cause the overexpression of extracellular matrix, PKC inhibitors have been shown both to inhibit TGF-β expression by hyperglycemia and to prevent the mesangial expansion observed in diabetic nephropathy (7,9,11).

C. Na^+-K^+ ATPase

Na^+-K^+ ATPase, an integral component of the sodium pump, is involved in the maintenance of cellular integrity and functions such as contractility, growth, and differentiation (5). It is well established that Na^+-K^+ ATPase activity is generally decreased in the vascular and neuronal tissues of diabetic patients and experimental animals (5,86–88). However, studies on the mechanisms by which hyperglycemia inhibited Na^+-K^+ ATPase activity have provided some conflicting results regarding the role of PKC.

Phorbol esters, activators of PKC, have been shown to prevent the inhibitory effect of hyperglycemia on Na^+-K^+ ATPase (5), which suggested that PKC activity might be decreased in diabetic conditions. Recently, however, we showed that elevated glucose level (20 mM) will increase PKC and $cPLA_2$ activities, leading to increases of arachadonic acid release and PGE_2 production resulting in decreases in Na^+-K^+ ATPase activity. Inhibitors of PKC or PLA_2 prevented glucose-induced reduction in Na^+-K^+ ATPase activities in aortic smooth muscle cells and mesangial cells (61). The apparent paradoxical effects of phorbol ester and hyperglycemia are probably due to both the quantitative and the qualitative differences of PKC stimulation induced by these stimuli. Phorbol ester, which is not a physiological activator, can increase the activity of many PKC isoforms and overall PKC activity by 5–10 times, whereas hyperglycemia only increases PKC by twofold, a physiological relevant change (61) that appears to affect only a few isoforms. Thus, the results derived from the studies using phorbol esters are difficult to interpret with respect to their physiological significance.

D. Extracellular Matrix Components

The thickening of the capillary basement membrane is one of the early structural abnormalities observed in almost all the tissues, including the vascular system, in diabetes (89). Because the basement membrane can affect numerous functions such as structural support, vascular permeability, cell adhesion, proliferation, differentiation, and gene expressions, alterations in its components may cause vascular dysfunction (90).

Histologically, increases in type IV and VI collagen, fibronectin, and laminin and decreases in proteoglycans are observed in the mesangium of diabetic patients (91,92). These observations can be replicated in mesangial cells incubated in media of increasing glucose levels (5–20 mM). These mesangium changes could be prevented by general PKC inhibitors (93–98). As described above, the increased expression of TGF-β has been implicated in the development of mesangial expansion and basement membrane thickening in diabetes (99–104). Ziyadeh et al. (105,106) reported that neutralizing TGF-β antibodies significantly reduced collagen synthesis and gene expression of type (IV) collagen and fibronectin in the renal cortex of diabetic rats and in cultured mesangial cells exposed to high glucose levels. Because PKC activation can increase the production of extracellular matrix and TGF-β expression, it is not surprising that several reports have shown that PKC inhibitors can also prevent hyperglycemia- or diabetes-induced increases in extracellular matrix and TGF-β in mesangial cells or renal glomeruli (32).

E. Selective PKCβ Isoform Inhibition

Numerous studies have used PKC inhibitors, such as staurosporine, H-7, and GF109203X, to characterize the role of PKC activation in diabetic vascular complications. Long-term studies involving PKC inhibitors, however, have not been possible due to their toxicity, which is associated with their nonspecificity with respect to inhibition of other kinases (19,107). Because analyses of retina, kidney, and cardiovascular tissues from diabetic rats showed that the PKCβ isoforms were preferentially activated (17,19,32), a specific inhibitor for the PKCβ isoforms could potentially be more effective and less toxic than the general isoform nonspecific PKC inhibitors.

Recently, we reported that increases in albuminuria and abnormal retinal and renal hemodynamics in diabetic rats can be ameliorated by an orally available PKCβ isoform selective inhibitor, LY333531. These physiological changes are concomitant with the inhibition of diabetes-induced PKC activation in retina and renal glomeruli (19). LY333531 prevented the overexpression of TGF-β, α1(IV) collagen, and fibronectin in renal glomeruli of diabetic rats (33). These results suggested that activation of PKCβ isoforms are involved in the development of some of the early abnormalities of diabetic vascular complications. PKC inhibitors could also mediate their effect by the inhibition of angiotensin actions. Angiotensin action appears to be increased because angiotensin-converting enzyme inhibitors have been shown to delay the progression of nephropathy (107). However, long-term studies are needed to clarify the usefulness of LY333531 to prevent the chronic pathological changes of diabetic vascular complications.

IV. VITAMIN E AND PKC INHIBITION

Oxidative stress has been postulated as an underlying cause of diabetic vascular complications (108–112). Antioxidants such as vitamin E have been the subject of considerable interest with respect to their potential ability to ameliorate diabetic complications. There has also been considerable interest in the use of vitamin E as an antioxidant agent for potential beneficial effects in coronary disease and cancers. Results from large multicenter clinical trials are now becoming available. A study on coronary heart disease in women (113) and in men (114) showed that increased vitamin E intake was associated with a significant risk reduction for coronary heart disease. Additionally, a recently published study involving male smokers in Finland (115) showed a 32% decrease in the incidence of prostate cancer in subjects taking 50 mg vitamin E/day. Interestingly, in this study there was a 23% increase in prostate cancer in those subjects randomized to β-carotene. Clinical studies aimed at characterizing the effect of vitamin E in the eye have focused primarily on the potential benefit of vitamin E in age-related macular degeneration (116,117), retinitis pigmentosa (118), and retinopathy of prematurity (119). The results from these studies are suggestive that vitamin E specifically and other antioxidants in general may be beneficial in treating macular degeneration and retinopathy of prematurity. There have been, however, no clinical studies aimed at investigating the effect of vitamin E in diabetes.

In the rat retina, vitamin E levels were fivefold higher than in other tissues such as the aorta (120). Vitamin E supplementation further increased these retinal vitamin E levels. Other investigators have shown that vitamin E is present in primate and human retinas (121–123), that the regional retinal distribution of vitamin E suggests an antioxidant protective effect against age-related macula degeneration, and that the level of vitamin E in the retina correlates with serum vitamin E levels (121).

Vitamin E, in addition to its antioxidant potential, has the other interesting property of being effective in inhibiting the activation of the DAG–PKC pathway in vascular tissues and cultured vascular cells exposed to high glucose levels (32,120). When retinal vascular endothelial cells exposed to high glucose were treated with vitamin E (*d*-α-tocopherol), DAG decreased and PKC activation was normalized (32,120). We reported that vitamin E can inhibit PKC activation, probably by decreasing DAG levels (32,120), because the direct addition of vitamin E to purified PKC α or β isoforms in vitro did not have any inhibitory effect (120). These results are consistent with other studies demonstrating that *d*-α-tocopherol will inhibit PKC activation (124–126). Boscoboinik et al. (124) first demonstrated in 1991 that PKC activation was inhibited by *d*-α-tocopherol in a manner unrelated to *d*-α-tocopherol's antioxidant action (124–127). They also showed that the magnitude of the inhibition was related to the level of PKC activation (128) with little effect of *d*-α-tocopherol if cellular PKC was not activated.

Recently, the activation of DAG kinase has been suggested to be one potential site of action for vitamin E to inhibit PKC. Results indicate an indirect effect through activation of DAG kinase and increased metabolic breakdown of DAG to phosphatidic acid that resulted in decreased DAG levels and decreased PKC activation (129). Koya et al. (130) confirmed these results in the kidney and showed that glomerular dysfunction in diabetic rats could be prevented by *d*-α-tocopherol treatment through PKC inhibition, most likely mediated through increased DAG kinase activity.

In vivo studies in the diabetic rat have shown that the decreased retinal blood flow is related to elevation of retinal DAG levels, inhibition of DAG kinase (131), and the activation of PKC (16,32), particularly the β isoform of PKC (19,131). The results from these studies showed that the effects of increased DAG levels and PKC activation on retinal hemodynamics in nondiabetic rats can mimic the hemodynamic changes measured in untreated diabetic rats.

In diabetic rats, vitamin E treatment through regular intraperitoneal injections prevented the increases in both DAG levels and the activation of PKC in the retina, aorta, heart, and renal glomeruli (120,131). Functionally, vitamin E treatment prevented the abnormal hemodynamics in retina and kidney of diabetic rats in parallel with the inhibition of DAG–PKC activation (120,131). In addition, increased albuminuria was prevented by vitamin E treatment in diabetic rats (131). Normalization of the physiological parameters studied in these diabetic rats was achieved despite chronically maintained elevated blood glucose levels. Thus, it is possible that some of the PKC activation induced by diabetes could also be the result of excessive oxidants, which are known to activate PKC and can be produced by hyperglycemia, leading to the development of vascular dysfunction in the early stages of diabetes (132).

In diabetic patients with no or minimal diabetic retinopathy, retinal blood flow was reduced to an extent comparable with that measured in diabetic rats (35,37). Studies have shown that the reduction in retinal blood flow in these patients is associated with the level of glycemic control (35). These clinical results combined with prior animal studies provide the support for performing clinical studies aimed at evaluating whether vitamin E treatment is also effective in normalizing retinal blood flow and renal function in patients with IDDM. Additionally, multicenter clinical trials will need to be initiated to answer the question of whether high doses of vitamin E can prevent the development of microvascular complications in diabetes.

V. SUMMARY

The results presented above are consistent with the activation of the DAG–PKC signal transduction pathway in diabetes. The initiating factors are chiefly metabolic with hyperglycemia as the main triggering element. Other metabolic changes such as those associated with free fatty acids are also potentially involved. The finding that the secondary metabolic products of glucose such as glycation products and oxidants can also increase DAG–PKC suggest that the activation of DAG–PKC could be a common downstream mechanism by which multiple byproducts of glucose are exerting their adverse effects. It is not surprising that changes in the DAG–PKC pathway can play a role in diabetic microvascular complications as this signal transduction pathway is known to regulate many vascular actions and functions as described above (11,12). It is also likely that hyperglycemia and diabetes may affect other signal transduction pathways besides the DAG–PKC pathway because a number of these other pathways can also regulate vascular functions.

Hyperglycemia or diabetes has also been associated with the activation of more than one PKC isoform. Again, this is not surprising because many isoforms are DAG sensitive and each cell usually contains several PKC isoforms (11,12). However, it is surprising that the results of immunoblotting and the use of PKCβ isoform inhibitor appear to suggest that PKCβ isoforms are predominantly activated in all vascular tissues and may be responsible for many of the vascular dysfunctions.

The correlation between the activation of DAG–PKC and diabetic vascular and neurological complications are substantial in rodent models of diabetes (7,8,17–19,31); however, limited data are available to indicate that DAG–PKC levels are increased in the vasculature of diabetic patients. This is primarily due to the difficulty of obtaining fresh human vascular or neurological tissues for the measurement of DAG–PKC levels. Thus, further studies are needed to confirm whether DAG–PKC activation plays a role in the development of diabetic complications. First, the activation of the DAG–PKC pathway needs to be chronically inhibited in a long-term animal model of diabetes to demonstrate which of the various retinal and renal pathologies can be prevented. Long-term experiments to chronically inhibit PKC can be accomplished through the use of specific PKC isoform inhibitors or by characterizing the pathologic changes in transgenic mice strains lacking a specific PKC isoform. These experimental approaches are now possible because a specific and relatively nontoxic oral inhibitor of PKCβ isoforms is now available and can be used to test which of the vascular dysfunctions are due to PKCβ isoform activation (19).

Second, most of the reported findings to date have been performed in animal tissues and not in human vascular tissues. Thus, there may be differences between human and animal vascular tissue responses in relation to glucose metabolism and PKC isoform expression. A PKCβ isoform inhibitor will only be useful in diabetic patients if the same profile of PKC isoforms are activated or expressed in diabetic patients as in the diabetic rodent models. In addition, the secondary markers of PKC activation need to be identified because they can be used to monitor the effectiveness of PKC inhibition when treated with intensive glycemic control or with PKC inhibitors. Progress has been made to identify some of these potential secondary parameters of vascular pathologies, such as the levels of VEGF, changes in retinal hemodynamics, and endothelial cell function (40,49,50,61).

The most important requirement for determining the role of activation of the DAG–PKC pathway in the vascular complication of diabetic patients has to be clinical trials using specific PKC isoform inhibitors. These trials are now in progress, specifically with the orally available PKCβ inhibitor. The need for clinical trials is vital as multiple agents have been shown to be capable of reversing vascular abnormalities induced by hyperglycemia in rodent models of diabetes. None of these agents, however, has been shown to be effective in clinical trials (133,134), clearly indicating the difficulties in extrapolating results to humans from those obtained using rodent models for diabetic complications. An additional potential problem with any therapeutic PKC inhibitor used clinically is the issue of toxicity because PKC activation is involved in so many vital functions of the cell. This is especially true in the clinical arena as these agents can be used by patients over long periods of time.

Thus, a large body of evidence has suggested that the activation of the DAG–PKC pathway by hyperglycemia and diabetes plays a role in the development of some vascular dysfunctions and neurovascular changes noted in diabetes. However, definitive studies as described above are ongoing and should determine clearly the role of DAG–PKC in the development of the various complications of diabetic patients.

REFERENCES

1. Brownlee M, Cerami A, Vlassara H. Advanced glycosylation end products in tissue and the biochemical basis of diabetic complications. N Engl J Med 1988; 318:1315–1321.
2. Vlassara H. Advanced glycation end-products and atherosclerosis. Ann Med 1996; 28:419–426.
3. Schmidt AM, Hori O, Cao R, Yan SD, Brett J, Wautier JL, Ogawa S, Kuwabara K, Matsumoto M, Stern D. RAGE: a novel cellular receptor for advanced glycation end products. Diabetes 1996; 45:S77–S80.
4. Kaiser N, Sasson S, Feener EP, Boukobza-Vardi N, Higashi S, Moller DE, Davidheiser S, Przybylski RJ, King GL. Differential regulation of glucose

transport and transporters by glucose in vascular endothelial and smooth muscle cells. Diabetes 1993; 42:80–89.

5. Greene D, Lattimer SA, Sima AAF. Sorbitol, phosphoinositides and sodium-potassium-ATPase in the pathogenesis of diabetic complications. N Engl J Med 1987; 316:599–606.
6. Williamson JR, Chang K, Frangos M, Hasan KS, Ido Y, Kawamura T, Nyengaard JR, Van den Enden M, Kilo C, Tilton RG. Hyperglycemic pseudohypoxia and diabetic complications. Diabetes 1993; 42:801–813.
7. King GL, Ishii H, Koya D. Diabetic vascular dysfunctions: a model of excessive activation of protein kinase C. Kidney Int 1997; 52:S77–S85.
8. Derubertis FR, Craven PA. Activation of protein kinase C in glomerular cells in diabetes. Mechanisms and potential link to the pathogenesis of diabetic glomerulopathy. Diabetes 1994; 43:1–8.
9. Sharma K, Ziyadeh FN. Hyperglycemia and diabetic kidney disease. The case for transforming growth factor-β as a key modulator. Diabetes 1995; 44:1139–1146.
10. Baynes JW, Thorpe SR. The role of oxidative stress in diabetic complications. Curr Opin Endocrinol 1996; 3:277–284.
11. Nishizuka Y. Intracellular signaling by hydrolysis of phospholipids and activation of protein kinase C. Science 1992; 258:607–614.
12. Nishizuka Y. Protein kinase C and lipid signaling for sustained cellular responses. FASEB J 1995; 9:484–496.
13. Liscovitch M, Cantley LC. Lipid second messengers. Cell 1994; 77:329–334.
14. Nakanishi H, Brewer KA, Exton JH. Activation of the zeta isozyme of protein kinase C by phosphatidylinositol 3,4,5-trisphosphate. J Biol Chem 1993; 268: 13–16.
15. Chang EY, Szallasi Z, Acs P, Raizada V, Wolfe PC, Fewtrell C, Blumberg PM, Rivera J. Functional effects of overexpression of protein kinase C-alpha, -beta, -delta, -epsilon, and -eta in the mast cell line RBL-2H3. J Immunol 1997; 159:2624–2632.
16. Shiba T, Inoguchi T, Sportsman JR, Heath W, Bursell S, King GL. Correlation of diacylglycerol and protein kinase C activity in rat retina to retinal circulation. Am J Physiol 1993; 265:E783–E793.
17. Inoguchi T, Battan R, Handler E, Sportsman JR, Heath W, King GL. Preferential elevation of protein kinase C isoform βII and diacylglycerol levels in the aorta and heart of diabetic rats: differential reversibility of glycemic control by islet cell transplantation. Proc Natl Acad Sci USA 1992; 89:11059–11063.
18. Craven PA, Davidson CM, DeRubertis FR. Increase in diacylglycerol mass in isolated glomeruli by glucose from de novo synthesis of glycerolipids. Diabetes 1990; 39:667–674.
19. Ishii H, Jirousek MR, Koya D, Takagi C, Xia P, Clermont A, Bursell S-E, Kern TS, Ballas LM, Heath WF, Stramm LE, Feener EP, King GL. Amelioration of vascular dysfunctions in diabetic rats by an oral PKC β inhibitor. Science 1996; 272:728–731.
20. Considine RV, Nyce MR, Allen LE, Morales LM, Triester S, Serrano J, Colberg

J, Lanza-Jacoby S, Caro JF. Protein kinase C is increased in the liver of humans and rats with non-insulin-dependent diabetes mellitus: an alteration not due to hyperglycemia. J Clin Invest 1995; 95:2938–2944.

21. Saha AK, Kurowski TG, Colca JR, Ruderman NB. Lipid abnormalities in tissues of the KKAy mouse: effects of pioglitazone on malonyl-CoA and diacylglycerol. Am J Physiol 1994; 267:E95–E101.
22. Xia P, Inoguchi T, Kern TS, Engerman RL, Oates PJ, King GL. Characterization of the mechanism for the chronic activation of diacylglycerol-protein kinase C pathway in diabetes and hypergalactosemia. Diabetes 1994; 43:1122–1129.
23. Craven PA, DeRubertis FR. Protein kinase C is activated in glomeruli from streptozotocin diabetic rats. J Clin Invest 1989; 83:1667–1675.
24. Yasanare K, Kahno M, Kano H, Yokokawa K, Horio T, Yoshikawa J. Possible involvement of phospholipase and protein kinase C in vascular growth induced by elevated glucose concentration. Hypertension 1996; 28:159–168.
25. Inoguchi T, Pu X, Kunisaki M, Higashi S, Feener EP, King GL. Insulin's effect on protein kinase C and diacylglycerol induced by diabetes and glucose in vascular tissues. Am J Physiol 1994; 267:E369–379.
26. Berne C. The metabolism of lipids in mouse pancreatic islets. The biosynthesis of triacylglycerol and phospholipids. Biochem J 1975; 152:667–673.
27. Dunlop ME, Larkins RG. Pancreatic islets synthesize phospholipids de novo from glucose via acyl-dihydroxyacetone phosphate. Biochem Biophys Res Commun 1985; 132:467–473.
28. Brindley DN, Sturton RG. Phosphatidate metabolism and its relation to triacylglycerol biosynthesis. In: Hawthorne JN, Ansel GB, eds. Phospholipids. New York: Elsevier, 1982:179–207.
29. Holub BJ, Kuksis A. Metabolism of molecular species of diacylglycerol phospholipids. Adv Lipid Res 1986; 16:1–125.
30. Ido Y, McHowat J, Chang KC, Arrogori-Martelli E, Orfaliam Z, Kilo C, Corr PB, Williamson JR. Neural dysfunction and metabolic imbalances in diabetic rats. Prevention by acetyl-L carritine. Diabetes 1994; 43:1469–1477.
31. Ayo SH, Radnik R, Garoni JA, Troyer DA, Kreisberg JI. High glucose increases diacylglycerol mass and activates protein kinase C in mesangial cell cultures. Am J Physiol 1991; 261:F571–577.
32. Kunisaki M, Bursell S-E, Umeda F, Nawata H, King GL. Normalization of diacylglycerol-protein kinase C activation by vitamin E in aorta of diabetic rats and cultured rat smooth muscle cells exposed to elevated glucose levels. Diabetes 1994; 43:1372–1377.
33. Koya D, Jirousek MR, Lin Y-W, Ishii H, Kuboki K, King GL. Characteristics of protein kinase C β isoform activation on the gene expression of transforming growth factor β, extracellular matrix components and prostanoids in the glomeruli of diabetic rats. J Clin Invest 1997; 100:115–126.
34. Kikkawa R, Haneda M, Uzu T, Koya D, Sugimoto T, Shigeta Y. Translocation of protein kinase α and ζ in rat glomerular mesangial cells cultured under high glucose conditions. Diabetologia 1994; 37:838–841.

35. Bursell S-E, Clermont AC, Kinsley BT, Simonson DC, Aiello LM, Wolpert HA. Retinal blood flow changes in patients with insulin-dependent diabetes mellitus and no diabetic retinopathy. Invest Ophthalmol Vis Sci 1996; 37:886–897.
36. Feke GT, Buzney SM, Ogasawara H, Fujio N, Goger DG, Spack NP, Gabbay KH. Retinal circulatory abnormalities in type 1 diabetes. Invest Ophthalmol Vis Sci 1994; 35:2968–2975.
37. Clermont AC, Aiello LP, Mori F, Aiello LM, Bursell SE. Vascular endothelial growth factor and severity of nonproliferative diabetic retinopathy mediate retinal hemodynamics in vivo: a potential role for vascular endothelial growth factor in the progression of nonproliferative diabetic retinopathy. Am J Ophthalmol 1997; 124:433–446.
38. Konno S, Feke GT, Yoshida A, Fujio N, Goger DG, Buzney SM. Retinal blood flow changes in type I diabetes: a long term follow-up study. Invest Ophthamol Vis Sci 1996; 37:1140–1148.
39. Small KW, Stefànsson E, Hatchell D. Retinal blood flow in normal and diabetic dogs. Invest Ophthalmol Vis Sci 1987; 28:672–675.
40. Clermont AC, Brittis M, Shiba T, McGovern T, King GL, Bursell S-E. Normalization of retinal blood flow in diabetic rats with primary intervention using insulin pumps. Invest Ophthalmol Vis Sci 1994; 35:981–990.
41. Miyamoto K, Ogura Y, Nishiwaki H, Matsuda N, Honda Y, Kato S, Ishida H, Seino Y. Evaluation of retinal microcirculatory alterations in the Goto-Kakizaki rat. Invest Ophthalmol Vis Sci 1996; 37:898–905.
42. Takagi C, King GL, Clermont AC, Cummins DR, Takagi H, Bursell SE. Reversal of abnormal retinal hemodynamics in diabetic rats by acarbose, an alpha-glucosidase inhibitor. Curr Eye Res 1995; 14:741–749.
43. Higashi S, Clermont AC, Dhir V, Bursell SE. Reversibility of retinal flow abnormalities is disease-duration dependent in diabetic rats. Diabetes 1998; 47: 653–659.
44. Kohner EM. Role of blood flow and impaired autoregulation in the pathogenesis of diabetic retinopathy. Diabetes 1995; 44:603–607.
45. Tesfayes S, Malik R, Ward JD. Vascular factors in diabetic neuropathy. Diabetologia 1994; 37:847–851.
46. Cameron NE, Cotter MA, Lai K, Hohman TC. Effect of protein kinase C inhibition on nerve function, blood flow and Na^+K^+ ATPase defects in diabetic rats. Diabetes 1997; 46(suppl 1):31A–0121.
47. Takagi C, Bursell S-E, Lin Y-W, Takagi H, Duh E, Jiang Z, Clermont AC, King GL. Regulation of retinal hemodynamics in diabetic rats by increased expression and action of endothelin-1. Invest Ophthalmol Vis Sci 1996; 37: 2504–2518.
48. Takagi C, King GL, Takagi H, Lin Y-W, Clermont AC, Bursell SE. Endothelin-1 action via endothelin receptors is a primary mechanism modulating retinal circulatory response to hyperoxia. Invest Ophthalmol Vis Sci 1996; 37: 2099–2109.

49. Aiello LP, Avery RL, Arrigg PG, Keyt BA, Jampel HD, Shah ST, Pasquale LR, Thieme H, Iwamoto MA, Park JE, Nguyen HV, Aiello LM, Ferrara N, King GL. Vascular endothelial growth factor in ocular fluids of patients with diabetic retinopathy and other retinal disorders. N Engl J Med 1994; 331:1480–1487.
50. Williams B, Gallachen B, Patel H, Orme C. Glucose-induced protein kinase C activation regulates vascular permeability factor mRNA expression and peptide production vascular smooth muscle cells in vitro. Diabetes 1997; 46:1497–1503.
51. Ditzel J, Schwartz M. Abnormally increased glomerular filtration rates in short-term insulin treated diabetic subjects. Diabetes 1967; 16:264–267.
52. Christiansen JS, Gammelgaard J, Frandsen M, Parving HH. Increased kidney size, glomerular filtration rate and renal plasma flow in short-term insulin-dependent diabetes. Diabetologia 1981; 20:451–456.
53. Hostetter TH, Troy JL, Brenner BM. Glomerular hemodynamics in experimental diabetes mellitus. Kidney Int 1981; 19:410–415.
54. Viberti GC. Early functional and morphological changes in diabetic nephropathy. Clin Nephrol 1979; 12:47–53.
55. O'Donnell MP, Kasiske BL, Keane WF. Glomerular hemodynamic structural alterations in experimental diabeties mellitus. FASEB J 1988; 2:2339–2347.
56. Anderson S, Jung FF, Ingelfinger JR. Renal renin-angiotensin system in diabetes: functional immunohistochemical and molecular biologica correlations. Am J Physiol 1993; 265:F477–F486.
57. Ruan X, Arendshorst WJ. Role of protein kinase C in angiotensin II-induced renal vasoconstriction in genetically hypertensive rats. Am J Physiol 1996; 270: F945–F952.
58. Craven PA, Caines MA, DeRubertis FR. Sequential alterations in glomerular prostaglandin and thromboxane synthesis in diabetic rats: relationship to the hyperfiltration of early diabetes. Metabolism 1987; 36:95–103.
59. Perico N, Benigni A, Gabanelli M, Piccinelli A, Ròg M, Riva CD, Remuzzi G. Atrial natriuretic peptide and prostacyclin synergistically mediate hyperfiltration and hyperperfusion of diabetic rats. Diabetes 1992; 41:533–538.
60. Williams B, Schrier RW. Glucose-induced protein kinase C activity regulates arachidonic acid release and eicosanoid production by cultured glomerular mesangial cells. J Clin Invest 1993; 92:2889–2896.
61. Xia P, Kramer RM, King GL. Identification of the mechanism for the inhibition of Na^+, K^+-adenosine triphosphatase by hyperglycemia involving activation of protein kinase C and cytosolic phospholipase A_2. J Clin Invest 1995; 96:733–740.
62. Haneda M, Arakis I, Togaro M, Sugimoto T, Isono M, Kikkawa R. Mitogen activated protein kinase C is activated in glomeruli of diabetic rats and glomerular mesangial cells cultured under high glucose conditions. Diabetes 1997; 46: 847–853.

63. Lin L-L, Wartmann M, Lin AY, Knopf JL, Seth A, Davis RJ. cPLA$_2$ is phosphorylated and activated by MAP kinase. Cell 1993; 72:269–278.
64. Bank N, Aynedjian HS. Role of EDRF (nitric oxide) in diabetic renal hyperfiltration. Kidney Int 1993; 43:1306–1312.
65. Tolins JP, Shultz PJ, Raij L, Brown DM, Mauer SM. Abnormal renal hemodynamic response to reduced renal perfusion pressure in diabetic rats: role of NO. Am J Physiol 1993; 265:F886–F895.
66. Komers R, Allen TJ, Cooper ME. Role of endothelium-derived nitric oxide in the pathogenesis of the renal hemodynamic changes of experimental diabetes. Diabetes 1994; 43:1190–1197.
67. Sharma K, Danoff TM, DePiero A, Ziyadeh FN. Enhanced expression of inducible nitric oxide synthase in murine macrophages and glomerular mesangial cells by elevated glucose levels: possible mediation via protein kinase C. Biochem Biophys Res Commun 1995; 207:80–88.
68. Graier WF, Simecek S, Kukovetz WR, Kostner GM. High D-glucose-induced changes in endothelial Ca^{2+}/EDRF signaling are due to generation of superoxide anions. Diabetes 1996; 45:1386–1395.
69. Craven PA, Studer RK, DeRubertis FR. Impaired nitric oxide-dependent cyclic guanosine monophosphate generation in glomeruli from diabetic rats. J Clin Invest 1994; 93:311–320.
70. Muniyappa R, Srinivas PR, Ram JL, Walsh MF, Sowers JR. Calcium and protein kinase C mediate high-glucose-induced inhibition of inducible nitric oxide synthase in vascular smooth muscle cells. Hypertension 1998; 31(1 Pt 2):289–295.
71. Nishio E, Watanabe Y. Glucose-induced down-regulation of NO production and inducible NOS expression in cultured rat aortic vascular smooth muscle cells: role of protein kinase C. Biochem Biophys Res Commun 1996; 229:857–863.
72. Kamata K, Miyata N, Kasuya Y. Involvement of endothelial cells in relaxation and contraction responses of the aorta to isoproterenol in native and streptozotocin-induced diabetic rats. J Pharmacol Exp Ther 1989; 249:890–894.
73. Mayhan WG. Impairment of endothelium-dependent dilatation cerebral arterioles during diabetes mellitus. Am J Physiol 1989; 256:H621–H625.
74. Tesfamariam B, Jakubowski JA, Cohen RA. Contraction of diabetic rabbit aorta caused by endothelium-derived PGH_2-TxA_2. Am J Physiol 1989; 257:H1327–H1333.
75. McVeigh GE, Brennan GM, Johnston GD, McDermott BJ, McGrath LT, Henry WR, Andrews JW. Impaired endothelium-dependent and independent vasodilation in patients with Type 2 (non-insulin-dependent) diabetes mellitus. Diabetologia 1992; 35:771–776.
76. Tesfamariam B, Brown ML, Cohen RA. Elevated glucose impairs endothelium-dependent relaxation by activating protein kinase C. J Clin Invest 1991; 87:1643–1648.
77. Williamson JR, Chang K, Tilton RG, Prater C, Jeffrey JR, Weigel C, Sherman

WR, Eades DM, Kilo C. Increased vascular permeability in spontaneously diabetic BB/W rats and in rats with mild versus severe streptozotocin-induced diabetes. Diabetes 1987; 36:813–821.

78. Oliver JA. Adenylate cyclase and protein kinase C mediate opposite actions on endothelial junctions. J Cell Physiol 1990; 145:536–542.
79. Lynch JJ, Ferro TJ, Blumenstock FA, Brockenauer AM, Malik AM. Increased endothelial albumin permeability mediated by protein kinase C activation. J Clin Invest 1990; 85:1991–1998.
80. Wolf BA, Williamson JR, Easom RA, Chang K, Sherman WR, Turk J. Diacylglycerol accumulation and microvascular abnormalities induced by elevated glucose levels. J Clin Invest 1991; 87:31–38.
81. Werth DK, Niedel JE, Pastan I. Vinculin, a cytoskeletal substrate of protein kinase C. J Biol Chem 1983; 258:11423–11426.
82. Stasek JE, Patterson CE, Garcia JGN. Protein kinase C phosphorylates caldesmon$_{77}$ and vimentin and enhances albumin permeability across cultured bovine pulmonary artery endothelial cell monolayers. J Cell Physiol 1992; 153:62–75.
83. Nagpala PG, Malik AB, Vuong PT, Lum H. Protein kinase C β_1 overexpression augments phorbol ester-induced increase in endothelial permeability. J Cell Physiol 1996; 166:249–255.
84. Xia P, Aiello LP, Ishii H, Jiang Z, Park DJ, Robinson GS, Takagi H, Newsome WP, Jirousek MR, King GL. Characterization of vascular endothelial growth factor's effect on the activation of protein kinase C, its isoforms, and endothelial cell growth. J Clin Invest 1996; 98:2018–2026.
85. Aiello LP, Bursell SE, Clermont A, Duh E, Ishii H, Takagi C, Mori F, Ciulla TA, Ways K, Jirousek M, Smith LE, King GL. Vascular endothelial growth factor-induced retinal permeability is mediated by protein kinase C in vivo and suppressed by an orally effective β-isoform-selective inhibitor. Diabetes 1997; 46:1473–1480.
86. King GL, Shiba T, Oliver J, Inoguchi T, Bursell S-E. Cellular and molecular abnormalities in the vascular endothelium of diabetes mellitus. Annu Rev Med 1994; 45:179–188.
87. Winegrad AI. Does a common mechanism induce the diverse complications of diabetes? Diabetes 1987; 36:396–406.
88. MacGregor LC, Matschinsky FM. Altered retinal metabolism in diabetes II: measurement of sodium-potassium ATPase and total sodium and potassium in individual retinal layers. J Biol Chem 1986; 261:4052–4058.
89. Williamson JR, Kilo C. Extracellular matrix changes in diabetes mellitus. In: Scarpelli DG, Migahi G, eds. Comparative pathobiology of major age-related diseases. New York: Liss, 1984:269–288.
90. Lu TT, Yan LG, Madri JA. Integrin engagement mediates tyrosine dephosphorylation on platelet-endothelial cell adhesion molecule 1. Proc Natl Acad Sci USA 1996; 93:11808–11813.
91. Scheinman JL, Fish AJ, Matas AJ, Michael AF. The immunohistopathology of

glomerular antigens. II. The glomerular basement membrane, actomyosin, and fibroblast surface antigens in normal, diseased and transplanted human kidneys. Am J Pathol 1978; 90:71–88.

92. Bruneval P, Foidart JM, Nochy D, Camilleri JP, Bariety J. Glomerular matrix proteins in nodular glomerulosclerosis in association with light chain deposition disease and diabetes mellitus. Hum Pathol 1985; 16:477–484.
93. Studer RK, Craven PA, DeRubertis FR. Role for protein kinase C in the mediation of increased fibronectin accumulation by mesangial cells grown in high-glucose medium. Diabetes 1993; 42:118–126.
94. Ayo SH, Radnik RA, Garoni J, Glass II WF, Kreisberg JI. High glucose causes an increase in extracellular matrix proteins in cultured mesangial cells. Am J Pathol 1990; 136:1339–1348.
95. Ayo SH, Radnik RA, Glass II WF, Garoni JA, Rampt ER, Appling DR, Kreisberg JI. Increased extracellular matrix synthesis and mRNA in mesangial cells grown in high-glucose medium. Am J Physiol 1991; 260:F185–F191.
96. Haneda M, Kikkawa R, Horide N, Togawa M, Koya D, Kajiwara N, Ooshima A, Shigeta Y. Glucose enhances type IV collagen production in cultured rat glomerular mesangial cells. Diabetologia 1991; 34:198–200.
97. Pugliese G, Pricci F, Pugliese F, Mene P, Lenti L, Andreani D, Galli G, Casini A, Bianchi S, Rotella CM, Mario UD. Mechanisms of glucose-enhanced extracellular matrix accumulation in rat glomerular mesangial cells. Diabetes 1994; 43:478–490.
98. Fumo P, Kuncio GS, Ziyadeh FN. PKC and high glucose stimulate collagen α_1 (IV) transcriptional activity in a reporter mesangial cell line. Am J Physiol 1994; 267:F632–F638.
99. MacKay K, Striker LJ, Stauffer JW, Doi T, Agodoa LY, Striker GE. Transforming growth factor β. Murine glomerular receptors and responses of isolated glomerular cells. J Clin Invest 1989; 83:1160–1167.
100. Suzuki S, Ebihara I, Tomino Y, Koide H. Transcriptional activation of matrix genes by transforming growth factor beta 1 in mesangial cells. Exp Nephrol 1993; 1:229–237.
101. Nakamura T, Miller D, Ruoslahti E, Border WA. Production of extracellular matrix by glomerular epithelial cells regulated by transforming growth factor-β1. Kidney Int 1992; 41:1213–1221.
102. Yamamoto T, Nakamura T, Noble NA, Ruoslahti E, Border WA. Expression of transforming growth factor β is elevated in human and experimental diabetic nephropathy. Proc Natl Acad Sci USA 1993; 90:1814–1818.
103. Sharma K, Ziyadeh FN. Renal hypertrophy is associated with upregulation of TGF-β1 gene expression in diabetic BB rat and NOD mouse. Am J Physiol 1994; 267:F1094–F1101.
104. Pankewycz OG, Guan J-X, Bolton WK, Gomez A, Benedict JF. Renal TGF-β regulation in spontaneously diabetic NOD mice with correlations in mesangial cells. Kidney Int 1994; 46:748–758.
105. Ziyadeh FN, Sharma K, Ericksen M, Wolf G. Stimulation of collagen gene

expression and protein synthesis in murine mesangial cells by high glucose is mediated by autocrine activation of transforming growth factor-β. J Clin Invest 1994; 93:536–542.

106. Sharma K, Jin Y, Guo J, Ziyadeh FN. Neutralization of TGF-β by anti-TGF-β antibody attenuates kidney hypertrophy and the enhanced extracellular matrix gene expression in STZ-induced diabetic mice. Diabetes 1996; 45:522–530.
107. Lewis EJ, Hunsicker LG, Bain RP, Rohde RD. The effect of angiotensin converting enzyme inhibitor on diabetic nephropathy. N Engl J Med 1993; 329: 1456–1462.
108. Baynes JW, Thorpe SR. The role of oxidative stress in diabetic complications. Curr Opin Endocrinol 1996; 3:277–284.
109. Giugliano D, Cerellio A, Paolisso G. Diabetes mellitus, hypertension and cardiovascular disease: which role for oxidative stress. Metabolism 1995; 44:363–368.
110. Giugliano D, Cerellio A, Paolisso G. Oxidative stress and diabetic vascular complications. Diabetes Care 1996; 19:257–265.
111. Asahina T, Kashiwagi A, Yoshihiko N, et al. Impaired activation of glucose oxidation and NADH supply in human endothelial cells exposed to H_2O_2 in high glucose medium. Diabetes 1995; 44:520–526.
112. Chappey O, Dosquet C, Wautier MP, Wautier JL. Advanced glycation end products, oxidant stress and vascular lesions. Eur J Clin Invest 1997; 27:97–108.
113. Stampfer MJ, Hennekens CH, Manson JE, Colditz GA, Rosner B, Willett WC. Vitamin E consumption and the risk of coronary disease in women. N Engl J Med 1993; 328:1444–1449.
114. Rimm EB, Stampfer MJ, Ascherio A, Giovannucci E, Colditz GA, Willett WC. Vitamin E consumption and the risk of coronary heart disease in men. N Engl J Med 1993; 328:1450–1456.
115. Heinonen OP, Albanes D, Virtamo J et al. Prostate cancer and supplementation with α-tocopherol and β-carotene: incidence and mortality in a controlled trial. J Natl Cancer Inst 1998; 90:440–446.
116. Mares-Perlman JA, Brady WE, Klein R et al. Serum antioxidants and age-related macular degeneration in a population-based case-control study. Arch Ophthalmol 1995; 113:1518–1523.
117. Snodderly DM. Evidence for protection against age-related macular degeneration by carotenoids and antioxidant vitamins. Am J Clin Nutr 1995; 62:1448S–1461S.
118. Berson EL, Rosner B, Sandberg MA et al. A randomized trial of vitamin A and vitamin E supplementation for retinitis pigmentosa. Arch Ophthalmol 1993; 111:761–772.
119. Johnson L, Quinn GE, Abbasi S, Gerdes J, Bowen FW, Bhutani V. Severe retinopathy of prematurity in infants with birth weights less than 1250 grams: incidence and outcome of treatment with pharmacologic serum levels of vita-

min E in addition to cryotherapy from 1985 to 1991. J Pediatr 1995; 127:632–639.
120. Kunisaki M, Bursell S-E, Clermont AC, Ishii H, Ballas LM, Jirousek MR, Umeda F, Nawata H, King GL. Vitamin E prevents diabetes-induced abnormal retinal blood flow via the diacylglycerol-protein kinase C pathway. Am J Physiol 1995; 269:E239–E246.
121. Crabtree DV, Snodderly DM, Adler AJ. Retinyl palmitate in macaque retina-retinal pigment epithelium-choroid: distribution and correlation with age and vitamin E. Exp Eye Res 1997; 64:455–463.
122. Crabtree DV, Adler AJ, Snodderly DM. Radial distribution of tocopherols in rhesus monkey retina and retinal pigment epithelium-choroid. Invest Ophthalmol Vis Sci 1996; 37:61–76.
123. Friedrichson T, Kalbach HL, Buck P, van Kuijk FJ. Vitamin E in macular and peripheral tissues of the human eye. Curr Eye Res 1995; 14:693–701.
124. Boscoboinik D, Szewczyk A, Hensey C, Azzi A. Inhibition of cell proliferation by alpha-tocopherol. Role of protein kinase C. J Biol Chem 1991; 266:6188–6194.
125. Boscoboinik DO, Chatelain E, Bartoli G-M, Stauble B, Azzi A. Inhibition of protein kinase C activity and vascular smooth muscle cell growth by d-α-tocopherol. Biochim Biophys Acta 1994; 1224:418–426.
126. Ozer NK, Palozza P, Boscoboinik D, Azzi A. *d*-α-Tocopherol inhibits low density lipoprotein induced proliferation and protein kinase C activity in vascular smooth muscle cells. FEBS Lett 1993; 322:307–310.
127. Boscoboinik D, Ozer NK, Moser U, Azzi A. Tocopherols and 6-hydroxy-chroman-2carbonitrile derivatives inhibit vascular smooth muscle cell proliferation by a nonantioxidant mechanism. Arch Biochem Biophys 1995; 318:241–246.
128. Tasinato A, Boscoboinik D, Bartoli GM, Maroni P, Azzi A. *d*-α-Tocopherol inhibition of vascular smooth muscle cell proliferation occurs at physiological concentrations, correlates with protein kinase C inhibition and is independent of its antioxidant properties. Proc Natl Acad Sci USA 1995; 92:12190–12194.
129. Tran K, Proulx PR, Chan AC. Vitamin E suppresses diacylglycerol (DAG) level in thrombin-stimulated endothelial cells through an increase of DAG kinase activity. Biochim Biophys Acta 1994; 1212:193–202.
130. Koya D, Lee I-K, Ishii H, Kanoh H, King GL. Prevention of glomerular dysfunctions in diabetic rats by treatment of d-α-tocopherol. J Am Soc Nephrol 1997; 8:426–35.
131. Bursell S-E, Takagi C, Clermont AC et al. Specific retinal DAG and PKC-β isoform modulation mimics abnormal retinal hemodynamics in diabetic rats. Invest Ophthalmol Vis Sci 1997; 38:2711–2720.
132. Konishi H, Tanaka M, Takemura Y, Matsuzaki H, Ono Y, Kikkawa U, Nishizuka Y. Activation of protein kinase C by tyrosine phosphorylation in response to H202. Proc Natl Acad Sci USA 1997; 94:11233–11237.

133. Porte D Jr, Schwartz MW. Diabetes complications: why is glucose potentially toxic? Science 1996; 272:699–700.
134. Nicolucci A, Carinci F, Cavaliere D, Scorpiglione N, Belfiglio M, Labbrozzi D, Mari E, Benedetti MM, Tognoni G, Liberati A. A meta-analysis of trials on aldose reductase inhibitors in diabetic peripheral neuropathy. The Italian Study Group. The St. Vincent Declaration. Diabetes Med 1996; 13:1017- 1026.

17

Oxidative Stress and Pancreatic β-Cell Destruction in Insulin-Dependent Diabetes Mellitus

Mizuo Hotta, Eiji Yamato, and Jun-ichi Miyazaki
Osaka University Medical School, Osaka, Japan

Insulin-dependent diabetes mellitus (IDDM) is considered to be an autoimmune disease (1,2). Recent reports suggest that reactive oxygen species (ROS) participate in the development of IDDM (3,4). Thioredoxin (TRX) is a small (12 kDa) reduction/oxidation (redox) protein (5,6) and has protective effects on cells against oxidative stress by scavenging ROS (5–7), by repairing DNA and proteins damaged by ROS (5–8), and by blocking apoptosis induced by ROS (6,9).

Nonobese diabetic (NOD) mice are well known as an excellent animal model for human IDDM (10–12). To elucidate the roles of oxidative stress in autoimmune diabetes, we generated NOD transgenic mice overexpressing TRX exclusively in pancreatic β-cells. Spontaneous diabetes was prevented or delayed in the NOD transgenic mice. The results indicate that ROS in pancreatic β-cells may play an essential role in the development of IDDM.

Here we describe the proposed mechanisms of the β-cell destruction by ROS in IDDM and the protective effects of the TRX system against β-cell destruction.

I. PATHOGENESIS OF IDDM PATIENTS AND NOD MICE

IDDM is caused by autoimmune destruction of pancreatic β-cells (1,2). Because β-cells are almost completely destroyed at clinical onset of this disease, the affected individuals require daily injection of insulin to prevent diabetic ketoacidosis and to sustain their lives.

NOD mice spontaneously develop autoimmune diabetes (10–12) after the infiltration of inflammatory cells into pancreatic islets, termed ''insulitis,'' and are known as an excellent animal model for studying human IDDM (10–12). Infiltrating cells are composed of T and B lymphocytes, macrophages (MΦ), and natural killer (NK) cells. The β cells are thought to be destroyed by these immunocytes directly or via cytotoxic cytokines such as interleukin-1 (IL-1), tumor necrosis factor-α(TNF-α), and interferon-γ (3,4,13).

II. OXIDATIVE STRESS AND IDDM

Recent studies have indicated that ROS such as nitric oxide (NO), superoxide anion radical (O_2^-), and hydrogen peroxide (H_2O_2) are generated by MΦ in islets or induced in β-cells by cytotoxic cytokines secreted from immunocytes (3,4) (Fig. 1). It has been shown that the expression of inducible nitric oxide

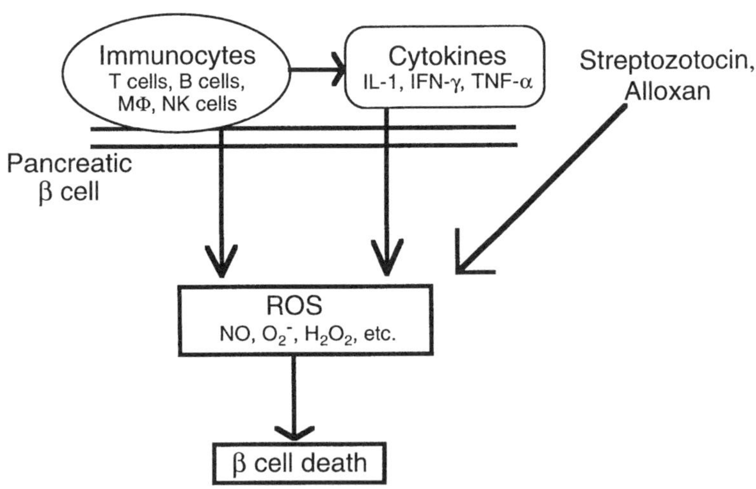

Figure 1 A proposed mechanism of pancreatic β-cell destruction by oxidative stress in autoimmune diabetes and drug-induced diabetes.

synthase (iNOS) is augmented in β-cells of NOD mice (14). It has also been suggested that NO was induced by iNOS in the β-cells of human IDDM patients (15). These data indicate that oxidative stress may be one of the effector mechanisms of β-cell destruction by infiltrating inflammatory cells in autoimmune diabetes.

It has previously been suggested that pancreatic β-cells are especially vulnerable to oxidative stress. In fact, β-cells are selectively destroyed by ROS-generating agents, streptozotocin (STZ) and alloxan (16–18). Such susceptibility to ROS is probably due to low levels of key enzymes scavenging ROS, such as superoxide dismutase (SOD), catalase, and glutathione peroxidase (19–22). Overexpression of *Drosophila* Cu/Zn SOD in β cells has been shown to confer resistance to alloxan-induced diabetes (23). Antioxidative agents such as nicotinamide (24,25) and vitamin E (26) have been shown to have protective effects against diabetes of NOD mice. Recently, it was reported that transgenic mice overexpressing iNOS in β cells develop insulin-dependent diabetes without insulitis (27). These results suggest that ROS and the antioxidative systems in β-cells play pivotal roles in the destruction of β-cells in the development of autoimmune diabetes.

III. OXIDATIVE STESS AND APOPTOSIS

Recent histochemical analysis suggested that apoptosis is the mechanism of β-cell destruction in autoimmune diabetes (28,29). The Fas/Fas ligand (FasL) system is profoundly related to apoptosis (30) (Fig. 2). Transgenic mice overexpressing FasL in β-cells were reported to be highly susceptible to autoimmune diabetes (31), whereas Fas deficient (lpr/lpr) mice were resistant to autoimmune diabetes (31,32). Fas/FasL system was also suggested to mediate β-cell destruction in human IDDM patients (15).

NF-κB has been implicated in apoptosis, although the functions of NF-κB are complicated and there is controversy about the functions of NF-κB in apoptosis (33,34). It has recently been reported that NF-κB is induced by IL-1 in rat islets and RINm5F cells (35). Because NF-κB is known to activate iNOS (33,34), these results indicate that excessive NO may be generated by IL-1 (36) via activation of NF-κB (33,34), resulting in β-cell destruction, possibly due to apoptosis (37).

IV. TRX AND ANTIOXIDATIVE EFFECTS

TRX is a small reduction/oxidation (redox) protein present in both prokaryotic and eukaryotic cells (5,6). In human, this protein was found as an adult T-

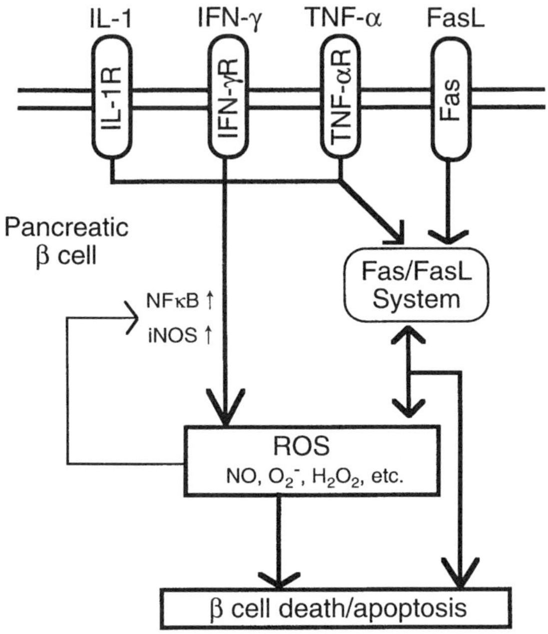

Figure 2 A proposed mechanism of pancreatic β-cell death/apoptosis by cytotoxic cytokines in autoimmune diabetes.

cell leukemia-derived factor (6). TRX is induced by various types of stress, such as viral infection, ischemic insult, ultraviolet light, x-ray irradiation, and H_2O_2 (5,6). Recently, TRX has been shown to have protective effects on cells against oxidative stress. TRX itself can function as an ROS scavenger (6,7). TRX, originally studied as a cofactor of ribonucleotide reductase in DNA synthesis, has been revealed to be a substrate of the antioxidative and antiapoptotic enzyme, TRX peroxidase (38). Recent studies have indicated that TRX plays essential roles in the repair of DNA and proteins damaged by ROS (5–8,39–43).

Augmented expression of TRX is often seen in neoplastic cells (5,6,44–46) and appears to protect neoplastic cells against the cytotoxicity of ROS-generating antineoplastic agents such as *cis*-diaminedichloroplatinum (II), adriamycin, etoposide, and mitomycin C (6,9,45,46). Recombinant TRX prevents cell death induced by ROS (6). TRX also protects cells against apoptosis induced by TNF and Fas-agonistic antibody (6,47). A number of in vitro studies have suggested that the TRX system plays an important role in the protection of cells against the cytotoxicity of oxidative stress (6,9,44–48).

V. TRX AS A REGULATOR OF INTRACELLULAR SIGNALING AGAINST OXIDATIVE STRESS

Recent reports revealed that TRX also functions as a regulator of intracellular signalings (6). NF-κB (6,49,50) and Ref-1 (6,8,43), which have TRX binding sites, are regulated by TRX. Ref-1 regulates activator factor (AP)-1 (6,8,43). NF-κB and AP-1 have been implicated in apoptosis (33,51), although the precise functions and mechanisms are complicated and still unknown. It has been reported that overexpression of TRX inactivates NF-κB and activates AP-1 (49). Inactivation of NF-κB by TRX overexpression may reduce excessive NO production under oxidative stress.

Very recently, mammalian TRX has been shown to function as a direct inhibitor of apoptosis signal-regulating kinase (ASK)-1 (52). Das et al. (53) suggested that TRX can induce antioxidative proteins such as MnSOD. These results indicate that TRX acts as a regulator of intracellular signalings against oxidative stress.

VI. ENDOGENOUS TRX EXPRESSION IN PANCREATIC β-CELLS

In our study using immunoblot analysis, we found the expression of endogenous TRX to be much lower in islet cells than in pancreatic exocrine cells. Based on immunohistochemical analysis, Hansson et al. (54) also suggested that TRX expression of islet cells was lower compared with pancreatic exocrine cells. Their result was consistent with our study. This attenuation of TRX expression in β-cells may be one of the reasons why β-cells are vulnerable to oxidative stress.

VII. PREVENTIVE EFFECTS OF TRX OVEREXPRESSION AGAINST AUTOIMMUNE DIABETES IN VIVO

To directly assess the roles of oxidative stress in β-cell destruction in autoimmune diabetes, we generated NOD transgenic mice overexpressing TRX exclusively in β-cells. The incidence of diabetes in NOD transgenic mice was

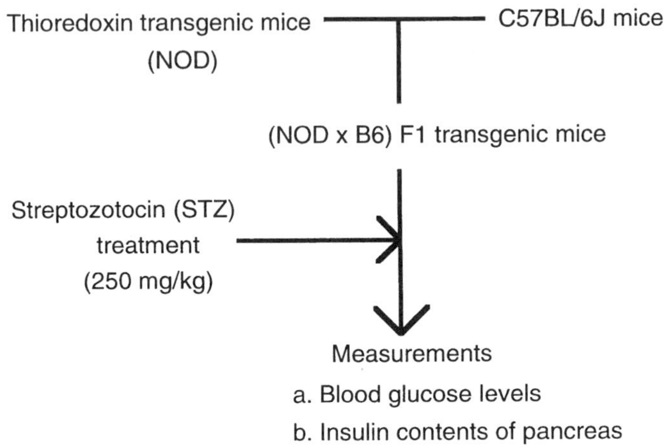

Figure 3 The generation of (NOD × B6) F1 transgenic mice and the evaluation of pancreatic β-cell damage after streptozotocin treatment.

remarkably reduced compared with their negative littermates. Although the incidence of diabetes was reduced, the severity of insulitis before overt diabetes was not significantly different between NOD transgenic mice and their negative littermates. To study the protective effects of TRX against ROS-generating agents, we produced (NOD × C57BL/6J (B6)) F1 transgenic mice and injected the ROS-generating agent STZ into them (Fig. 3). The elevation of blood glucose levels in (NOD × B6) F1 transgenic mice was reduced and the reduction of insulin contents was suppressed compared with their negative littermates. These results suggest that ROS play pivotal roles in β-cell destruction, in autoimmune diabetes and in STZ-induced diabetes.

VIII. SUMMARY

TRX overexpression has preventive effects on both autoimmune diabetes and ROS-generating agent-induced diabetes as described. Our data suggest that the pancreatic β-cell-targeted control of redox systems utilizing TRX and/or the antioxidative therapies targeted to β-cells are anticipated to prevent or delay the overt diabetes even after the development of insulitis.

REFERENCES

1. Gepts W. Pathologic anatomy of the pancreas in juvenile diabetes mellitus. Diabetes 1965; 14:619–633.

2. Foulis AK, Clark A. Pathology of the pancreas in diabetes mellitus. In: Kahn CR, Weir GC, eds. Joslin's diabetes mellitus, 13th ed. Philadelphia: Lea & Febiger, 1994:265–281.
3. Mandrup-Poulsen T. The role of interleukin-1 in the pathogenesis of IDDM. Diabetologia 1996; 39:1005–1029.
4. Eizirik DL, Flodstrom M, Karlsen AE, et al. The harmony of the spheres: inducible nitric oxide synthase and related genes in pancreatic beta cells. Diabetologia 1996; 39:875–890.
5. Holmgren A. Thioredoxin. Annu Rev Biochem 1985; 54:237–271.
6. Nakamura H, Nakamura K, Yodoi J. Redox regulation of cellular activation. Annu Rev Immunol 1997; 15:351–369.
7. Mitsui A, Hirakawa T, Yodoi J. Reactive oxygen-reducing and protein-refolding activities of adult T cell leukemia-derived factor/human thioredoxin. Biochem Biophys Res Commun 1992; 186:1220–1225.
8. Hirota K, Matsui M, Iwata S, et al. AP-1 transcriptional activity is regulated by a direct association between thioredoxin and Ref-1. Proc Natl Acad Sci USA 1997; 94:3633–3638.
9. Baker A, Payne CM, Briehl MM, et al. Thioredoxin, a gene found overexpressed in human cancer, inhibits apoptosis in vitro and in vivo. Cancer Res 1997; 15: 5162–5167.
10. Makino S, Kunimoto K, Muraoka Y, et al. Breeding of a non-obese, diabetic strain of mice. Jikken Dobutsu 1980; 29:1–13.
11. Kikutani H, Makino S. The murine autoimmune diabetes model: NOD and related strains. Adv Immunol 1992; 51:285–322.
12. Andre I, Gonzalez A, Wang B, et al. Checkpoints in the progression of autoimmune disease: lessons from diabetes models. Proc Natl Acad Sci USA 1996; 93: 2260–2263.
13. Pujol-Borrell R, Todd I, Doshi M, et al. HLA class II induction in human islet cells by interferon gamma plus tumour necrosis factor or lymphotoxin. Nature 1987; 326:304–306.
14. Rabinovitch A, Suarez-Pinzon WL, Sorensen O, et al. Inducible nitric oxide synthase (iNOS) in pancreatic islets of nonobese diabetic mice: identification of iNOS-expressing cells and relationships to cytokines expressed in the islets. Endocrinology 1996; 137:2093–2099.
15. Stassi G, Maria RD, Trucco G, et al. Nitric oxide primes pancreatic beta cells for Fas-mediated destruction in insulin-dependent diabetes mellitus. J Exp Med 1997; 186:1193–1200.
16. Grankvist K, Marklund S, Sehlin J, et al. Superoxide dismutase, catalase and scavengers of hydroxyl radical protect against the toxic action of alloxan on pancreatic islet cells in vitro. Biochem J 1979; 182:17–25.
17. Malaisse WJ, Malaisse-Lagae F, Sener A, et al. Determinants of the selective toxicity of alloxan to the pancreatic beta cell. Proc Natl Acad Sci USA 1982; 79:927–930.
18. Takasu N, Komiya I, Asawa T, et al. Streptozocin- and alloxan-induced H_2O_2

generation and DNA fragmentation in pancreatic islets. H_2O_2 as mediator for DNA fragmentation. Diabetes 1991; 40:1141–1145.

19. Grankvist K, Marklund SL, Taljedal IB. CuZn-superoxide dismutase, Mn-superoxide dismutase, catalase and glutathione peroxidase in pancreatic islets and other tissues in the mouse. Biochem J 1981; 199:393–398.
20. Gandy SE 3d, Galbraith RA, Crouch RK, et al. Superoxide dismutase in human islets of Langerhans. N Engl J Med 1981; 304:1547–1548.
21. Cornelius JG, Luttge BG, Peck AB. Antioxidant enzyme activities in IDD-prone and IDD-resistant mice: a comparative study. Free Radic Biol Med 1993; 14: 409–420.
22. Lenzen S, Drinkgern J, Tiedge M. Low antioxidant enzyme gene expression in pancreatic islets compared with various other mouse tissues. Free Radic Biol Med 1996; 20:463–466.
23. Kubisch HM, Wang J, Bray TM, et al. Targeted overexpression of Cu/Zn superoxide dismutase protects pancreatic beta-cells against oxidative stress. Diabetes 1997; 46:1563–1566.
24. Yamada K, Nonaka K, Hanafusa T, et al. Preventive and therapeutic effects of large-dose nicotinamide injections on diabetes associated with insulitis. Diabetes 1982; 31:749–753.
25. Elliott RB, Pilcher CC, Stewart A, et al. The use of nicotinamide in the prevention of type 1 diabetes. Ann NY Acad Sci 1993; 696:333–341.
26. Beales PE, Williams AJ, Albertini MC, et al. Vitamin E delays diabetes onset in the non-obese diabetic mouse. Horm Metab Res 1994; 26:450–452.
27. Takamura T, Kato I, Kimura N, et al. Transgenic mice overexpressing type 2 nitric-oxide synthase in pancreatic beta cells develop insulin-dependent diabetes without insulitis. J Biol Chem 1998; 273:2493–2496.
28. Kurrer MO, Pakala SV, Hanson HL, et al. Beta cell apoptosis in T cell-mediated autoimmune diabetes. Proc Natl Acad Sci USA 1997; 94:213–218.
29. O'Brien BA, Harmon BV, Cameron DP, et al. Apoptosis is the mode of beta cell death responsible for the development of IDDM in the nonobese diabetic (NOD) mouse. Diabetes 1997; 46:750–757.
30. Nagata S, Golstein P. The Fas death factor. Science 1995; 267:1449–1456.
31. Chervonsky AV, Wang Y, Wong FS, et al. The role of Fas in autoimmune diabetes. Cell 1997; 89:17–24.
32. Itoh N, Imagawa A, Hanafusa T, et al. Requirement of Fas for the development of autoimmune diabetes in nonobese diabetic mice. J Exp Med 1997; 186:613–618.
33. Sonenshein GE. Rel/NF-kappa B transcription factors and the control of apoptosis. Semin Cancer Biol 1997; 8:113–119.
34. Sibenlist U, Franzoso G, Brown K. Structure, regulation and function of NFκB. Annu Rev Cell Biol 1994; 10:405–455.
35. Kwon G, Corbett JA, Hauser S, et al. Evidence for involvement of the proteosome complex (26S) and NFκB in IL-1β-induced nitric oxide and prostaglandin production by rat islets and RINm5F cells. Diabetes 1998; 47:583–591.
36. Corbett JA, Wang JL, Sweetland MA, et al. Interleukin-1 beta induces the forma-

tion of nitric oxide by beta-cells purified from rodent islets of Langerhans. Evidence for the beta-cell as a source and site of action of nitric oxide. J Clin Invest 1992; 90:2384–2391.
37. Kaneto H, Fujii J, Seo HG, et al. Apoptotic cell death triggered by nitric oxide in pancreatic beta-cells. Diabetes 1995; 44:733–738.
38. Zhang P, Liu B, Kang SW, et al. Thioredoxin peroxidase is a novel inhibitor of apoptosis with a mechanism distinct from that of Bcl-2. J Biol Chem 1997; 272: 30615–30618.
39. Laurent TC, Moore EC, Reichard P. Enzymatic synthesis of deoxyribonucleotides. IV. Isolation and characterzation of thioredoxin, the hydrogen donor from Escherichia coli B. J Biol Chem 1964; 239:3436–3444.
40. Huber HE, Russel M, Model P, et al. Interaction of mutant thioredoxins of Escherichia coli with the gene 5 protein of phage T7: the redox capacity of thioredoxin is not required for stimulation of DNA polymerase activity. J Biol Chem 1986; 261:15006–15012.
41. Steitz TA. A mechanism for all polymerases. Nature 1998; 391:231–232.
42. Ramana CV, Boldogh I, Izumi T, et al. Activation of apurinic/apyrimidinic endonuclease in human cells by reactive oxygen species and its correlation with their adaptive response to genotoxicity of free radicals. Proc Natl Acad Sci USA 1998; 95:5061–5066.
43. Qin J, Clore GM, Kennedy WP, et al. The solution structure of human thioredoxin complexed with its target from Ref-1 reveals peptide chain reversal. Structure 1996; 4:613–620.
44. Berggren M, Gallegos A, Gasdaska JR, et al. Thioredoxin and thioredoxin reductase gene expression in human tumors and cell lines, and the effects of serum stimulation and hypoxia. Anticancer Res 1996; 16:3459–3466.
45. Sasada T, Iwata S, Sato N, et al. Redox control of resistance to cis diamminedichloroplatinum (II) (CDDP): protective effect of human thioredoxin against CDDP-induced cytotoxicity. J Clin Invest 1996; 97:2268–2276.
46. Yokomizo A, Ono M, Nanri H, et al. Cellular levels of thioredoxin associated with drug sensitivity to cisplatin, mitomycin C, doxorubicin, and etoposide. Cancer Res 1995; 55:4293–4296.
47. Matsuda M, Masutani H, Nakamura H, et al. Protective activity of adult T cell leukemia-derived factor (ADF) against tumor necrosis factor-dependent cytotoxicity on U937 cells. J Immunol 1991; 147:3837–3841.
48. Gallegos A, Berggren M, Gasdaska JR, et al. Mechanisms of the regulation of thioredoxin reductase activity in cancer cells by the chemopreventive agent selenium. Cancer Res 1997; 57:4965–4970.
49. Schenk H, Klein M, Erdbrugger W, et al. Distinct effects of thioredoxin and antioxidants on the activation of transcription factors NF-kappa B and AP-1. Proc Natl Acad Sci USA 1994; 91:1672–1676.
50. Qin J, Clore GM, Kennedy WM, et al. Solution structure of human thioredoxin in a mixed disulfide intermediate complex with its target peptide from the transcription factor NF kappa B. Structure 1995; 3:289–297.

51. Karin M, Liu Zg, Zandi E. AP-1 function and regulation. Curr Opin Cell Biol 1997; 9:240–246.
52. Saitoh M, Nishitoh H, Fujii M, et al. Mammalian thioredoxin is a direct inhibitor of apoptosis signal-regulating kinase (ASK-1). EMBO J 1998; 17:2596–2606.
53. Das KC, Lewis-Molock Y, White CW. Elevation of manganese superoxide dismutase gene expression by thioredoxin. Am J Respir Cell Mol Biol 1997; 17: 713–726.
54. Hansson HA, Holmgren A, Rozell B, et al. Immunohistochemical localization of thioredoxin and thioredoxin reductase in mouse exocrine and endocrine pancreas. Cell Tissue Res 1986; 245:189–195.

18

Interrelationship Between Oxidative Stress and Insulin Resistance

Karen Yaworsky, Romel Somwar, and Amira Klip
The Hospital for Sick Children and University of Toronto, Toronto, Ontario, Canada

I. INSULIN RESISTANCE: A KEY FACTOR IN TYPE 2 DIABETES

Insulin is the predominant hormone responsible for the maintenance of glucose homeostasis through its regulation of metabolic activites in muscle, liver, and adipose tissue. Insulin causes an increase in glucose uptake into peripheral tissues, specifically muscle and fat cells; conversely, in the liver, the hormone decreases gluconeogenesis, thereby reducing hepatic glucose output. Insulin is also responsible for the promotion of protein synthesis. These effects result from both rapid and long-term metabolic actions of the hormone (1).

One hundred million people worldwide suffer from type 2 diabetes (2), yet despite intense research, the primary lesion(s) responsible for type 2 diabetes remains unknown. The genetic susceptibility of this disease fails to follow simple Mendelian inheritance but is of a polygenic nature with superimposed environmental influences (3). An aggregation of small genetic effects rather than the effect of one single gene, gene-to-gene, and gene-to-environment interactions are thought to contribute to the development of this disease, yet most genes involved in the origin of type 2 diabetes remain unknown (R. Heggele, personal communication). The environmental factors that favor the development of this disease in genetically predispositioned individuals include high-fat diets, low levels of physical activity, and increasing age (3).

Type 2 diabetes is characterized by resistance to the insulin stimulation of glucose uptake in skeletal muscle and adipose tissue, by impaired insulin-dependent inhibition of hepatic glucose production, and by dysregulated insulin secretion (3). Both the insulin resistance and insulin secretory defects appear to be the result of genetic and environmental factors associated with the disease.

It is largely acknowledged that insulin resistance is a primary factor responsible for glucose intolerance in the prediabetic state. Initially, to compensate for the insulin resistance, insulin secretion increases to maintain normal glycemic levels. However, when the insulin secretory capacity fails to adequately compensate for the impaired insulin action, hyperglycemia ensues. This in turn further exacerbates the primary insulin resistance through the effects of high glucose (collectively known as glucose toxicity) and through the increased circulation of fatty acids and triglycerides (4). Hence, insulin resistance has primary and secondary causes in type 2 diabetes (Fig. 1).

A. Molecular Basis of Insulin Action and Insulin Resistance in Peripheral Tissues

To understand the molecular basis of insulin resistance (whether primary or secondary) in muscle and fat cells, it is imperative to gain knowledge of the normal mechanisms of insulin action. In these tissues, insulin stimulates glucose uptake by rapidly mobilizing preexisting glucose transporters (primarily the GLUT4 isoform) from an intracellular storage organelle (or vesicle) to the plasma membrane (5,6). This is achieved by a series of signals elicited from the receptor, which are detected in an unknown fashion by the intracellular organelle. The latter is then free to find and interact with docking sites on the plasma membrane (7) that will ultimately enable fusion of the two membranes to provide functional glucose transporters. Detailed knowledge has emerged on the signals emanating from the receptor that are essential for GLUT4 translocation and the nature of the proteins engaged in vesicle docking and fusion with the plasma membrane.

The signaling events involved in the insulin-mediated GLUT4 translocation include autophosphorylation of the insulin receptor, tyrosine phosphorylation of docking proteins known as insulin receptor substrates (IRS 1–4), their subsequent binding to the enzyme phosphatidylinositol 3-kinase (PI 3-kinase), and the resultant activation of PI 3-kinase to produce phosphorylated phosphoinositides. How these signals then translate into translocation of the GLUT4 vesicle is the subject of vigorous study. A serine/threonine kinase identified

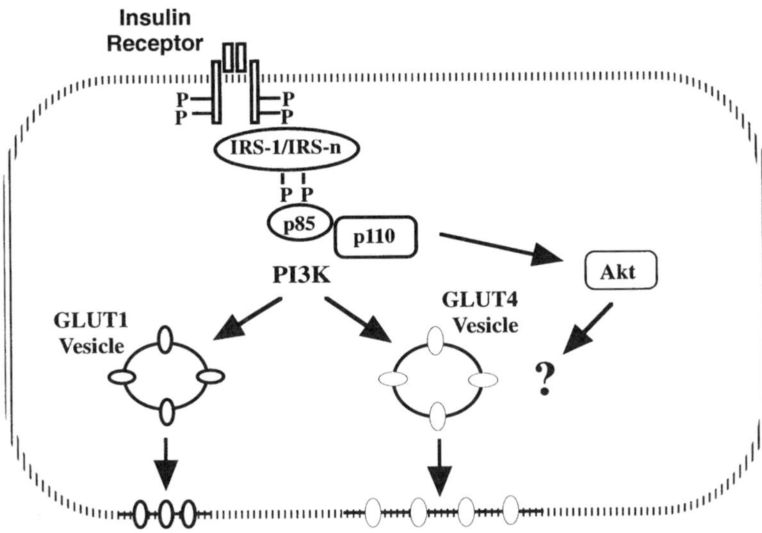

Figure 1 Proposed model for the development of insulin resistance and type 2 diabetes. It is proposed that elevations in insulin levels, as a result of genetic defects and excess carbohydrate and fat intake, lead to increased levels of nonesterified fatty acids (NEFA) and hyperlipidemia. These elevated levels of lipids result in impaired β-cell function and induce insulin resistance through changes in glucose metabolism in skeletal muscle and in the liver. These changes in metabolism in insulin responsive tissues lead to hyperglycemia and the diabetic state ensues.

as protein kinase B, also referred to as Akt, has been shown to be activated by these phosphoinositides in vitro (8,9) and in response to insulin in vivo (10) and has been proposed to be a mediator of GLUT4 translocation (11,12) (Fig. 2).

Among the proteins involved in vesicle docking and fusion with the target plasma membrane are the vesicular proteins of the synaptobrevin family and the plasma membrane proteins syntaxin4 and SNAP23 (13–17). These proteins are isoforms of functional equivalents that participate in synaptic vesicle docking and fusion with the presynaptic plasma membrane of neurons. In contrast to this knowledge, little is known about how the glucose transporter-containing vesicles sense the insulin signal or travel to the plasma membrane.

It follows that the diminished response to insulin of glucose uptake into muscle and fat could result from any of the following possibilities: defects in

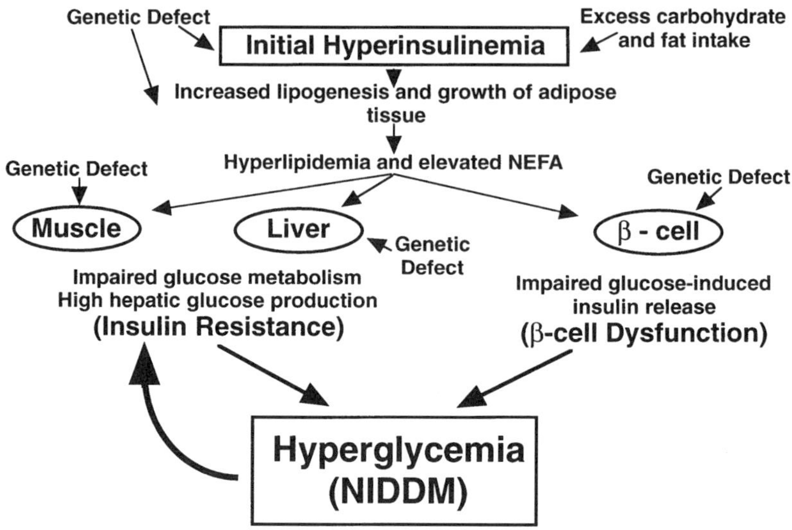

Figure 2 Schematic diagram of the glucose transporter translocation hypothesis. Insulin-responsive tissues, specifically adipose tissue and skeletal muscle, contain intracellular stores of glucose transporter proteins (GLUT). The binding of insulin and the subsequent increase in tyrosine kinase activity of the insulin receptor initiates a signaling cascade, which results in the tyrosine phosphorylation of insulin receptor substrates (IRS 1-n), their binding to the enzyme phosphatidylinositol 3-kinase (PI 3-kinase), and the resultant activation of PI 3-kinase to produce phosphorylated phosphoinositides. This signaling cascade leads to the mobilization and insertion of stored glucose transporters into the plasma membrane, allowing for increased glucose influx into the cell in response to insulin.

insulin signals, defects in detecting/transducing the signal, a reduction in the total amount of glucose transporters, and/or inability of the transporters to properly dock with and incorporate into the plasma membrane. Of these, defects in insulin signaling and glucose transporter levels have been amply explored, and emerging evidence is being provided for defects in glucose transporter translocation. No studies have examined the mechanism of glucose transporter interaction with the plasma membrane in either humans or animals with diabetes. Finally, because the mechanism whereby the intracellular organelle detects the insulin signal is largely unknown, the possibility that this step is defective remains unexplored. A brief account of the status of glucose transporter levels, GLUT4 translocation, and defects in the insulin signaling pathway in diabetes is provided below. It is important to realize that, for the most part, these studies do not distinguish whether the defects found relate to the primary or secondary insulin resistance.

1. GLUT4 Expression

The levels of expression of the GLUT4 glucose transporter have been analyzed in a variety of animal models of type 2 diabetes and in tissue from individuals with type 2 diabetes (for review see 18,19). GLUT4 protein content is markedly diminished in adipose tissues of human and most animal models. It has been found that GLUT4 expression in adipocytes decreases as diabetes develops in older Zucker rats (18,19), and adipose cells taken from humans with type 2 diabetes also show a reduction in GLUT4 content (20). However, this change in GLUT4 levels is restricted to adipose tissue and is not seen in skeletal muscle of these animal models of type 2 diabetes as normal expression of GLUT4 is observed in muscle of *db/db* mice and Zucker rats (21–24). Muscle biopsies taken from individuals with type 2 diabetes also show normal skeletal muscle GLUT4 content (25). However, a small number of studies have examined the amount of GLUT4 protein on the plasma membrane of muscle from diabetic animals, and it was found to be abnormal (18,19). This may suggest that sorting of the transporter is a key factor in muscle, whereas net synthesis of the transporter is more pertinent in fat. Whether these changes cause the diabetic state or ensue from hyperglycemia, hyperinsulinemia, and/or hypertriglyceridemia remains to be established. In a study attempting to shed light on this question, brown adipose tissue was ablated in transgenic mice, resulting in a decrease in the total GLUT4 protein in adipocytes. This led to the development of diabetes, suggesting that a reduction in the level of GLUT4 could be causative in this disease (26). However, genetic knockout of the GLUT4 gene in muscle and fat did not create a phenotype of diabetes, although glucose intolerance was generated (27).

2. GLUT4 Translocation

In skeletal muscle of humans with type 2 diabetes, the plasma membrane does not show a reduction and in fact may show a small increase in the amount of GLUT4 transporters. Yet the stimulation of glucose uptake by insulin is totally blunted. Zierath et al. (28) showed that the membranes of these muscles display a diminished gain in glucose transporters in response to an insulin clamp. A similar observation was also made in two animal models of diabetes (24,29). Defective GLUT4 translocation is also seen in fat cells from these animals (30) and in fat cells from humans with type 2 diabetes (20). As a result, several explanations have been put forward to account for this reduced translocation of GLUT4 to the cell surface in skeletal muscle and adipocytes. These include topics that have been briefly mentioned, such as impaired translocation machinery and an inability of the transporters to functionally incorporate into the plasma membrane, in addition to the next topic to be discussed, an alteration in the signaling emerging from the insulin receptor.

3. Insulin Signaling

In animal models of type 2 diabetes and in humans with type 2 diabetes, there is considerable evidence for defects in the early stages of insulin action (31–33). There is an approximately 50% decrease in insulin receptor phosphorylation and an 80% decrease in IRS-1 phosphorylation in liver and skeletal muscle of *ob/ob* mice (34). This was associated with a more than 90% decrease in insulin-stimulated PI 3-kinase activity associated with IRS-1 and no detectable stimulation of total PI 3-kinase activity. In addition, insulin-stimulated Akt kinase activity in skeletal muscle of the lean diabetic Goto-Kakizaki rat was reduced by 68% (35). Skeletal muscle isolated from individuals with type 2 diabetes also show defects at the level of the insulin receptor tyrosine kinase activity, IRS-1 expression and phosphorylation, and IRS-1-associated PI 3-kinase activity (36). A reduction in IRS-1 expression (by 70%) and IRS-1-associated PI 3-kinase activity has also been reported in adipose cells isolated from individuals with type 2 diabetes (20). Thus, in type 2 diabetes, there are defects at four early steps of insulin action. Whether there are also defects distal to the initial signaling events that contribute to impaired translocation of GLUT4 remains to be determined.

In addition to alterations in the level of expression or activation of the signaling molecules in type 2 diabetes, the isoform selectivity of signaling also changes. In adipose cells isolated from humans with type 2 diabetes, IRS-2 becomes the main docking protein for PI 3-kinase and Grb2 in response to insulin (20). This is not surprising because expression of IRS-2 increases, and this protein predominates as the main insulin receptor substrate in mice lacking IRS-1 (37,38). Importantly, mice genetically manipulated to lack IRS-1 do not develop diabetes (38), whereas mice lacking IRS-2 do (39).

In summary, changes in the levels of glucose transporter expression, defects in the insulin signaling pathway, and alterations in pattern of signaling molecules may all contribute to either or both primary and secondary insulin resistance in type 2 diabetes.

B. Factors That May Trigger Insulin Resistance

It has been suggested that circulating and metabolic factors could play an important role in the etiology of insulin resistance. This is supported by the observation that insulin resistance of in vitro muscle preparations can be reversed by incubation in solutions of normal insulin and glucose levels (40). Circulating factors, such as tumor necrosis factor-α (TNF-α) and free fatty acids (FFA), and intracellular metabolites, such as glucosamine, can induce an insulin-resistant state in vitro and may contribute to the development of insulin resistance in vivo.

1. Tumor Necrosis Factor-α

The level of expression of adipose tissue TNF-α, a multifunctional cytokine, rises as a consequence of obesity. It is also closely correlated with circulating insulin levels, which serve as an index of insulin resistance, (41) and is expressed in increased levels in skeletal muscle of individuals with insulin resistance (42). Mice homozygous for a targeted null mutation in the TNF-α gene were significantly less insulin resistant compared with normal obese mice (43), suggestive of a causative role of TNF-α in obesity-related insulin resistance. The mechanism by which TNF-α exerts an impairment of insulin action remains incompletely understood. In adipocytes, chronic TNF-α exposure induced serine phosphorylation of IRS-1, inhibiting the insulin receptor tyrosine kinase (44). However, acute exposure of TNF-α in rat hepatoma cells induced serine phosphorylation of IRS-1 without any inhibitory effect on the insulin receptor tyrosine kinase, yet IRS-1 tyrosine phosphorylation and association with the p85 regulatory subunit of PI 3-kinase was blunted (45). Greater confusion on the TNF-α mechanism of action was seen in 3T3-L1 adipocytes, whereby TNF-α increased IRS-1 tyrosine phosphorylation and association with p85 (46). Further studies are required to elucidate the mechanism by which TNF-α acts as a mediator, directly or indirectly, of obesity-related insulin resistance.

2. Free Fatty Acids

It has been demonstrated that increased levels of circulating FFA correlate with peripheral insulin resistance in humans (47,48). Animal models of hyperlipidemia lend support to a correlation between increased FFA and insulin resistance (49,50). In addition, infusion of intralipid in vivo was shown to inhibit insulin-stimulated glucose uptake (48,51), and numerous studies also demonstrate that elevated plasma FFA levels decrease insulin-stimulated glucose uptake in skeletal muscle (48,51,52). However, the underlying mechanism of how FFA induce insulin resistance remains unknown. Elevated plasma FFA levels have been suggested to have an inhibitory effect on glucose oxidation, via the classic glucose–fatty acid cycle (53) and have been linked to impaired glycogen synthesis (54). It has also been suggested that the decrease in insulin-stimulated glucose uptake in skeletal muscle mediated by elevated FFA occurs at early steps in glucose utilization, specifically at the level of glucose transport and/or glucose phosphorylation (51,55). In support of a mechanism whereby elevated FFA induces insulin resistance through inhibition of glucose transport/phosphorylation, it was recently reported that elevations in FFA induce insulin resistance in vivo via inhibition of components of the insulin signaling cascade, specifically inhibition of IRS-1-associated PI 3-kinase activity (56). Overall, these results suggest that elevated FFA may contribute to insulin resistance by action at several cellular processes that control glucose uptake.

3. Glucosamine

An intracellular mechanism that has received much attention lately as a possible generator of insulin resistance is increased flux of glucose through the hexosamine pathway (57). This pathway utilizes intracellular glucose and the amino acid glutamine to produce glucosamine, which is a precursor of UDP-*N*-acetylglucosamine (UDP-GlcNAc) and UDP-*N*-acetylgalactosamine (UDP-GalNAc) used in protein glycosylation. How glycosylation leads to insulin resistance is not known, but increasing evidence supports the concept that a rise in *N*-acetylglucosamine is linked to insulin resistance. The first observations were made in primary cultures of rat adipocytes, in which it was observed that increased glucose flux through the hexosamine biosynthetic pathway is the mechanism by which prolonged exposure to high levels of glucose and insulin resulted in impaired glucose transport (58,59). Induction of insulin resistance via increased glucosamine flux can be reproduced by administration of glucosamine in vitro and in vivo and is associated with increased accumulations of UDP-GlcNAc and UDP-GalNAc (60,61). These serve as an index of the amount of carbon flux through the pathway. Impaired insulin-mediated glucose disposal induced by elevated glucosamine levels is associated with decreased muscle GLUT4 translocation to the sarcolemmal fraction in response to insulin (62). Furthermore, overexpression of glucosamine fructose amido transferase, the rate-limiting enzyme for the hexosamine biosynthetic pathway, resulted in decreased GLUT4 translocation to the plasma membrane in response to insulin (63). Increased glucose flux though the hexosamine biosynthetic pathway could therefore be responsible for inducing insulin resistance through the downregulation of the glucose transport system.

In contrast to the evidence presented whereby circulating factors such as TNF-α, FFA, and the metabolite glucosamine may be involved in the induction of insulin resistance, there is no formal evidence to support or discard a role of oxidative stress in the origin of insulin resistance. The folllowing section examines thc possibility that a link might exist between them.

II. OXIDATIVE STRESS IN RELATION TO DIABETES AND INSULIN RESISTANCE

A. Methods of Detection of Oxidative Stress

Oxidative stress is defined as the oxidative damage inflicted by an excess of reactive oxygen species (ROS) on a cell or organ (64). As the natural balance between toxic oxidants and protective antioxidant defenses is altered, oxidative stress results. Such conditions include an increase in free radical concentration or a decrease in the antioxidant capacity—or oxidant scavenging ability—of the cell (65).

Free radicals are highly reactive atoms or molecules containing one or more unpaired electrons (64). These toxic metabolites, such as peroxides, superoxides, and hydroxyl radicals, can be generated through both essential and nonessential oxidation-reduction reactions of the cytosol and mitochondria (66). Free radical-mediated oxidative damage has been observed in a variety of pathological conditions, including type 2 diabetes. However, difficulties arise in measuring oxygen radicals due to the highly reactive nature of these species, because they rapidly react with various substrates, including themselves, and have short lifespans (10^{-6}, 10^{-9} s) in aqueous systems (65). Nonetheless, measurements of free radicals via direct and indirect measures, although complicated, allow for an approximate assessment of oxidative stress. These measurements include spin trapping to directly measure the levels of free radicals (65), direct measurement of superoxide radicals in plasma (64), and identification of products of the oxidation of polyunsaturated fatty acids (PUFA) by lipid hydroperoxide assays (65). In addition, the plasma GSH/GSSG ratio (reduced glutathione/oxidized glutathione) serves as an indirect measurement of free radical reactions and as an indicator of the oxidative stress that may occur under physiological and pathological conditions (65).

Several of these methods have been used to measure oxidative stress in diabetes (67), as discussed elsewhere in this book. A few examples follow.

Animal models have been used to address the possible in vivo relationship between oxidative stress and diabetes. Accelerated accumulation of advanced glycation end products (AGEs) was measured as the amount of fluorescent protein adducts with lipoperoxidative aldehydes (malondialdehyde [MDA] and 4-hydroxynonenal [HNE]) in rat skin collagen of diabetic BB rats

(68). The diabetic rats had significantly higher levels of autoantibody against albumin modified by the lipoperoxidative aldehydes, MDA, and HNE, in addition to reactive oxygen species ROS (69). This suggests an increased generation of oxygen free radicals and lipoperoxidative aldehydes in these diabetic rats. Also, the duration of diabetes correlated significantly with the development of antibodies directed against MDA and HNE. The presence of antibodies against oxidatively modified proteins in spontaneously diabetic rats provides indirect evidence of the occurrence of oxidative modification of proteins in vivo (69). In addition, decreased plasma concentrations of ascorbic acid (AA) have been reported in individuals with diabetes (70). In a recent study, lens and renal AA levels were partially restored when normal glycemia was approached by insulin treatment in streptozotocin-diabetic BB rats (71). These in vivo studies provide evidence for the coexistence of oxidative stress associated with the increased level of oxidative damage in diabetes.

Studies of humans with type 2 diabetes also reveal the coexistence of oxidative stress with the disease. Serum has antioxidant activity against transition metal ion-catalyzed reactions, a result of the ferrous iron oxidizing (ferroxidase) activity of caeruloplasmin and of the iron-free fraction of transferrin (72). Increased levels of transferrin, ferritin, ferroxidase activity of caeruloplasmin, and iron-binding capacity were described in the serum of 67 subjects with type 2 diabetes (73). This observation has been interpreted to represent a protective response to the increased level of oxidative stress in subjects with diabetes.

Free radical-mediated oxidative stress has been implicated in the pathogenesis of complications associated with type 2 diabetes. This wide field is not discussed here because it is treated amply elsewhere in this book. The following paragraphs address the origin of oxidative stress in diabetes and its possible link to insulin resistance.

B. Origin of Oxidative Stress in Type 2 Diabetes

Suspected causative agents of the increased level of oxidative stress associated with type 2 diabetes are hyperglycemia, hyperinsulinemia, and an alteration of serum antioxidant activity (Fig. 3).

1. Hyperglycemia

Hyperglycemia has been strongly implicated in the development of diabetic complications, an effect also known as glucose toxicity. The mechanisms of glucose toxicity are the subject of extensive investigation and include glucose

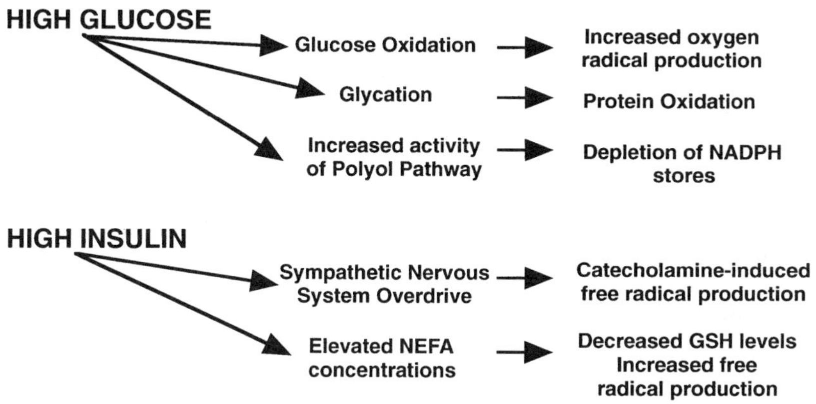

Figure 3 How oxidative stress may arise in diabetes. The characteristic high levels of glucose and insulin observed in type 2 diabetes may contribute to oxidative stress through the production of free radicals, protein oxidation, and by depletion of intracellular reductants and antioxidants. This increased level of oxidative stress may be attributed to the increased levels of glucose oxidation, glycation, increased activity of the polyol pathway, sympathetic nervous system overdrive, and elevated nonesterified free fatty acid (NEFA) concentrations resulting from high levels of glucose and insulin.

oxidation, glycation, increased levels of polyols, and elevation of the hexosamine biosynthetic pathway. Most of these actions can contribute to oxidative stress.

Glucose Enolization. Glucose enolizes in vitro, reducing molecular oxygen catalyzed by transition metals, to yield oxidizing intermediates and α-ketoaldehydes (74) (Fig. 4). Hydroxyl radicals, superoxide anions, and hydrogen peroxide are the reduced oxygen products formed in this glucose oxidation reaction, all of which are capable of protein damage through cross-linking, fragmentation, and lipid oxidation (64,75).

Glycation and AGEs. The protein reactive α-ketoaldehydes, which are formed via protein glycation, are in turn protein reactive and are thus responsible for the formation of AGEs and protein cross-linking (74) (Fig. 4). AGEs have been implicated in the generation of ROS, activation of the transcription factor NF-κB, and in modulation of endothelial physiology (66).

Sorbitol and Fructose Levels. Intracellularly, elevated glucose levels can promote glucose reduction into sorbitol and fructose due to increased free glucose and an elevation in aldose-reductase and sorbitol-dehydrogenase activities (76). The rise in aldose-reductase activity diminishes NADPH cellular

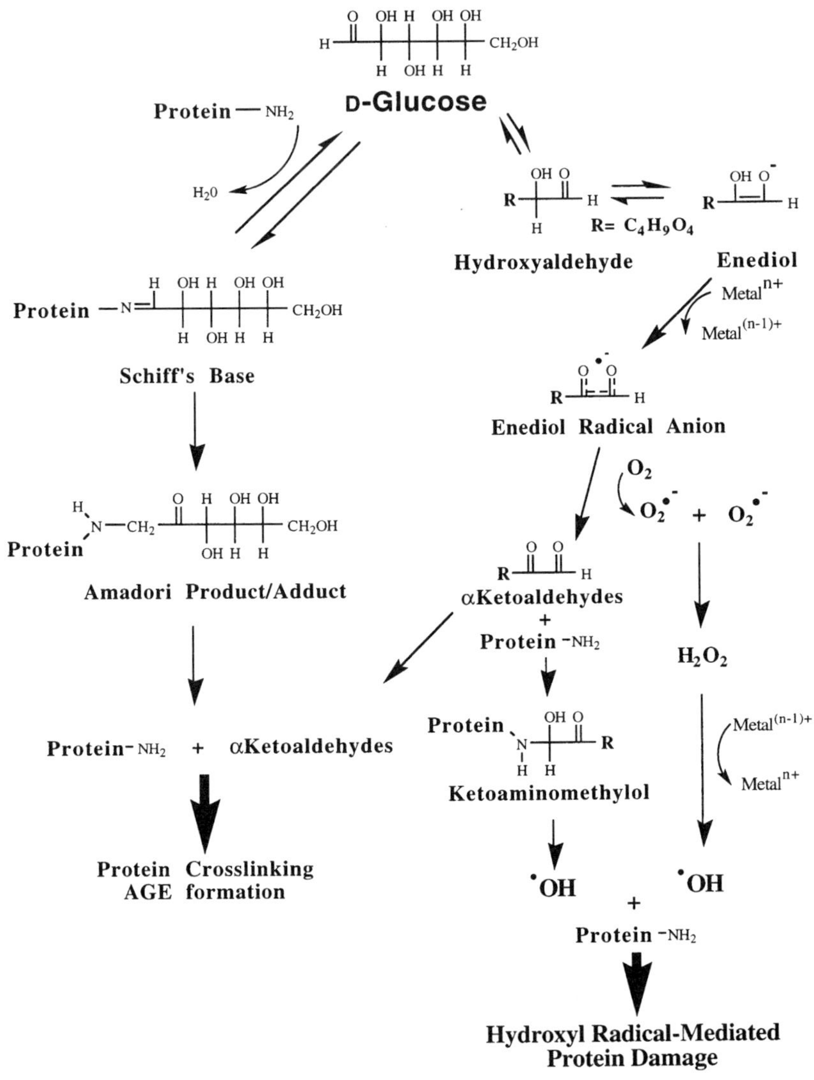

Figure 4 Glucose oxidation and glycation: glucose-induced protein damage and increased oxidative stress. Glucose, via glycative and oxidative processes, can result in protein damage and increased levels of oxidative stress as a result of the increased production of advanced glycation end products (AGEs) and hydroxyl radicals. These processes can therefore be attributed to type 2 diabetes due to the increased glucose levels (hyperglycemia) associated with this disease. (From Hunt JV, Dean RT, Wolff SP. Hydroxyl radical production and autoxidative glycosylation: glucose autoxidation as the cause of protein damage in the experimental glycation model of diabetes mellitus and ageing. Biochem J 1998; 256:205–212. Copyright 1988 by The Biochemical Society and Portland Press.)

levels, thereby lowering the reducing power of the cell. It has been proposed that this leads to inhibition of the activity of NADPH-requiring enzymes including nitric oxide synthase and glutathione reductase (64). Vasoconstriction and tissue injury can result from the diminished nitric oxide synthase activity (77), and the low glutathione reductase activity could result in an increased cellular susceptibility to free radical damage (78) and oxidative stress.

2. *Hyperinsulinemia*

Hyperinsulinemia, a hallmark of insulin resistance, has recently been invoked as a plausible causative agent in the development of oxidative stress-induced diabetic complications. Experimental evidence suggests a relationship between hyperinsulinemia and increased free radical production (79). In human fat cells, increased accumulation of hydrogen peroxidase occurs upon exposure to elevated insulin levels (79). It has been hypothesized that the increase in free radical production associated with elevated levels of insulin may result from heightened sympathetic nervous system activity and from elevated FFA concentrations (64). High insulin leads to an overdrive of the sympathetic nervous system that results in increased catecholamine release (80,81). Catecholamines have been associated with an augmented production of free radicals in diabetic animals through a rise in metabolic rate and autooxidation (82).

In vitro and in vivo studies suggest that the hyperinsulinemia-induced rise in fasting FFA concentrations may be associated with oxidative stress. An in vitro study with cultured endothelial cells showed an association between increased fatty acid levels in the medium with both an increase in oxidative stress and a decrease in initial glutathione levels (83). Further studies in humans have supported a relationship between increased FFA levels and free radical-associated oxidative stress; the latter was inferred from the lower GSH/GSSG ratio in the plasma of subjects with diabetes compared with controls (64).

3. *Natural Antioxidant Activities*

A brief summary of certain properties of selected antioxidants is addressed in the following section. Antioxidants are scavengers of free radicals that constitute an important component of the cellular defense mechanism against oxidative stress. As a result, reduction or changes in the activity of these compounds result in deleterious effects to the cell due to the development of free radical-mediated oxidative stress. In previous and in following sections, evidence is provided to discuss the status of antioxidants in diabetes.

Vitamin E (tocopherol) is the predominant lipophilic antioxidant and is localized to the plasma membrane (66). It is one of the most important chain-breaking antioxidants responsible for the prevention of the propagation of free radical-induced reactions (84). Interestingly, vitamin E has been shown to decrease the covalent linking of glucose to serum proteins in vitro and to inhibit the glycation of serum proteins in vivo (85).

Glutathione is one of the most important water-soluble antioxidants. It is a tripeptide, and the reduced form is the major hydrophilic intracellular reductant responsible for protection and repair against oxidant damage (66).

Ascorbate (vitamin C), a key aqueous phase antioxidant, is involved in vitamin E reduction (86), thereby promoting many of the antioxidant properties of vitamin E, including the ability to prevent the propagation of free radical-induced chain reactions.

α-Lipoic acid is the most potent endogenous antioxidant and is also a natural cofactor of mitochondrial dehydrogenase complexes. The redox potential of the dihydrolipoate (DHLA)/α-lipoic acid couple is −0.32 mV (87). This strong reductant is responsible for the regeneration of reduced glutathione and vitamin E. It can also prevent lipid peroxidation, possibly through its ability to scavenge superoxide and hydroxyl radicals, and is involved in the inhibition of the activation of NF-κB by directly preventing its translocation from the cytoplasm to the nucleus (66). The ability of α-lipoic acid to protect against oxidative stress is an important feature that might be applied to counteract the oxidative stress-mediated diabetic complications. This approach is discussed elsewhere in this book.

C. Can Oxidative Stress Cause Insulin Resistance?

The question of precedence between hyperinsulinemia and oxidative stress into the subsequent development of diabetes remains unanswered (64). The studies mentioned above suggest that at least the secondary hyperinsulinemia could plausibly precede or cause increased free radical production and the resulting oxidative stress. Further studies are necessary to address whether oxidative stress, as a result of hyperinsulinemia-mediated increased free radical production, could precede insulin resistance and lead to the onset of diabetes. To date there is no evidence that primary insulin resistance is linked to oxidative effects. The following sections analyze two emerging lines of study in this direction.

1. Oxidative Stress, Antioxidants, and Insulin Resistance In Vivo

There is little evidence for a role of antioxidant therapy in the prevention of insulin resistance and type 2 diabetes. Serum of individuals with type 2 diabetes have a lower vitamin E level and a higher GSH/GSSG ratio compared with control subjects (88). Individuals with type 2 diabetes who received vitamin E supplementation had improved metabolic control, as indicated by the significant drop in circulating levels of glycosylated hemoglobin (89). In a small randomized trial with humans with or without type 2 diabetes, vitamin E supplementation reduced oxidative stress and improved insulin action (64,88), verifying an important role for antioxidant therapy in diabetes. This study involved the use of a euglycemic hyperinsulinemic clamp to study the effects of vitamin E supplementation on insulin sensitivity (90). The results showed a significant gain in insulin-mediated nonoxidative glucose disposal after supplementation of 900 mg vitamin E (90). In addition, the vitamin E supplementation significantly increased plasma vitamin E levels and significantly reduced GSH/GSSG ratios in all subjects (90). It was proposed that the mechanism by which vitamin E improves insulin responsiveness in individuals with and without diabetes was related to its role as an antioxidant (88). The hypothesis was put forward that increased lipid peroxidation, as a result of increased free radical-induced oxidative stress or a reduction in the antioxidant capacity of the cell, could cause changes in the fluidity of the membrane; this in turn would purportedly lower glucose uptake (91). The ability of an antioxidant to quench free radicals and reduce lipid peroxidation could presumably provide protection from changes to membrane fluidity and restore normal glucose transporter function.

The first prospective population study undertaken to address the role of free radical stress and antioxidants in relation to the incidence of diabetes examined whether low vitamin E concentrations are a risk factor for the incidence of type 2 diabetes (92). The authors computed the levels of plasma vitamin E and the incidence of developing diabetes over a 4-year period in 944 men aged 42–60 who were determined not to have diabetes at baseline examination (92). Type 2 diabetes was defined by either a fasting blood glucose concentration of $\geq$6.7 mM, a blood glucose concentration $\geq$ 10.0 mM 2 h after a glucose load, or by a clinical diagnosis of diabetes with either dietary, oral, or insulin treatments. Forty-five men developed diabetes over the 4-year follow-up period (92). However, these 45 men also had a raised baseline body mass index, elevated blood glucose and serum fructosamine concentrations, a higher ratio of saturated fatty acids to the sum of monounsaturated and polyunsaturated fatty acids, and a higher serum triglyceride concentration (92). From the multivariate logistic regression model used in this study, it was found that the baseline body mass index was the strongest predictor of diabetes. Other factors with significant associations to an excess risk of diabetes included low plasma vitamin E concentrations, a high ratio of saturated to other fatty acids in serum, and a high socioeconomic status (92).

From this multivariate logistic regression model, a 3.9-fold risk of developing diabetes was associated with a low lipid standardized plasma vitamin E concentration (below median) (92). In addition, another model was used whereby lipid standardized vitamin E concentrations were replaced by unstandardized vitamin E concentrations when other risk factors such as serum low-density-lipoprotein cholesterol and triglyceride concentrations were taken as the strongest predictors of diabetes. From this model, a decrease of 1 μmol/L of uncategorized vitamin E concentration was associated with an increment of 22% in the risk of developing diabetes (92). Hence, a significant relationship was proposed to exist between low vitamin E concentrations and an increased risk of diabetes. Clinical trials are needed to support the effect of antioxidants in the prevention of diabetes. It has been suggested that these trials should address the need for a ''free radical initiative'' (93) to understand how free radicals could affect the intrinsic mechanisms of diabetes (65). Also, trials are necessary to confirm a role of vitamin E, or other antioxidants, in the prevention of type 2 diabetes (92).

2. *Oxidative Stress and Insulin Resistance In Vitro*

In vitro, insulin resistance can be induced by prolonged insulin treatment, exposure of cells to high glucose concentrations, or by the preexposure of cells to glucosamine (Fig. 5). Insulin resistance at the level of glucose transport can result from various signaling defects as previously mentioned, including alterations in insulin receptor function, depletion of the GLUT4 transporter pool, and alterations in the postreceptor signaling pathway (94).

Prolonged insulin treatment of 3T3-L1 adipocytes induced an insulin-resistant state as a result of changes in the insulin signal transduction cascade (95). Treatment of 3T3-L1 adipocytes with 500 nM insulin for 24 h increased basal glucose transport and led to an insulin-resistant state for this transport (5,96,97). This treatment did not modify the insulin receptor or levels of GLUT4; however, it prevented GLUT4 translocation in response to acute insulin stimulation (95). Prolonged insulin treatment also induced a decrease in the level of IRS-1 expression and phosphorylation and a reduced ability of insulin to stimulate PI 3-kinase and MAP kinase (98). Thus, insulin resistance induced by prolonged insulin treatment of 3T3-L1 adipocytes is associated with multiple signaling defects, including defects at the level of IRS-1, PI 3-kinase, MAP kinase, and impaired GLUT4 translocation (98). These defects are similar to those observed in the hyperinsulinemic states of obese humans and rodents (98), validating this insulin-resistant model as an effective approach to study alterations of the insulin signaling pathway and insulin resistance.

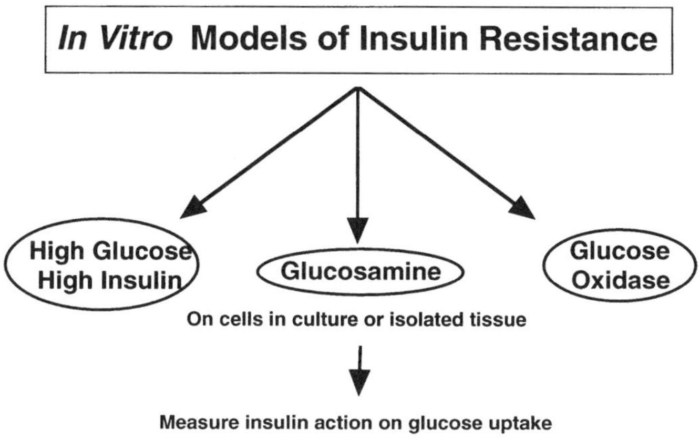

Figure 5 In vitro models of insulin resistance provide an effective tool to study alterations in the insulin signaling pathway and insulin resistance. Treatment of cells in culture or tissue with high levels of glucose, insulin, glucosamine, or glucose oxidase gnerate systems of insulin resistance, thus enabling further studies of insulin action in the insulin-resistant state.

Hyperglycemia has been linked to a worsening of insulin resistance (99–101) attributed to a disruption of normal cellular metabolism and of insulin-induced glucose disposal (102). In vitro, adipocytes exposed to high concentrations of glucose develop impaired insulin signaling, reduced insulin responsiveness, and diminished recruitment of glucose transporters to the plasma membranes in response to insulin (58,103). These alterations may be a result of the adverse metabolic consequences of the hyperglycemia.

Furthermore, it was discovered that an additional factor, glucosamine, was necessary for the glucose-induced desensitization of the insulin-stimulated glucose transport system (104). Glucosamine was also found to be more potent than glucose in the ability to induce insulin resistance and to decrease insulin responsiveness (104). It has been hypothesized from these findings that hexosamine metabolism may be the pathway by which cells sense and respond to ambient glucose levels and, when glucose flux is excessive, downregulation of glucose transport occurs and insulin resistance results (102,104). Thus, these models may lead to a better understanding of the mechanisms involved in the alterations of glucose metabolism seen in the insulin-resistant state.

To assess the role of oxidant stress and insulin resistance in vitro, Rudich et al. (105) used 3T3-L1 adipocytes preexposed to an enzymatic system capable of generating ROS. Exposure of the 3T3-L1 adipocytes to 25 mU/mL glucose oxidase for 18 h resulted in steady production of H_2O_2, with a concomitant threefold increase in basal 2-deoxyglucose uptake activity and a reduction in insulin-dependent 2-deoxyglucose uptake (105). The increase in basal transport as a result of increased oxidative stress was associated with an increase in GLUT1 mRNA and protein level (105). A reduction in GLUT4 protein and mRNA content was also observed, and this may account for a portion of the reduced insulin-stimulated glucose transport in the glucose oxidase-treated adipocytes (105). Basal lipogenesis was also enhanced by this treatment, whereas acute insulin stimulation of glucose oxidase-treated adipocytes significantly reduced lipogenesis activity (105). A further alteration of insulin-stimulated metabolism was also observed in these adipocytes as exposure to glucose oxidase lowered both the basal and insulin-stimulated glycogen synthase *a* activity (105). Recently, Rudich et al. (106) observed that GLUT4 translocation was selectively impaired in glucose oxidase-treated 3T3-L1 adipocytes as there was impaired redistribution of PI 3-kinase to the LDM fraction of cells upon insulin stimulation. This suggests that oxidative stress could impair the insulin-mediated PI 3-kinase cellular redistribution, which results in the impaired GLUT4 translocation.

D. α-Lipoic Acid: Stimulation of Glucose Uptake via Components of the Insulin Signaling Pathway

As previously mentioned, α-lipoic acid is a naturally occurring cofactor of oxidative metabolism, which is found as lipoamide covalently bound to a lysyl residue in five eukaryotic proteins, including mitochondrial dehydrogenase complexes (107). A natural antioxidant, lipoic acid has been used for the treatment of diabetic neuropathy (108) and ischemia-reperfusion injury (109) and has been indicated to improve glucose metabolism (110). In vitro and in vivo studies have demonstrated that exogenously supplied α-lipoic acid is taken up and reduced to DHLA by NADH- or NADPH-dependent enzymes in a variety of cells and tissues (111,112). Furthermore, α-lipoic acid has the ability to decrease the $NADH/NAD^+$ ratios elevated as a result of sorbitol oxidation to fructose under hyperglycemic conditions by the consumption of NADH (113). Further antioxidant properties attributed to α-lipoic acid include its ability to directly scavenge ROS and to recycle thioredoxin, glutathione, vitamin E, and vitamin C (114). However, it is not known whether these potent antioxidant properties of α-lipoic acid contribute to its ability to improve glucose utilization.

α-Lipoic acid has been shown in vitro to stimulate glucose utilization in isolated rat diaphragms (115), to enhance insulin-stimulated glucose metabolism in insulin-resistant skeletal muscle of obese Zucker rats (116), and to stimulate glucose transport activity in skeletal muscle isolated from both lean and obese Zucker rats (117). In streptozotocin-diabetic rats, chronic α-lipoic acid treatment reduced blood glucose concentrations by enhancement of muscle GLUT4 content and increased muscle glucose utilization (118). In addition, acute and repeated parenteral administration of α-lipoic acid improved insulin-stimulated glucose disposal in individuals with type 2 diabetes (110,119), strengthening its therapeutic value as an antidiabetic agent. Estrada et al. (120) established the ability of α-lipoic acid to stimulate glucose uptake into the insulin-responsive L6 skeletal muscle cells and 3T3-L1 adipocytes in culture. The naturally occurring (R)+ isoform of lipoic acid was shown to have a significantly greater effect on the stimulation of glucose uptake in L6 cells in comparison with the (S)− isoform or the racemic mixture (120). In addition, (R)+ lipoic acid had a positive effect on both basal and insulin-stimulated glucose uptake but did not improve the sensitivity of glucose uptake to submaximal concentrations of insulin (120). It was suggested that this increase in glucose uptake could not be entirely attributed to the antioxidant abilities of this agent alone. The increase in glucose uptake was mediated by a rapid translocation of the GLUT1 and GLUT4 glucose transporter isoforms from the internal membrane fraction to the plasma membrane of L6 myotubes (120).

We have recently shown that α-lipoic acid similarly stimulates the translocation of GLUT1 and GLUT4 from the internal membrane fractions to the plasma membrane in 3T3-L1 adipocytes (K. Yaworsky, unpublished data). To account for the mechanism by which α-lipoic acid could stimulate this increase in glucose uptake via rapid glucose transporter translocation, an inhibitor of PI 3-kinase, wortmannin, was used. As stated earlier, PI 3-kinase activity is essential for the propagation of the insulin signal responsible for the mediation of insulin-stimulated glucose uptake as a result of the translocation of glucose transporters (121). Wortmannin significantly lowered the α-lipoic acid stimulated increase in glucose uptake in L6 myotubes, suggesting the involvement of PI 3-kinase in lipoic acid's mechanism of action (120). More recent evidence has shown that α-lipoic acid directly stimulates IRS-1 immunoprecipitated PI 3-kinase activity in L6 myotubes, and this increase in PI 3-kinase activity is wortmannin sensitive (R. Somwar, K. Yaworsky, and A. Klip, unpublished data). These data suggest that α-lipoic acid engages components of the insulin signaling pathway in its ability to stimulate glucose uptake in L6 myotubes. This differs from other stimuli of glucose uptake such as the exercise and/or hypoxia pathway that do not use PI 3-kinase in their ability to stimulate glucose uptake, although they require glucose transporter translocation (122,133). The unique action of α-lipoic acid to increase glucose uptake

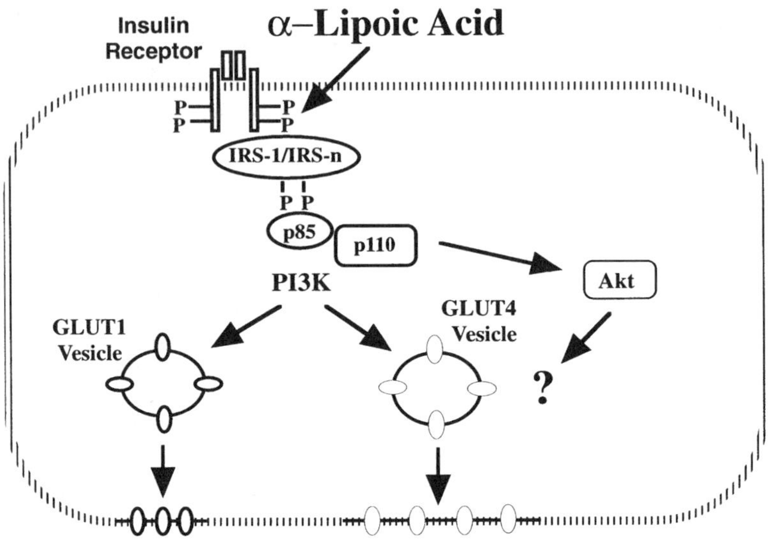

Figure 6 Schematic diagram of the proposed α-lipoic acid signaling mechanism. α-Lipoic acid uses components of the insulin signaling pathway in its ability to stimulate glucose uptake via the rapid translocation of GLUT1 and GLUT4 to the plasma membrane. In L6 myotubes, it has been shown that lipoic acid activates phosphatidylinositol 3-kinase (PI3K) and Akt in a wortmannin-sensitive fashion. These results indicate that lipoic acid uses components of the insulin signal transduction cascade in its ability to increase glucose uptake into insulin-responsive cells in culture.

via an insulin-sensitive pathway was further exemplified by studies whereby α-lipoic acid increased Akt activity in L6 myotubes (R. Somwar, K. Yaworsky, and A. Klip, unpublished data) (Fig. 6). These actions of α-lipoic acid are distinctive from other currently used antidiabetic agents and highlight α-lipoic acid as an attractive therapeutic strategy for the treatment of insulin resistance in type 2 diabetes.

REFERENCES

1. Heesom K, Harbeck M, Kahn C, Denton R. Insulin action on metabolism. Diabetologia 1997; 40:B3–B9.
2. Groop LC, Tuomi T. Non-insulin dependent diabetes mellitus—a collision between thrifty genes and an affluent society. Ann Med 1997; 29:37–53.

3. Kahn BB. Type 2 diabetes: when insulin secretion fails to compensate for insulin resistance. Cell 1998; 92:593–596.
4. Day C, Grove J, Daly A, Stewart M, Avery P, Walker M. Tumour necrosis factor-alpha gene promoter polymorphism and decreased insulin resistance. Diabetologia 1998; 41:430–434.
5. Cushman S, Wardzala L. Potential mechanism of insulin action on glucose transport in the isolated rat adipose cell. Apparent translocation of intracellular transport systems to the plasma membrane. J Biol Chem 1980; 255:4758–4762.
6. Suzuki K, Kono T. Evidence that insulin causes translocation of glucose transport activity to the plasma membrane from an intracellular storage site. Proc Natl Acad Sci USA 1980; 77:2542–2545.
7. Rea S, James D. Moving GLUT4 the biogenesis and trafficking of GLUT4 storage vesicles. Diabetes 1997; 46:1667–1677.
8. Franke TF, Yang SI, Chan TO, et al. The protein kinase encoded by the Akt proto-oncogene is a target of the PDGF-activated phosphatidylinositol 3-kinase. Cell 1995; 81:727–736.
9. Franke TF, Kaplan DR, Cantley LC, Toker A. Direct regulation of the Akt proto-oncogene product by phosphatidylinositol-3,4-bisphosphate [see comments]. Science 1997; 275:665–668.
10. Kohn AD, Kovacina KS, Roth RA. Insulin stimulates the kinase activity of RAC-PK, a pleckstrin homology domain containing ser/thr kinase. EMBO 1995; 14:4288–4295.
11. Kohn AD, Summers SA, Birnbaum MJ, Roth RA. Expression of a constitutively active Akt Ser/Thr kinase in 3T3-L1 adipocytes stimulates glucose uptake and glucose transporter 4 translocation. J Biol Chem 1996; 271:1372–1378.
12. Cong L, Chen H, Li Y, et al. Physiological role of Akt in insulin-stimulated translocation of GLUT4 in transfected rat adipose cells. Mol Endocrinol 1997; 11:1881–1890.
13. Sollner T, Whiteheart S, Brunner M, et al. SNAP receptors implicated in vesicle targeting and fusion. Nature 1993; 362:318–324.
14. Volchuk A, Ewart HS, et al. Syntaxin 4 in 3T3-L1 adipocytes: regulation by insulin and participation in insulin-dependent glucose transport. Mol Biol Cell 1996; 7:1075–1082.
15. Sudhof T, De Camilli P, Niemann H, Jahn R. Membrane fusion machinery: insights from synaptic proteins. Cell 1993; 75:1–4.
16. Rothman J. Mechanisms of intracellular protein transport. Nature 1994; 372: 55–63.
17. Wong P, Daneman N, Volchuk A, et al. Tissue distribution of SNAP-23 and its subcellular localization in 3T3-L1 cells. Biochem Biophys Res Commun 1997; 230:64–68.
18. Klip A, Tsakiridis T, Marette A, Ortiz PA. Regulation of expression of glucose transporters by glucose—a review of studies in vivo and in cell cultures. FASEB J 1994; 8:43–53.

19. Tsakiridis T, Marette A, Klip A. Glucose transporters in skeletal muscle of animal models of diabetes. In: Shafrir E, ed. Lessons from Animal Models of Diabetes 1994:141–159.
20. Rondinone CM, Wang L-M, Lonnroth P, Wesslau C, Pierce JH, Smith U. Insulin receptor substrate (IRS) 1 is reduced and IRS-2 is the main docking protein for phosphatidylinositol 3-kinase in adipocytes from subjects with non-insulin-dependent diabetes mellitus. Proc Natl Acad Sci USA 1997; 94:4171–4175.
21. Friedman JE, Sherman WM, Reed MJ, Elton CW, Dohm GL. Exercise training increases glucose transporter protein GLUT-4 in skeletal muscle of obese Zucker (fa/fa) rats. FEBS Lett 1990; 268:13–16.
22. Koranyi L, James D, Mueckler M, Permutt MA. Glucose transporter levels in spontaneously obese (db/db) insulin-resistant mice. J Clin Invest 1990; 85:962–967.
23. Kahn BB, Rossetti L, Lodish HF, Charron MJ. Decreased in vivo glucose uptake but normal expression of GLUT1 and GLUT4 in skeletal muscle of diabetic rats. J Clin Invest 1991; 87:2197–2206.
24. King PA, Horton ED, Hirshman MF, Horton ES. Insulin resistance in obese Zucker rat (fa/fa) skeletal muscle is associated with a failure of glucose transporter translocation. J Clin Invest 1992; 90:1568–1575.
25. Pedersen O, Bak JF, Andersen PH, et al. Evidence against altered expression of GLUT1 or GLUT4 in skeletal muscle of patients with obesity or NIDDM. Diabetes 1990; 39:865–870.
26. Hamann A, Benecke H, et al. Characterization of insulin resistance and NIDDM in transgenic mice with reduced brown fat. Diabetes 1995; 44:1266–1273.
27. Katz E, Stenbit A, Hatton K, DePinho R, Charron M. Cardiac and adipose tissue abnormalities but not diabetes in mice deficient in GLUT4. Nature 1995; 377:151–155.
28. Zierath JR, He L, Guma A, Odegoard Wahlstrom E, Klip A, Wallberg-Henriksson H. Insulin action on glucose transport and plasma membrane GLUT4 content in skeletal muscle from patients with NIDDM. Diabetologia 1996; 39: 1180–1189.
29. Gibbs EM, Stock JL, McCoid SC, et al. Glycemic improvement in diabetic *db/db* mice by overexpression of the human insulin-regulatable glucose transporter (GLUT4). J Clin Invest 1995; 95:1512–1518.
30. Kahn B. Glucose transport: pivotal step in insulin action. Diabetes 1996; 45: 1644–1654.
31. Kahn CR. Insulin action, diabetogenes, and the cause of type II diabetes. Diabetes 1994; 43:1066–1084.
32. Saad MJA, Araki E, Miralpeix M, Rothenberg PL, White MF, Kahn CR. Regulation of insulin receptor substrate-1 in liver and muscle of animal models of insulin resistance. J Clin Invest 1992; 90:1839–1849.
33. Le Marchand-Brustel Y, Gremeaux T, Ballotti R, Van Obberghen E. Insulin receptor tyrosine kinase is defective in skeletal muscle of insulin-resistant obese mice. Nature 1985; 315:676–678.

34. Folli F, Saad MJA, Backer JM, Kahn CR. Regulation of phosphatidylinositol 3-kinase activity in liver and muscle of animal models of insulin-resistant and insulin-deficient diabetes-mellitus. J Clin Invest 1993; 92:1787–1794.
35. Krook A, Kawano Y, Song XM, et al. Improved glucose tolerance restores insulin-stimulated Akt kinase activity and glucose transport in skeletal muscle from diabetic Goto-Kakizaki rats. Diabetes 1997; 46:2110–2114.
36. Bjornholm M, Kawano Y, Lehtihet M, Zierath JR. Insulin receptor substrate-1 phosphorylation and phosphatidylinositol 3-kinase activity in skeletal muscle from NIDDM subjects after in vivo insulin stimulation. Diabetes 1997; 46:524–527.
37. Tamemoto H, Kadowaki T, Tobe K, et al. Insulin resistance and growth retardation in mice lacking insulin receptor substrate-1. Nature 1994; 372:182–186.
38. Araki E, Lipes MA, Patti M-E, et al. Alternative pathway of insulin signaling in mice with targeted disruption of the IRS-1 gene. Nature 1994; 372:186–190.
39. Withers DJ, Gutierrez JS, Towery H, et al. Disruption of IRS-2 causes type 2 diabetes in mice. Nature 1998; 391:900–904.
40. Zierath J, Galuska D, Nolte A, Thorne A, Kristensen J, Wallberg-Henriksson H. Effects of glycaemia on glucose transport in isolated skeletal muscle from patients with NIDDM—in vitro reversal of muscular insulin resistance. Diabetologia 1994; 37:270–277.
41. Hotamisligil G, Arner P, Caro J, Atkinson R, Spiegelman B. Increased adipose tissue expression of tumour necrosis factor alpha in human obesity and insulin resistance. J Clin Invest 1995; 95:2409–2415.
42. Saghizadeh M, Ong J, Garvey W, Henry R, Kern P. The expression of TNF alpha by human muscle. J Clin Invest 1996; 97:1111–1116.
43. Uysal K, Weisbrock S, Marino M, Hotamisligil G. Protection from obesity-induced insulin resistance in mice lacking TNF-alpha function. Nature 1997; 389:610–614.
44. Hotamisligil G, Peraldi P, Budavari A, Ellis R, White M, Spiegelman B. IRS-1-mediated inhibition of insulin receptor tyrosine kinase activity in TNF-alpha and obesity-induced insulin resistance. Science 1996; 271:665–668.
45. Kanety H, Hemi R, Papa M, Karasik A. Sphingomyelinase and ceramide suppress insulin-induced tyrosine phosphorylation of the insulin receptor substrate-1. J Biol Chem 1996; 271:9895–9897.
46. Guo D, Donner D. Tumour necrosis factor promotes phosphorylation and binding of insulin receptor substrate-1 to phosphatidylinositol 3-kinase in 3T3-L1 adipocytes. J Biol Chem 1996; 271:615–618.
47. Falholt K, Jensen I, Lindkaer Jensen S, et al. Carbohydrate and lipid metabolism of skeletal muscle in type 2 diabetic patients. Diabetic Med 1988; 5:27–31.
48. Kelley D, Mokan M, Simoneau J-A, Mandarino L. Interaction between glucose and free fatty acid metabolism in human skeletal muscle. J Clin Invest 1993; 92:91–98.
49. Shillabeer G, Chamoun C, Hatch G, Lau DCW. Exogenous triacylglycerol in-

hibits insulin-stimulated glucose transport in L6 muscle cells in vitro. Biochem Biophys Res Commun 1995; 207:768–774.

50. Zarjevski N, Doyle P, Jeanrenaud B. Muscle insulin resistance may not be a primary etiological factor in the genetically obese fa/fa rat. Endocrinology 1992; 130:1564–1570.
51. Boden G, Jadali F, White J, et al. Effects of fat on insulin-stimulated carbohydrate metabolism in normal men. J Clin Invest 1991; 88:960–966.
52. Vaag A, Handberg A, Skott P, Richter E, Beck-Nielson H. Glucose-fatty acid cycle operates in humans at the levels of both whole body and skeletal muscle during low and high physiological plasma insulin concentrations. Eur J Endocrinol 1994; 130:70–79.
53. Randle P, Garland P, Hales C, Newsholme E. The glucose-fatty acid cycle: its role in insulin sensitivity and the metabolic disturbances of diabetes mellitus. Lancet 1963: 785–789.
54. Shagro E, Woldegiorgis G, Ruoho A, DiRusso C. Fatty acyl-CoA esters as regulators of cell metabolism. Prostaglandins Leukot Essent Fatty Acids 1995; 52:163–166.
55. Hargreaves M, Kiens B, Richter E. Effect of increased plasma free fatty acid concentrations on muscle metabolism in exercising men. J Appl Physiol 1991; 70:194–201.
56. Marcucci M, Griffin M, Estrada P, Barucci N, Cline G, Shulman G. Elevations in free fatty acids induce insulin resistance via inhibition of IRS-1-associated PI 3-kinase activity in vivo. Diabetes 1998; 47(suppl 1):A284.
57. O'Doherty R, Stein D, Foley J. Insulin resistance. Diabetologia 1997; 40:B10–B15.
58. Garvey W, Olefsky J, Matthaei S, Marshall S. Glucose and insulin coregulated the glucose transport system in primary cultured adipocytes. J Biol Chem 1987; 262:189–197.
59. Marshall S, Bacote V, Traxinger R. Discovery of a metabolic pathway mediating glucose-induced desensitization of the glucose transport system. Role of hexosamine biosynthesis in the induction of insulin resistance. J Biol Chem 1991; 266:4706–4712.
60. Rossetti L, Hawkins M, Chen W, Gindi J, Barzilai N. In vivo glucosamine infusion induces insulin resistance in normoglycemic but not in hyperglycemic conscious rats. J Clin Invest 1995; 96:132–140.
61. Hawkins M, Angelov I, Liu R, Barzilai N, Rossetti L. The tissue concentration of UDP-*N*-acetylglucosamine modulates the stimulatory effect of insulin on skeletal muscle glucose uptake. J Biol Chem 1997; 272:4889–4895.
62. Baron A, Zhu J-S, Zhu J-H, Weldon H, Maianu L, Garvey W. Glucosamine induces insulin resistance in vivo by affecting GLUT 4 translocation in skeletal muscle. Implications for glucose toxicity. J Clin Invest 1995; 96:2792–2801.
63. Chen H, Ing B, Robinson K, Feagin A, Buse M, Quon M. Effects of overexpression of glutamine: fructose-6-phosphate amidotransferase (GFAT) and glucos-

amine treatment on translocation of GLUT4 in rat adipose cells. Mol Cell Endocrinol 1997; 135:67–77.

64. Paolisso G, Giugliano D. Oxidative stress and insulin action: is there a relationship? Diabetologia 1996; 39:357–363.
65. Cominacini L, Garbin U, Cascio V. The need for a ''free radical initiative.'' Diabetologia 1996; 39:364–366.
66. Hofmann M, Bierhaus A, Ziegler R, Wahl P, Nawroth P, Tritschler H. Lipoate effects on atherogenesis. In: Fuchs J, Packer L, Zimmer G, eds. Lipoic Acid in Health and Disease. New York: Marcel Dekker, 1997.
67. Cross C, Halliwell B, Borish E. Oxygen radicals and human disease. Ann Intern Med 1987; 107:526–545.
68. Odetti P, Traverso N, Cosso L, Noberasco G, Pronzato M, Marinari U. Good glycemic control reduces oxidation and glycation end-products in collagen of diabetic rats. Diabetologia 1996; 39:1440–1447.
69. Traverso N, Menini S, Cosso L, et al. Immunological evidence for increased oxidative stress in diabetic rats. Diabetologia 1998; 41:365–370.
70. Paolisso G, D'Amore A, Balbi V, et al. Plasma vitamin C affects glucose homeostasis in healthy subjects and in non-insulin-dependent diabetics. Am J Physiol 1994; 266:E261–E268.
71. Lindsay R, Jamieson N, Walker S, McGuigan C, Smith W, Baird J. Tissue ascorbic acid and polyol pathway metabolism in experimental diabetes. Diabetologia 1998; 41:516–523.
72. Stocks J, Gutteridge J, Sharp R, Dormandy T. The inhibition of lipid autoxidation by human serum and its relationship to serum proteins and tocopherol. Clin Sci Mol Med 1974; 47:223–233.
73. Jones A, Winkles J, Jennings P, Florkowski C, Lunec J, Barnett A. Serum antioxidant activity in diabetes mellitus. Diabetes Res 1988; 7:89–92.
74. Wolff S, Jiang Z, Hunt J. Protein glycation and oxidative stress in diabetes mellitus and ageing. Free Radic Biol Med 1991; 10:339–352.
75. Brownlee M, Cerami A, Vlassara H. Advanced glycosylation end products in tissue and biochemical basis of diabetic complication. N Engl J Med 1988; 318: 1315–1322.
76. Hohman T, Beg M. Diabetic complication: progress in the development of treatments. Exp Opin Invest Drugs 1994; 3:1041–1049.
77. Lowenstein C, Dinerman J, Snyder S. Nitric oxide: a physiologic messenger. Ann Intern Med 1994; 120:227–237.
78. Chari S, Noth N, Rothi A. Glutathione and its redox system in diabetic polymorphonuclear leukocytes. Am J Med Sci 1984; 297:14–15.
79. Krieger-Brauer H, Kather K. Human fat cells possess a plasma membrane bound H2O2 generating system that is activated by insulin via a mechanism bypassing the receptor kinase. J Clin Invest 1992; 89:1006–1013.
80. DeFronzo R, Ferrannini E. Insulin resistance: a multifaceted syndrome responsible for NIDDM, obesity, hypertension and atherosclerotic cardiovascular disease. Diabetes Care 1991; 14:173–194.

81. Rowe J, Young J, Minaker K, Stevens A, Pallotta J, Landsberg L. Effect of insulin and glucose infusion on sympathetic nervous system activity in normal men. Diabetes 1981; 30:219–225.
82. Singal P, Beamish R, Dhalla N. Potential oxidative pathways of catecholamines in the formation of lipid peroxides and genesis of heart disease. Adv Exp Med Biol 1983; 161:391–401.
83. Henning B, Enoch C, Chow C. Protection by vitamin E against endothelial cell injury by linoleic acid hydroperoxides. Nutr Res 1983; 7:1253–1259.
84. Young I, Torney J, Trimble E. The effect of ascorbate supplementation on oxidative stress in the streptozotocin diabetic rat. Free Radic Biol Med 1992; 13: 41–46.
85. Ceriello A, Quatraro A, Giugliano D. New insights on non-enzymatic glycosylation may lead to therapeutic approaches for the prevention of diabetic complications. Diabet Med 1992; 9:297–299.
86. Sies H. Strategies of antioxidant defense. Eur J Biochem 1993; 215:213–219.
87. Jocelyn P. The standard redox potential of cysteine-cystine from the thioldisulphide exchange reaction with glutathione and lipoic acid. Eur J Biochem 1967; 2:327–331.
88. Caballero B. Vitamin E improves the action of insulin. Nutr Rev 1993; 51: 339–340.
89. Cerierro A, Giugliano D, Quatraro A, Donzella C, Dipalo G, Lefebvre P. Vitamin E reduction of protein glycosylation in diabetics: new prospect for prevention of diabetic complications. Diabetes Care 1991; 14:68–72.
90. Paolisso G, D'Amore A, Giugliano D, Ceriello A, Vericchio M, D'Onofrio F. Pharmacologic doses of vitamin E improve insulin action in healthy subjects and noninsulin-dependent diabetic patients. Am J Clin Nutr 1993; 57:650–656.
91. Whitesell R, Reyen D, Meth A, Pelletier D, Abumrad N. Activation energy of slowest step in the glucose carrier cycle: correlation with membrane lipid fluidity. Biochemistry 1989; 28:5818–5825.
92. Salonen J, Nyyssonen K, Tuomainen T, et al. Increased risk of non-insulin dependent diabetes mellitus at low plasma vitamin E concentrations: a four year follow up study in men. Br Med J 1995; 311:1124–1127.
93. Meshnick S. Oxidant stress distressed. Redox Rep 1995; 1:77–78.
94. Kahn B. Facilitative glucose transporters: regulatory mechanisms and dysregulation in diabetes. J Clin Invest 1992; 89:1367–1374.
95. Kozka I, Clark A, Holman G. Chronic treatment with insulin selectively down regulates cell-surface GLUT4 glucose transporters in 3T3-L1 adipocytes. J Biol Chem 1991; 266:11726–11731.
96. Tordjman K, Leingang K, James D, Mueckler M. Differential regulation of two distinct glucose transporter species expressed in 3T3-L1 adipocytes: effect of chronic insulin and tolbutamide treatment. Proc Natl Acad Sci USA 1989; 86: 7761–7765.

97. Rosen O, Simith C, Fung C, Rubins C. Development of hormone receptors and hormone responsiveness in vitro. Effect of prolonged insulin treatment on hexose uptake in 3T3-L1 adipocytes. J Biol Chem 1978; 253:7579–7583.
98. Ricort J-M, Tanti J-F, Van Obberghen E, Le Marchand-Brustel Y. Alterations in insulin signaling pathway induced by prolonged insulin treatment of 3T3-L1 adipocytes. Diabetologia 1995; 38:1148–1156.
99. Yki-Jarvinen H, Helve E, Koivisto V. Hyperglycemia decreases glucose uptake in type I diabetes. Diabetes 1987; 36:892–896.
100. Unger R, Grundy S. Hyperglycemia as an inducer as well as a consequence of impaired islet cell function and insulin resistance. Diabetologia 1985; 28:119–121.
101. DelPrato S, Sheehan P, Leonetti F, Simonson D. Effect of chronic physiologic hyperglycemia on insulin secretion and glucose metabolism (Abstr). Diabetes 1986; 35(suppl 1):196A.
102. McClain DA, Crook ED. Hexosamines and insulin resistance. Diabetes 1996; 45:1003–1009.
103. Garvey W, Huecksteadt T, Birnbaum M. Pretranslational suppression of an insulin-responsive glucose transporter in rats with diabetes mellitus. Science 1989; 245:60–63.
104. Marshall S, Bacote V, Traxinger R. Discovery of a metabolic pathway mediating glucose-induced desensitization of the glucose transport system. J Biol Chem 1991; 266:4706–4712.
105. Rudich A, Kozlovsky N, Potashnik R, Bashan N. Oxidant stress reduces insulin responsiveness in 3T3-L1 adipocytes. Am J Physiol 1997; 272:E935–E940.
106. Rudich A, Kozlovsky N, Potashnik R, Tirosh A, Pessler D, Bashan N. Regulation of glucose transporters gene expression and protein function in oxidative stress induced insulin resistance. VII International Symposium on Insulin Receptor & Insulin Action: Molecular and Clinical Aspects, Jerusalem, Israel, 1998.
107. Packer L, Roy S, Sen C. Alpha-lipoic acid: a metabolic antioxidant and potential redox modulator of transcription. Adv Pharmacol 1996; 38:79–101.
108. Ziegler D, Hanefeid M, Ruhnau K, et al. Treatment of symptomatic diabetic peripheral neuropathy with the anti-oxidant alpha-lipoic acid. Diabetologia 1996; 38:1425–1433.
109. Panigrahi M, Sadguna Y, Shivakumar B, et al. Alpha lipoic acid protects against reperfusion injury following cerebral ischemia in rats. Brain Res 1996; 717: 79–101.
110. Jacob S, Henriksen E, Schiemann A, et al. Enhancement of glucose disposal in patients with type 2 diabetes by alpha-lipoic acid. Drug Res 1995; 45:872–874.
111. Handleman G, Han D, Tritschler H, Packer L. Alpha-lipoic acid reduction by mammalian cells to the dithiol form, and release into the culture medium. Biochem Pharmacol 1994; 47:1725–1730.

112. Haramaki N, Han D, Handelman G, Tritschler H, Packer L. Cytosolic and mitochondrial systems for NADH- and NADPH-dependent reduction of alpha-lipoic acid. Free Radic Biol Med 1997; 22:535–542.
113. Roy S, Sen C, Tritschler H, Packer L. Modulation of cellular reducing equivalent homeostasis by alpha lipoic acid. Biochem Pharmacol 1997; 53:393–399.
114. Packer L, Witt E, Tritschler H. Alpha-lipoic acid as a biological antioxidant. Free Radic Biol Med 1995; 19:227–250.
115. Haugaard N, Haugaard E. Stimulation of glucose utilization by thioctic acid in rat diaphragm incubated in vitro. Biochim Biophys Acta 1970; 222:583–586.
116. Jacob S, Streeper R, Fogt D, et al. The antioxidant alpha lipoic acid enhances insulin-stimulated glucose metabolism in insulin-resistant rat skeletal muscle. Diabetes 1996; 45:1024–1029.
117. Henriksen E, Jacob S, Streeper R, Fogt D, Hokama J, Tritschler H. Stimulation by alpha lipoic acid of glucose transport activity in skeletal muscle of lean and obese Zucker rats. Life Sci 1997; 61:805–812.
118. Khamaisi M, Potashnik R, Tirosh A, et al. Lipoic acid reduces glycaemia and increases muscle GLUT4 content in streptozotocin-diabetic rats. Metabolism 1997; 46:763–768.
119. Jacob S, Henriksen E, Tritschler H, Augustin H, Dietze G. Improvement of insulin-stimulated glucose disposal in type 2 diabetes after repeated parenteral administration of thioctic acid. Exp Clin Endocrinol Diabetes 1996; 104:284–288.
120. Estrada D, Ewart H, Tsakiridis T, et al. Stimulation of glucose uptake by the natural coenzyme alpha-lipoic acid/thioctic acid. Diabetes 1996; 45:1798–1804.
121. Cheatham B, Vlahos C, Cheatham L, Wang L, Blenis J, Kahn C. Phosphatidylinositol 3-kinase activation is required for insulin stimulation of pp70 S6 kinase, SNA synthesis and glucose transporter translocation. Mol Cell Biol 1994; 14: 4902–4911.
122. Lee A, Hansen P, Holloszy J. Wortmannin inhibits insulin-stimulated but not contraction-stimulated glucose transport activity in skeletal muscle. FEBS Lett 1995; 361:51–54.
123. Yeh J, Gulve E, Rameh L, Birnbaum M. The effects of wortmannin on rat skeletal muscle: dissociation of signaling pathways for insulin- and contraction-activated hexose transport. J Biol Chem 1995; 270:2107–2111.

19

Oxidative Stress and Antioxidant Treatment: Effects on Muscle Glucose Transport in Animal Models of Type 1 and Type 2 Diabetes

Erik J. Henriksen
University of Arizona, Tucson, Arizona

By definition, diabetes mellitus is a group of pathophysiological conditions of varying etiologies that has as a common denominator—the derangement of blood glucose regulation (i.e., hyperglycemia). Two major forms of diabetes mellitus exist: type 1, a less common form in which there is an absolute deficiency of circulating insulin due to destruction of the β-cells of the pancreas, and type 2, the most common form, characterized primarily by a decreased ability of insulin to stimulate skeletal muscle glucose transport and metabolism. Although there is increasing information that oxidative stress, characterized by the localized production of free radicals and other reactive oxygen species, may be associated with metabolic abnormalities present in both type 1 and type 2 diabetes and several studies have been published recently supporting the effectiveness of antioxidant interventions in improving the defective metabolic state characteristic of diabetes, the relationship between oxidative stress and insulin resistance remains controversial (1,2).

The purpose of this chapter is to briefly review the regulation of skeletal muscle glucose transport by insulin under normal conditions and the underlying defects in this regulation present in type 1 and type 2 diabetes and the available information regarding the role of oxidative stress in diabetes and the utility of antioxidant interventions, with a focus on the water-soluble antioxidant lipoic acid (3), in ameliorating these metabolic abnormalities associated with type 1 and type 2 diabetes. In this context, I discuss primarily evidence from animal model studies because Chapter 20 specifically addresses clinical investigations involving diabetes and antioxidant interventions.

I. REGULATION OF MUSCLE GLUCOSE TRANSPORT

Skeletal muscle is the major tissue responsible for the peripheral disposal of glucose in the face of a glucose or insulin challenge or during exercise (4,5). Skeletal muscle glucose transport activity is acutely regulated by insulin through the activation of a series of intracellular proteins, including insulin receptor autophosphorylation and tyrosine kinase activation, tyrosine phosphorylation of insulin receptor substrate-1 (IRS-1), and activation of phosphotidylinositol 3-kinase (PI 3-kinase), ultimately resulting in the translocation of a glucose transporter protein isoform, the GLUT4 protein, to the sarcolemmal membrane where glucose transport takes place via a facilitative diffusion process (for a review, see 6). Recent evidence from rodent studies indicates that the amount of GLUT4 protein incorporated into the sarcolemmal membrane correlates closely with the degree of insulin-stimulated glucose transport (7,8) and supports the idea that GLUT4 translocation represents the major mechanism for insulin stimulation of glucose transport in skeletal muscle.

Skeletal muscle glucose transport is also stimulated by an insulin-independent process that is activated by contractions (9–11) via a GLUT4 translocation mechanism (7,12). Evidence that these insulin-dependent and insulin-independent pathways for stimulation of glucose transport are mediated by different mechanisms came initially from studies demonstrating that the maximal effects of the two pathways are completely additive (11,13–15). Moreover, the additive effect of insulin and contractions in combination is due to an additivity of the effects of these stimuli on GLUT4 translocation into the sarcolemma (7). More recently, studies by Goodyear et al. (16) have provided a molecular basis for these two distinct pathways for activation of glucose transport in skeletal muscle. Although insulin increases tyrosine phosphorylation of the insulin receptor and IRS-1 and activates IRS-1-associated PI 3-kinase, muscle contraction alone has no effect on these factors, indicating that distinct intracellular pathways exist in muscle for activation of GLUT4 translocation and glucose transport by insulin and contractions (16).

II. INSULIN RESISTANCE IN DIABETES

Insulin resistance is defined as a reduced ability of insu'ʼn to activate specific insulin-dependent biological processes in cells of target organs. In poorly controlled type 1 diabetes, insulin resistance is thought to be a secondary effect of the dyslipidemic state (elevated free fatty acids) and the prolonged hyperglycemic state. In type 2 diabetes, insulin resistance of skeletal muscle glucose disposal is generally considered to be a primary factor in the etiology of this disease. In this latter state, the skeletal muscle insulin resistance is often accompanied by a variety of other metabolic abnormalities, including obesity, dyslipidemia, hypertension, and atherosclerosis (17–19), a condition referred to variously as ''syndrome X'' (18,19) or the ''insulin resistance syndrome'' (17). The link among these disorders has been attributed to hyperinsulinemia, a consequence of the insulin resistance (17). Indeed, the increased cardiovascular mortality associated with this condition has been directly attributed by some leading investigators to the hyperinsulinemia itself (20–22).

Interventions that improve insulin action on skeletal muscle glucose metabolism in insulin-resistant individuals are therefore expected to decrease conversion rates to overt diabetes and to reduce cardiovascular mortality in diabetic populations. Therefore, an understanding of the pathophysiology underlying this insulin resistance and the search for optimal interventions for improving insulin action on skeletal muscle are of substantial interest.

III. ANIMAL MODELS OF TYPE 1 AND TYPE 2 DIABETES

A. Type 1 Diabetes

The most widely used animal model of type 1 diabetes is the streptozotocin-induced diabetic rat. Streptozotocin is a compound that causes hypersecretion of insulin from the pancreatic β-cells, resulting in their eventual dysfunction and leading to a hypoinsulinemic state (23). The streptozotocin-diabetic rat is characterized by marked postprandial hyperglycemia and by an elevation in free fatty acids without ketoacidosis (23). Skeletal muscle from the streptozotocin-diabetic rat is markedly insulin resistant for stimulation of glucose transport (24,25) and expresses a significantly reduced protein expression of the GLUT4 glucose transporter isoform (24,25).

B. Type 2 Diabetes

Although numerous rodent models of type 2 diabetes exist, the focus here is on the obese Zucker (*fa/fa*) rat. The obese Zucker rat is an animal model of severe skeletal muscle insulin resistance also characterized by marked hyperinsulinemia (26), glucose intolerance (27,28), dyslipidemia (26), moderate hypertension (29), and central adiposity (30). It is therefore an excellent model with which to study the underlying pathophysiology and potential interventions in the insulin-resistance syndrome. Studies have identified at least one cellular locus for the insulin resistance of glucose transport in this animal model. Insulin-stimulated GLUT4 protein translocation (8,31) and glucose transport activity (8,32,33) are substantially impaired in isolated skeletal muscle from these obese animals.

Anai et al. (34) have very recently shown that in skeletal muscle from obese Zucker rats, there are significant defects in crucial aspects of the insulin signaling cascade. Compared with age-matched lean Zucker rats, in hindlimb muscle from the obese Zucker rats, there is a 60% smaller IRS-1 protein level, and insulin-stimulated IRS-1 phosphorylation is only 72% of control values, despite elevated basal levels. The amount of the regulatory subunit of PI 3-kinase (detected using a p85α antibody) associated with the tyrosine-phosphorylated IRS-1 in the insulin-stimulated state is only 29% of control. Finally, IRS-1-associated PI 3-kinase activity in muscle immunoprecipitates from the obese animals is 54% of the level observed in lean animals (34). These findings likely represent the molecular basis for the skeletal muscle insulin resistance present in the obese Zucker rat.

IV. OXIDATIVE STESS, INSULIN RESISTANCE, AND ANTIOXIDANT TREATMENT IN DIABETES

A. Streptozotocin-Diabetic Rat

There is ample evidence that markers of oxidative stress are increased in the most widely accepted rodent model of type 1 diabetes, the streptozotocin-diabetic rat. For example, plasma and liver lipid peroxides, as measured by the thiobarbituric acid reactive substances assay, are elevated in the streptozotocin-diabetic rat (35). In addition, recent evidence indicates that in this model of type 1 diabetes, sciatic nerve levels of reduced glutathione (GSH) are lower and the ratio of oxidized to reduced glutathione (GSSG/GSH) is elevated compared with tissue from normoglycemic control animals (36). Chronic treatment with the antioxidant lipoic acid brings about a nearly complete normalization of the GSH and GSSG/GSH profiles in sciatic nerve from the streptozotocin-diabetic rats and also significantly improves nerve blood flow and conduction velocity (36).

Plasma glucose is markedly elevated and insulin action on skeletal muscle glucose transport activity is substantially reduced in the streptozotocin-diabetic rat, possibly as a result of reduced muscle GLUT4 protein levels (25). Acutely, lipoic acid can cause a marked lowering of plasma glucose in these diabetic animals (25). Chronically, a 10-day treatment period of these diabetic animals with lipoic acid also results in a significant lowering of plasma glucose levels and causes profound increases in both skeletal muscle GLUT4 protein levels and insulin-stimulated glucose transport activity (25). Collectively, these results provide evidence that the beneficial metabolic effects of lipoic acid in this severely hyperglycemic diabetic animal model may be associated with an improvement in the oxidant/antioxidant status of the animal.

B. Obese Zucker Rat

Much less information regarding the oxidant/antioxidant status is presently available for the obese Zucker rat. It should be stressed that this animal model displays only mild fasting hyperglycemia, with more severe abnormalities observed when the animal is presented with a glucose load (27,37,38). Nevertheless, Nourooz-Zadeh (39) reported that the isoprostane 8-epi-$PGF_{2\alpha}$, a marker of oxidative stress, is elevated in the plasma of the diabetic Zucker rat compared with lean controls. Interestingly, these elevated levels of oxidative stress are significantly reduced with antioxidant treatment, such as α-tocopherol (39). These results concerning oxidative stress in the diabetic Zucker rat are consistent with observations of human type 2 diabetes. During a euglycemic hyperinsulinemic clamp, a significant inverse relationship has been observed between insulin action on nonoxidative glucose disposal and plasma superoxide ion, and a significant positive relationship has been seen between insulin action on nonoxidative glucose disposal and plasma GSH/GSSG ratio in type 2 diabetic patients (40). Patients with impaired glucose tolerance (a prediabetic state) or overt type 2 diabetes have significantly reduced erythrocyte levels of the antioxidant enzymes catalase and superoxide dismutase and diminished plasma GSH (41). Decreased serum vitamin E content, a marker of impaired oxidant/antioxidant status, was recently reported to be associated with increased risk of developing type 2 diabetes in a Finnish population (42), and type 2 diabetic patients themselves display significantly reduced plasma vitamin E levels (43). Finally, plasma hydroperoxides, another marker of oxidative stress, are higher in subjects with type 2 diabetes compared with healthy control subjects and are significantly inversely correlated with the degree of metabolic control (43).

The effectiveness of antioxidant interventions, particularly chronic treatment with lipoic acid, in ameliorating the metabolic abnormalities present in the obese Zucker rat has been demonstrated in a series of studies from our laboratory. The results of these studies are summarized below. In these studies, the obese Zucker rats were treated intraperitoneally with a racemic mixture (50% R- and 50% S-enantiomers) of lipoic acid for 10–12 days and were investigated after an overnight fast (food restricted to 4 g at 5 P.M. of the previous evening). As shown in Figure 1, the obese Zucker rat displays only mild hyperglycemia, and this slight elevation in plasma glucose is completely reversed with chronic lipoic acid treatment (30 mg/kg) (44,45). More striking is the marked hyperinsulinemia and dyslipidemia of the obese Zucker rat compared with the lean Zucker rat (44,45). Chronic lipoic acid treatment leads to significant reductions in both plasma insulin (~20%) and free fatty acids (~15%) (Fig. 1). It should be noted that these alterations due to the racemic mixture of lipoic acid are entirely due to the R-enantiomer, as treatment with the S-enantiomer actually exacerbates the hyperinsulinemia and has no significant effect in lowering plasma free fatty acids (45).

More recently, we have shown that glucose tolerance after a 1-g/kg oral glucose feeding is improved by lipoic acid in a dose-dependent fashion (Fig.

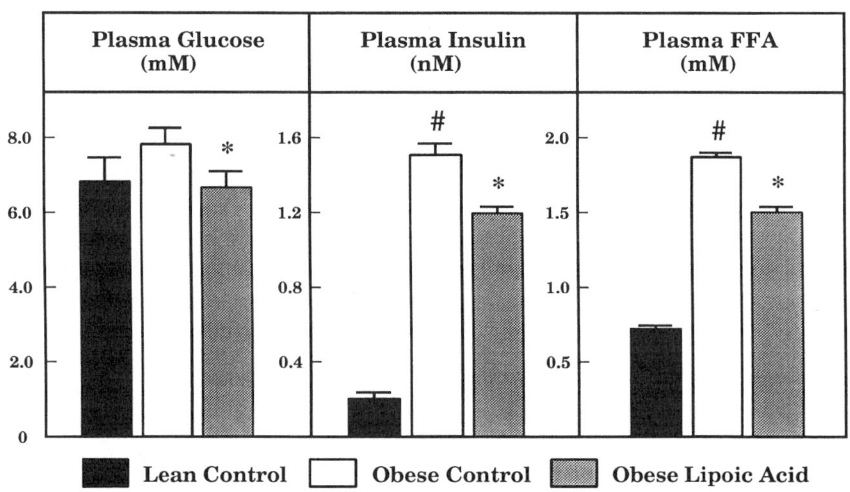

Figure 1 Effect of chronic treatment of obese Zucker rats with lipoate on plasma glucose, insulin, and free fatty acids. Values are means ± SE. $*p < 0.05$ vs. obese vehicle-treated control; $\#p < 0.05$ vs. lean control. (From Ref. 44.)

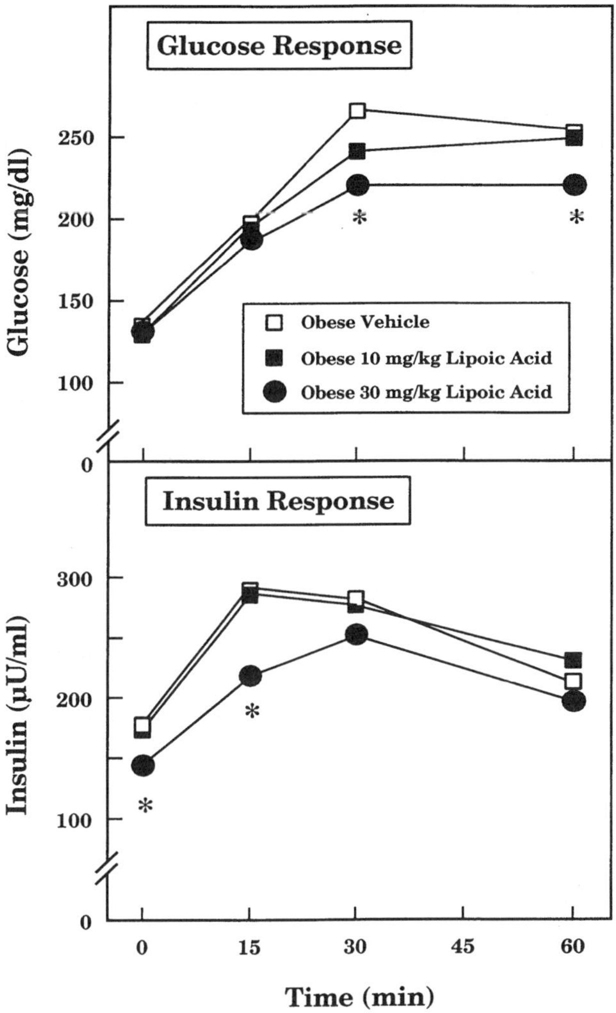

Figure 2 Effect of chronic treatment of obese Zucker rats with lipoate on glucose and insulin responses to a 1-g/kg oral glucose tolerance test. Values are means ± SE. $*p < 0.05$ vs. obese vehicle-treated control.

2), with a significantly smaller area under the curve (AUC) of the glucose response in a group of obese animals treated for 10 days with 30 mg/kg lipoic acid compared with control (Fig. 3, left). Moreover, this improved glucose response was seen in the face of a reduced insulin response during the test (Fig. 2) and a smaller insulin AUC (Fig. 3, middle). The glucose–insulin index, the product of the glucose and insulin AUCs and an indirect index of in vivo insulin action, was significantly lower in the 30 mg/kg lipoic acid-treated obese group compared with the obese control group, implying that peripheral insulin action was enhanced by lipoic acid. Consistent with this finding was our observation that insulin-mediated glucose transport activity in both fast glycolytic muscle (m. epitrochlearis, Fig. 4) and slow oxidative muscle (m. soleus, Fig. 5) was improved in the 30 mg/kg lipoic acid-treated obese group compared with the obese control group.

To determine the functional relevance of this improvement of insulin-mediated glucose transport, we assessed the correlation between insulin-mediated glucose transport activity in either the epitrochlearis or the soleus and the glucose-insulin index in obese animals treated with either vehicle, 10 mg/kg lipoic acid, or 30 mg/kg lipoic acid (Fig. 6). The correlation coefficients between the glucose–insulin index and insulin action on glucose transport in the epitrochlearis ($r = -0.598$, $p < 0.05$) and in the soleus ($r = -0.654$, $p < 0.05$) were statistically significant, indicating that the improved insulin action on muscle glucose transport was, at least in part, responsible for the improvement in whole-body glucose tolerance observed after lipoic acid treatment.

Because the whole homogenate level of GLUT4 protein in skeletal muscle from lipoic acid-treated obese Zucker rats is not significantly elevated compared with obese controls (44), this would imply that lipoic acid enhances the ability of insulin to activate translocation of intracellular GLUT4 protein into the sarcolemmal membrane, a process that is defective in obese Zucker rats (8,31). This hypothesis, however, remains to be tested experimentally.

V. PERSPECTIVES: ANTIOXIDANTS AND INSULIN RESISTANCE

A growing body of knowledge supports a role of oxidative stress in the complications associated with the hyperglycemic state of diabetes. Moreover, increasing evidence, though still fairly limited at this point, indicates that oxidative stress may be associated with the skeletal muscle insulin resistance inherent to both type 1 and type 2 diabetes. Therefore, interventions that can

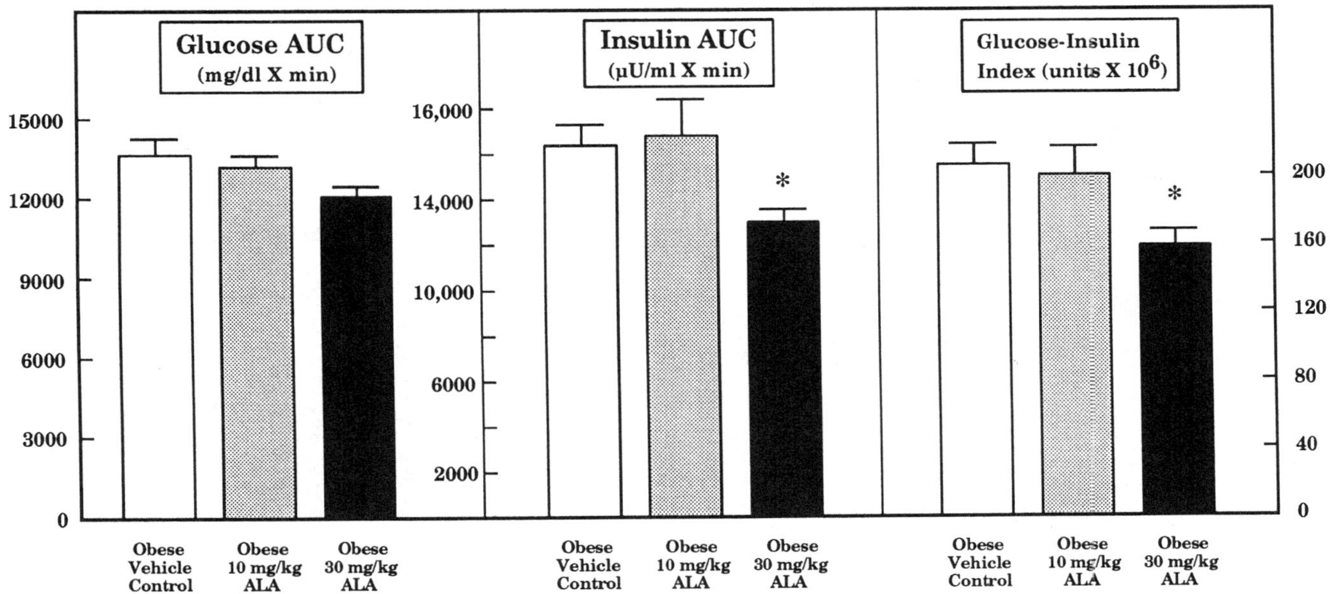

Figure 3 Areas under the curve (AUC) for the glucose and insulin responses to an oral glucose tolerance test in control and chronic lipoate-treated obese Zucker rats. The glucose-insulin index represents the product of the glucose AUC and the insulin AUC. Values are means ± SE. $*p < 0.05$ vs. obese vehicle-treated control.

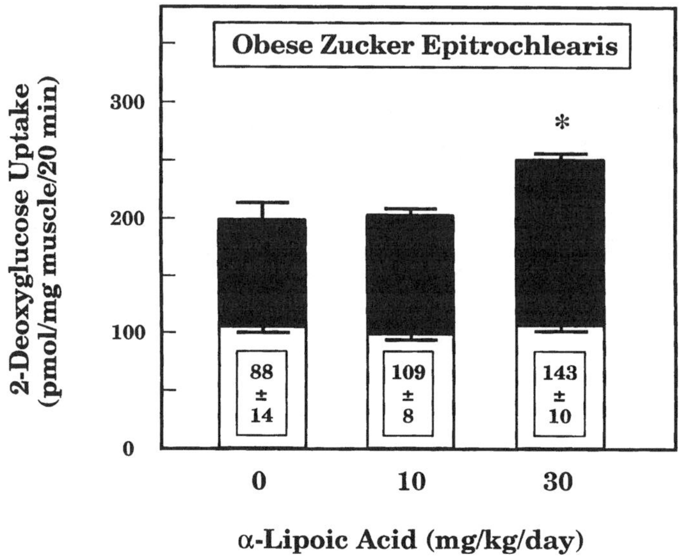

Figure 4 Effect of chronic treatment of obese Zucker rats with lipoate on in vitro insulin-stimulated glucose transport activity in the isolated epitrochlearis muscle. □, Basal 2-deoxyglucose uptake; ■, increase in 2-deoxyglucose uptake due to insulin (2 mU/mL). This increase is shown in the box for each bar. Values are means ± SE. $*p < 0.05$ vs. 0 mg/kg lipoate.

ameliorate the oxidant/antioxidant imbalance in this condition will be helpful in improving peripheral insulin action on glucose transport and metabolism in skeletal muscle. Indeed, several animal model and clinical investigations support the beneficial effects of antioxidants, particularly lipoic acid, in the diabetic state.

Ample evidence now exists in the literature indicating that one locus of action of lipoic acid in improving metabolic control in animal models of insulin resistance is at the level of the skeletal muscle itself. Chronic treatment of the streptozotocin-diabetic rat, a model of type 1 diabetes, leads to a reduction in blood glucose that is associated with an increase in muscle GLUT4 protein expression and insulin-stimulated muscle glucose transport. Likewise, chronic treatment of obese Zucker rats, an animal model of the insulin resistance syndrome, with lipoic acid enhances whole body glucose tolerance and is associated with significant improvements in insulin action on skeletal muscle glu-

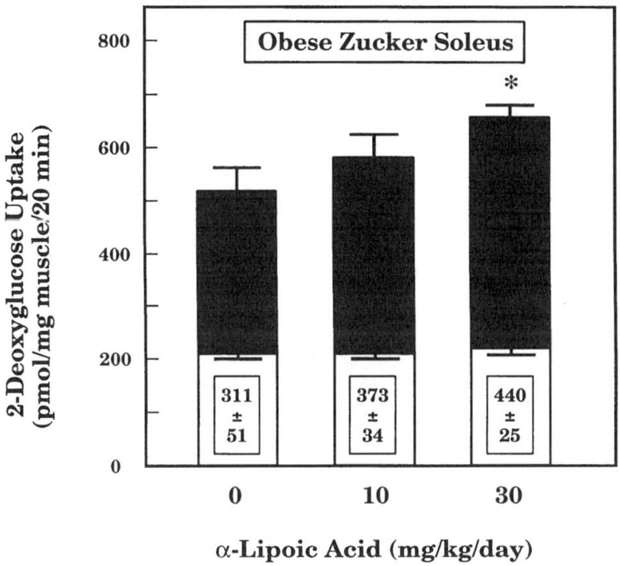

Figure 5 Effect of chronic treatment of obese Zucker rats with lipoate on in vitro insulin-stimulated glucose transport activity in the isolated soleus muscle strips. □, basal 2-deoxyglucose uptake; ■, increase in 2-deoxyglucose uptake due to insulin (2 mU/mL). This increase is shown in the box for each bar. Values are means ± SE. $*p < 0.05$ vs. 0 mg/kg lipoate.

cose transport and metabolism, and with reductions in plasma insulin and free fatty acids.

There are, however, areas where our knowledge of lipoic acid action on metabolism is incomplete. For example, we still need more information on the underlying molecular mechanism(s) responsible for the lipoic acid-induced improvement in insulin action. Some limited evidence indicates that there may be some interaction between lipoic acid and the insulin signaling cascade in the L6 muscle cell line (46) and in isolated muscle from the Zucker rat (47); however, a more complete characterization of this interaction in skeletal muscle is necessary. In addition, the relationship between lipoic acid action on skeletal muscle metabolism and its effects on cell oxidant/antioxidant status need to be more thoroughly investigated. It is clear that although investigations of the metabolic actions of lipoic acid have yielded much important information over the last few years, there is still much more work to be done

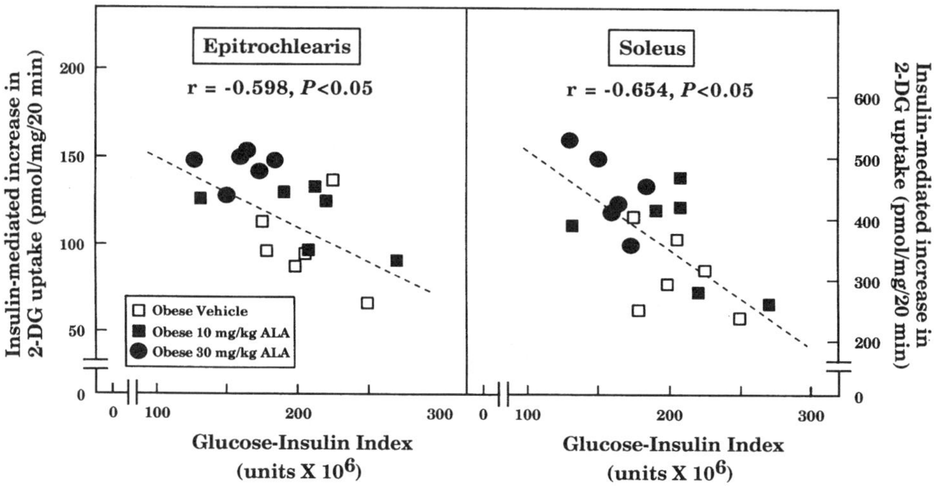

Figure 6 Correlations between the glucose-insulin index and skeletal muscle insulin-mediated glucose transport activity in epitrochlearis (left) or soleus (right) muscles from obese Zucker rats treated chronically with lipoate.

in the future to further our understanding of this important antioxidant compound.

ACKNOWLEDGMENTS

I would like to thank Dr. Stephan Jacob and Dr. Hans Tritschler for their intellectual contributions to the lipoic acid studies conducted in my laboratory and ASTA Medica AWD GmbH for continued financial support of these studies.

REFERENCES

1. Paolisso G, Giugliano D. Oxidative stress and insulin action: is there a relationship? Diabetologia 1996; 39:357–364.
2. Cominacini L, Garbin U, Cascio L. The need for a free radical initiative. Diabetologia 1996; 39:364–366.
3. Packer L, Witt EH, Tritschler HJ. Alpha-lipoic acid as a biological antioxidant. Free Radic Biol Med 1995; 19:227–250.

4. DeFronzo RA, Ferrannini E, Hendler R, Felig P, Wahren J. Regulation of splanchnic and peripheral glucose uptake by insulin and hyperglycemia in man. Diabetes 1983; 32:32–45.
5. Baron AD, Brechtel G, Wallace P, Edelman SV. Rates and tissue sites of non-insulin- and insulin-mediated glucose uptake in humans. Am J Physiol 1988; 255:E769–E774.
6. Cheatham B, Kahn CR. Insulin action and the insulin signaling network. Endocrine Rev 1995; 16:117–142.
7. Gao J, Ren J, Gulve EA, Holloszy JO. Additive effect of contractions and insulin on GLUT-4 translocation into the sarcolemma. J Appl Physiol 1994; 77:1587–1601.
8. Etgen GJ, Wilson CM, Jensen J, Cushman SW, Ivy JL. Glucose transport and cell surface GLUT-4 protein in skeletal muscle of the obese Zucker rat. Am J Physiol 1996; 271:E294–E301.
9. Holloszy JO, Narahara HT. Studies of tissue permeability. X. Changes in permeability to 3-methylglucose associated with contraction of frog muscle. J Biol Chem 1965; 240:3493–3500.
10. Garetto LP, Richter EA, Goodman MN, Ruderman NB. Enhanced muscle glucose metabolism after exercise in the rat: the two phases. Am J Physiol 1984; 246:E471–E475.
11. Nesher R, Karl IE, Kipnis DM. Dissociation of effects of insulin and contraction on glucose transport in rat epitrochlearis muscle. Am J Physiol 1985; 249:C226–C232.
12. Goodyear LJ, Hirshman MF, Horton ES. Exercise-induced translocation of skeletal muscle glucose transporters. Am J Physiol 1991; 261:E795–E799.
13. Richter EA, Garetto LP, Goodman MN, Ruderman NB. Enhanced muscle glucose metabolism after exercise: modulation by local factors. Am J Physiol 1984; 246:E476–E482.
14. Wallberg-Henriksson H, Constable SH, Young DA, Holloszy JO. Glucose transport into rat skeletal muscle: interaction between exercise and insulin. J Appl Physiol 1988; 65:909–913.
15. Henriksen EJ, Bourey RE, Rodnick KJ, Koranyi L, Permutt MA, Holloszy JO. Glucose transporter protein content and glucose transport capacity in rat skeletal muscles. Am J Physiol 1990; 259:E593–E598.
16. Goodyear LJ, Giorgino F, Balon TW, Condorelli G, Smith RJ. Effects of contractile activity on tyrosine phosphoproteins and PI 3-kinase activity in rat skeletal muscle. Am J Physiol 1995; 268:E987–E995.
17. DeFronzo RA, Ferrannini E. Insulin resistance. A multifaceted syndrome responsible for NIDDM, obesity, hypertension, dyslipidemia, and atherosclerotic cardiovascular disease. Diabetes Care 1991; 14:173–194.
18. Reaven GM. Role of insulin resistance in human disease. Diabetes 1988; 37:1595–1607.
19. Reaven GM. Role of insulin resistance in human disease (syndrome X): an expanded definition. Annu Rev Med 1993; 44:121–131.

20. Ferrannini E, Haffner SM, Mitchell BD, Stern MP. Hyperinsulinaemia: the key feature of a cardiovascular and metabolic syndrome. Diabetologia 1991; 34:416–422.
21. Reaven GM. The fourth Musketeer—from Alexander Dumas to Claude Bernard. Diabetologia 1995; 38:3–13.
22. King GL. The role of hyperglycaemia and hyperinsulinaemia in causing vascular dysfunction in diabetes. Ann Med 1996; 28:427–432.
23. Asayama K, Nakane T, Uchida N, Hayashibe H, Dobashi K, Nakazawa S. Serum antioxidant status in streptozotocin induced diabetic rats. Horm Metab Res 1994: 26:313–315.
24. Kainulainen H, Breiner M, Schurmann A, Marttinen A, Virjo A, Joost HG. In vivo glucose uptake and glucose transporter proteins GLUT1 and GLUT4 in heart and various types of skeletal muscle from streptozotocin-diabetic rats. Biochem Biophys Acta 1994; 1225:275–282.
25. Khamaisi M., Potashnik R, Tirosh A, Demshchak E, Rudich A, Tritschler H, Wessel K, Bashan N. Lipoic acid reduces glycemia and increases muscle GLUT4 content in streptozotocin-diabetic rats. Metabolism 1997; 46:763–768.
26. Bray GA. The Zucker-fatty rat: a review. Federation Proc 1977; 36:148–153.
27. Becker-Zimmerman K, Berger M, Berchtold P, Gries FA, Herberg L, Schwenen M. Treadmill training improves intravenous glucose tolerance and insulin sensitivity in fatty Zucker rats. Diabetologia 1982; 22:468–474.
28. Ionescu E, Sauter JF, Jeanrenaud B. Abnormal oral glucose tolerance in genetically obese (fa/fa) rats. Am J Physiol 1985; 248:E500–E506.
29. Turner NC, Gudgeon C, Toseland N. Effects of genetic hyperinsulinemia on vascular reactivity, blood pressure, and renal structure in the Zucker rat. J Cardiovasc Pharmacol 1995; 26:714–720.
30. Mathe D. Dyslipidemia and diabetes: animal models. Diab Metabol 1995; 21: 106–111.
31. King PA, Horton ED, Hirshman MF, Horton ES. Insulin resistance in obese Zucker rat (fa/fa) is associated with a failure of glucose transporter translocation. J Clin Invest 1993; 90:1568–1575.
32. Crettaz M, Prentki M, Zaninetti D, Jeanrenaud B. Insulin resistance in soleus muscle from obese Zucker rats: involvement of several defective sites. Biochem J 1980; 186:525–534.
33. Henriksen EJ, Jacob S. Effects of captopril on glucose transport activity in skeletal muscle of obese Zucker rats. Metabolism 1995; 44:267–272.
34. Anai M, Funaki M, Ogihara T, Terasaki J, Inukai K, Katagiri H, Fukushima Y, Yazaki Y, Kikuchi M, Oka Y, Asano T. Altered expression levels and impaired steps in pathways to phosphotidylinositol-3-kinase activation via insulin receptor substrates 1 and 2 in Zucker fatty rats. Diabetes 1998; 47:13–23.
35. Pritchard KA Jr, Patel ST, Karpen CW, Newman HA, Panganamala RV. Triglyceride-lowering effect of dietary vitamin E in stroptozotocin-induced diabetic rats: increased lipoprotein lipase activity in livers of diabetic rats fed high dietary vitamin E. Diabetes 1986; 35:278–281.

36. Nagamatsu M, Nickander KK, Schmelzer JD, Raya A, Wittrock DA, Tritschler H, Low PA. Lipoic acid improves nerve blood flow, reduces oxidative stress, and improves distal nerve conduction in experimental diabetic neuropathy. Diabetes Care 1995; 18:1160–1167.
37. Cortez MY, Torgan CE, Brozinick JT, Ivy JL. Insulin resistance of obese Zucker rats exercise trained at two different intensities. Am J Physiol 1991; 261:E613–E619.
38. Henriksen EJ, Jacob S, Fogt DL, Youngblood EB, Gödicke J. Antihypertensive agent moxonidine enhances muscle glucose transport in insulin-resistant rats. Hypertension 1997; 30:1560–1565.
39. Nourooz-Zadeh J. Antioxidant and prooxidant profile in diabetes mellitus and its relevance to the onset of the syndrome. Proceedings of the 1998 Oxygen Club of California World Congress, Santa Barbara, California, February 6–8, 1998.
40. Paolisso G, D'Amore A, Volpe C, Balbi V, Saccomanno F, Galzerano D, Giugliano D, Varricchio M, D'Onofrio F. Evidence for a relationship between oxidative stress and insulin action in NIDDM patients. Metabolism 1994; 43:1426–1429.
41. Vijayalingam S, Parthiban A, Shanmugasundaram KR, Mohan V. Abnormal antioxidant status in impaired glucose tolerance and non-insulin-dependent diabetes mellitus. Diabet Med 1996; 13:715–719.
42. Salonen JT, Nyyssonen K, Tuomainen TP, Maenpaa PH, Korpela H, Kaplan G, Lynch J, Helmrich SP, Salonen R. Increased risk of non-insulin-dependent diabetes mellitus at low plasma vitamin E concentrations: a four-year follow-up study in men. Br Med J 1995; 311:1124–1127.
43. Nourooz-Zadeh J, Rahimi A, Tajaddini-Sarmadi J, Tritschler H, Rösen P, Halliwell B, Betteridge DJ. Relationships between plasma measures of oxidative stress and metabolic control in NIDDM. Diabetologia 1997; 40:647–653.
44. Jacob S, Streeper RS, Fogt DL, Hokama JY, Tritschler HJ, Dietze GJ, Henriksen EJ. The antioxidant alpha-lipoic acid enhances insulin-stimulated glucose metabolism in insulin-resistant skeletal muscle. Diabetes 1996; 45:1024–1029.
45. Streeper RS, Henriksen EJ, Jacob S, Hokama JY, Fogt DL, Tritschler HJ, Dietze GJ. Differential effects of stereoisomers of alpha-lipoic acid on glucose metabolism in insulin-resistant rat skeletal muscle. Am J Physiol 1997; 273:E185–E191.
46. Tsakiridis T, Estrada DE, Tritschler H, Klip A. Thioctic (lipoic acid) induces protein tyrosine phosphorylation and phosphotidylinositol 3-kinase activation in muscle cells (abstr). Diabetologia 1995; 38:A132.
47. Henriksen EJ, Jacob S, Streeper RS, Fogt DL, Hokama JY, Tritschler HJ. Stimulation by alpha-lipoic of glucose transport activity in skeletal muscle of lean and obese Zucker rats. Life Sci 1997; 61:805–812.

20

Oxidative Stress and Insulin Action: A Role for Antioxidants?

Stephan Jacob, Rainer Lehmann, Kristian Rett, and Hans-Ulrich Häring

University of Tübingen, Tübingen, Germany

There is increasing evidence that alterations in the capacity to reduce oxidants, like superoxide anion radical (O_2^-), hydrogen peroxide (H_2O_2), hydroxyl radical (OH^-), nitric oxide (NO), and alkyl or peroxyl radicals, could play an important role in the pathogenesis of various diseases. The imbalance between oxidants and antioxidants in favor of the oxidants, so-called oxidative stress, results in a nonenzymatic free radical-mediated oxidation of biological molecules, membranes, and tissues associated with a variety of pathological events.

Although it is generally acknowledged that oxidative stress plays a role in the development of angiopathy in diabetes mellitus and its vascular complications (1–4), there is little information available about the impact of radical oxygen species in the pathogenesis of insulin resistance and the development of diabetes mellitus (5). Several groups have shown that the levels of free radicals are increased when metabolic control is poor. This is found in both type 1 (6) and type 2 diabetes (7,8).

Indices of this augmented oxidative stress are reduced or even reversed to normal when glycemia is well controlled, and this can be shown even after a very short period of time of improved glycemic control (9). Better metabolic control was also clearly shown to be associated with a drastic reduction of diabetic complications (10–12). These observations could suggest that oxidative stress does not play a role in the nonhyperglycemic/euglycemic state.

However, oxidative stress also seems to be present in uncomplicated type 2 (8,13) or type 1 (6) diabetes.

Furthermore, few reports describe increased radical formation in several conditions without clinical diabetes mellitus, such as dyslipidemia, impaired glucose tolerance, hypertension, coronary artery disease, aging, and smoking (1,2,14–20). These conditions have also been found to be associated with a decrease in insulin sensitivity (21–24), but contrary to the diabetic state, effects mediated by hyperglycemia can be excluded. Therefore, it seems that the origin of oxidative stress cannot be solely explained by hyperglycemia.

I. OXIDATIVE STRESS AND INSULIN SENSITIVITY—CLINICAL OBSERVATIONS

Paolisso et al. (25) demonstrated close correlations between the presence of O_2^- and insulin sensitivity in an elderly nondiabetic population. Epidemiological studies found a close correlation between low levels of antioxidants, such as vitamin E or vitamin C, and a high risk of developing frank type 2 diabetes (26,27). Several groups report a higher prevalence of radical oxygen species in prediabetic individuals who had an impaired oral glucose tolerance test (17–19).

An increase in plasma thiobarbituric acid reactive substance (TBARS) was found in healthy subjects when free fatty acids (FFA) were experimentally kept elevated by an infusion of intralipid and heparin (28); under these experimental conditions, insulin sensitivity was markedly reduced (28). It could thus be speculated that the elevation of FFA seen in patients with type 2 diabetes or with insulin resistance (29) could be a source for such an augmented oxidative stress.

II. ROLE OF IMPAIRED INSULIN ACTION IN THE PATHOGENESIS OF TYPE 2 DIABETES MELLITUS

In type 2 diabetes mellitus, plasma glucose levels are elevated as a result of an impairment of several metabolic pathways (29–31) (Table 1). Skeletal muscle is the principal organ for postprandial glucose uptake (29,30). In the pathogenesis of diabetes mellitus type 2, reduced insulin-stimulated glucose disposal (insulin resistance) plays a key role (21,29). When clearance of plasma glucose is impaired, blood glucose after a meal will remain slightly elevated

Table 1 Metabolic Alterations in Type 2 Diabetes

Diminished insulin-mediated peripheral glucose disposal and metabolism (insulin resistance)
Impaired insulin secretion (reduced first-phase response, prolonged second phase)
Decreased insulin-mediated inhibition of lipolysis
Increased gluconeogenesis

and will thus induce hyperinsulinemia to overcome resistance (Fig. 1). Hyperinsulinemia, however, will evoke an alteration of the insulin-signaling cascade, which will further augment insulin resistance, thus leading to a vicious cycle (29,30).

There is an ongoing scientific discussion as to whether insulin resistance of skeletal muscle or an impairment of insulin secretion is the first and principal disorder. However, epidemiological data indicate that reduced insulin sensitivity can already be demonstrated when insulin secretion is still adequate

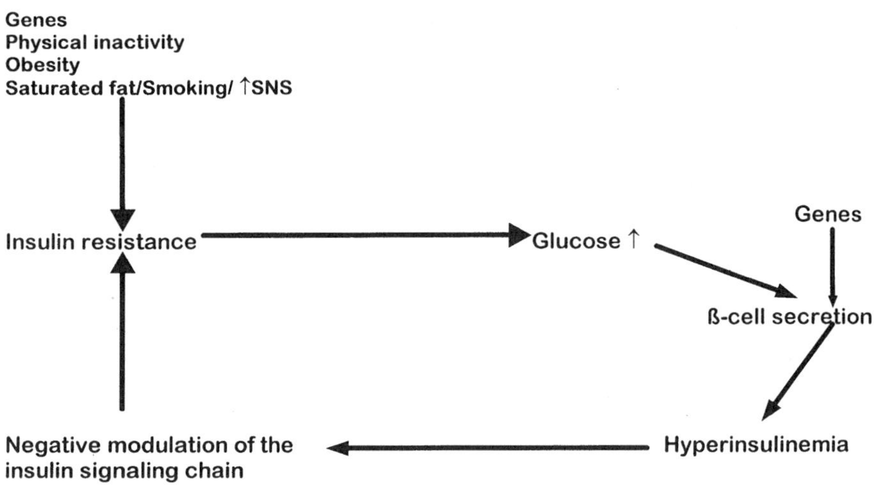

Figure 1 Vicious cycle of insulin resistance and hyperinsulinemia. Due to the reduced insulin sensitivity, peripheral glucose uptake is diminished. Therefore, plasma glucose clearance is reduced, and postprandial blood glucose will remain slightly higher. This will consequently induce hyperinsulinemia to overcome the insulin resistance. Hyperinsulinemia, however, will evoke a negative modulation of the insulin signaling chain, which will further exacerbate the insulin resistance, hence leading to a vicious cycle. SNS, sympathetic nervous system.

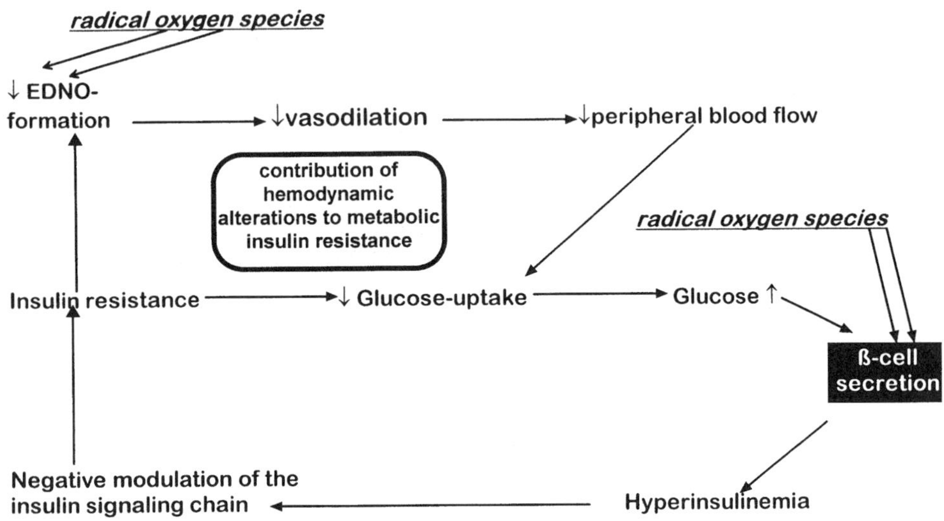

Figure 2 Model of the potential pathomechanism induced by oxidative stress. Interplay between hemodynamic and metabolic alterations. EDNO, endothelium-derived nitric oxide.

(29). Thus, it is currently believed that as long as hyperinsulinemia can compensate for insulin resistance, glucose tolerance will be normal; with progressive impairment of β-cell function, impaired glucose tolerance (iGT) or frank type 2 diabetes will be the consequence (29) (Fig. 2).

III. NITRIC OXIDE AND INSULIN SENSITIVITY

A. Nitric Oxide and Endothelial Dysfunction

Several groups have shown that insulin-resistant subjects have a reduced insulin-stimulated increase in leg blood flow; the changes in peripheral blood flow were closely associated with the degree of insulin resistance (22,32–35). This endothelial dysfunction is demonstrated not only in patients with type 2 diabetes but also in nondiabetic subjects, such as obese adolescents or first-degree relatives of patients with type 2 diabetes (33,35,36).

It seems that peripheral blood flow is augmented via an insulin-mediated NO-dependent process (Fig. 3), and inhibition of NO formation prevents the

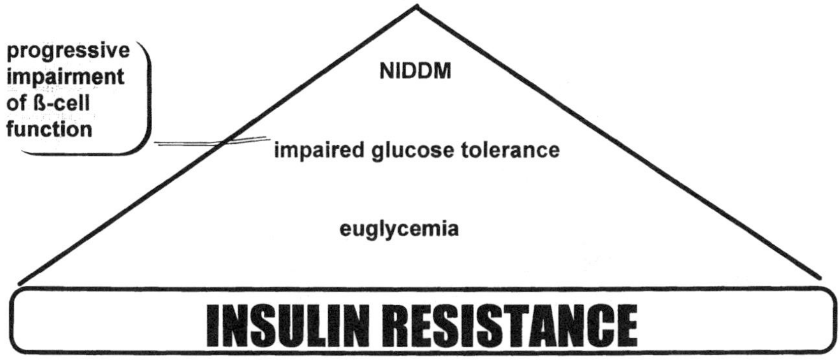

Figure 3 Progress from insulin resistance to type 2 diabetes mellitus.

insulin-induced increase in blood flow (37). Thus, NO could indirectly affect insulin sensitivity as it increases peripheral blood flow and subsequent substrate delivery to the skeletal muscle. However, there is still a debate about the clinical relevance of these findings.

B. Intracellular NO—A Direct Modulator of Glucose Uptake?

Very recently it was shown that NO synthase is also present within the skeletal muscle (38,39), and NO was found to increase glucose uptake by an insulin-independent mechanism (40–43). Furthermore, Roberts et al. (40) reported that exercise-stimulated glucose transport in the skeletal muscle of rats is NO dependent; this group provides evidence that NO is markedly involved in the regulation of exercise-induced glucose uptake. Exercise-induced skeletal muscle glucose uptake is normal, even in insulin-resistant animals (44). Thus, the exercised-induced elevation of NO availability (40,42) seems to provide an important alternative pathway. Animal studies indicate an improvement of endothelial function after exercise training (45).

C. NO—A Radical Scavenger

NO is also known to act as a radical scavenger itself (46,47). An increased availability of NO was associated with a decrease in the levels of superoxide

(47). Furthermore, exercise training was not only found to improve metabolism and endothelial function (40,42,45) but also antioxidant defense (48); therefore, one of the beneficial effects of exercise could be mediated by the increase of antioxidant defense mechanism. Indirect support for the association between NO availability and insulin sensitivity emerges from a clinical study, in which L-arginine, the substrate required for NO synthesis, was infused and insulin sensitivity and endothelial function was improved (49); the increase of insulin sensitivity, however, remained significant after adjustment for changes in blood flow (49).

It is thus conceivable that an increase in radical oxygen species may reduce the availability of NO, and this consequently would contribute to the endothelial dysfunction and possibly to the development of insulin resistance (Fig. 3).

D. Homocysteine, NO, and Insulin Sensitivity

Homocysteine levels were found to be significantly higher in patients with coronary artery disease and in those with diabetes mellitus (50–54). Elevated homocysteine levels induce oxidative stress and reduce NO availability (55); this can contribute to endothelial dysfunction. It seems possible that hyperhomocysteinemia could also alter insulin sensitivity by this mechanism. Therefore, it remains to be clarified whether there are any interactions between elevated homocysteine levels and the development of insulin resistance in nondiabetic subjects.

The interesting observation of an augmented oxidative stress, insulin resistance, and elevated homocysteine levels in smokers (14,23,24,50) suggests some interactions. However, this still remains to be evaluated.

IV. INTERVENTIONS KNOWN TO ALTER RADICAL OXYGEN SPECIES

A. Lifestyle

A diet high in saturated fat and low in fiber and a low level of physical activity are associated with an increased risk of developing type 2 diabetes mellitus (26,27). Modifications of these factors are known to improve metabolic control and insulin sensitivity (56) but should be also expected to reduce oxidative stress. Experimental data suggest that exercise training can improve insulin resistance in parallel with a better antioxidant defense (45). One explanation for this could be the improvement of NO availability in the skeletal muscle (see above).

Epidemiological data support the protective role of regular exercise: Greater physical activity (57–60) reduces the risk of developing type 2 diabetes mellitus, even in those with a family history of type 2 diabetes. Because smoking is known to be associated with an increased oxidative stress (14) and insulin resistance (23,24), this association could be one mechanism by which smoking cessation improves insulin sensitivity (61).

B. Pharmacological Intervention

Several compounds with an antioxidant potential were found to modify insulin sensitivity.

1. *Troglitazone*

Troglitazone, a thiazolidinedione which is the first compound of the new class of insulin sensitizers (62,63), improves glycemia and dyslipidemia by reducing insulin resistance and hyperinsulinemia in type 2 diabetes mellitus (64) and also in normoglycemic subjects with insulin resistance (65,66). Experimental data indicate that troglitazone improves insulin action by various mechanisms (67–69) (Table 2).

Troglitazone has a similar structure to vitamin E and is also known to be a potent radical scavenger (70–72). At present, it is not known whether the radical scavenging ability of troglitazone is relevant for its beneficial effect on insulin resistance. Pioglitazone, another thiazolidinedione, is also a potent insulin sensitizer, but an experimental study recently reported that it had no radical scavenging property (72).

2. *Glutathione*

Administration of glutathione was found to be advantageous in type 2 diabetics and those with impaired glucose tolerance (Table 2). Glutathione improved insulin secretion in patients with iGT (73). Because insulin secretion is impaired in type 2 diabetes (29) and because recent data suggest that lipotoxicity might play a role in decreasing β-cell function (74,75), glutathione could improve β-cell function by protecting the β-cell. However, this hypothesis still needs to be tested.

Glutathione also improves insulin sensitivity in patients with type 2 diabetes after acute (76) and chronic administration (49). In type 2 diabetes, a

Table 2 Synopsis of the Effects of Interventions Improving Antioxidant Capacity and Insulin Sensitivity

Intervention	Direct	Indirect	Other effects	Ref.
Diet	yes			1
Exercise	yes	endothelial function	↑ NO-availability	2–9
Smoking cessation	?	endothelial function		10,11
Troglitazone	yes	?endothelial function	PPARγ ↓ glucose toxicity ↑ LDL-oxidation	12–19
Glutathione	?yes	endothelial function	↑ insulin secretion in iGT ↑ microviscosity ↓ "lipotoxicity"	20–24
Vitamin E	?	endothelial function	↑ vasodilation no effect on insulin secretion	25–32
Vitamin C	?	endothelial function	↑ insulin-stimulated glucose uptake ↑ vasodilation no effect on insulin secretion	31,33–35
Thioctic acid	? yes	↑ insulin-independent glucose uptake endothelial function ↓ of adhesion molecules NF-κ B↓	↑ insulin-stimulated glucose uptake ↑ vasodilation ↑ microcirculation	36–45
Others				
ACE inhibitors	yes	endothelial function	insulin-stimulated glucose uptake is kinin-mediated	46–48
Vasodilating beta-blockers	?	endothelial function		49,50

reduced plasma GSH/GSSG ratio was found; this was negatively associated with the levels of fasting FFA ($r = -0.53$; $p < 0.05$) (49). In an experimental study with healthy volunteers, ''metabolic oxidative stress'' was induced by infusion of intralipid and heparin, resulting in a marked rise of FFA levels. This was associated with an increase of indicators of oxidative stress, as reflected by increased TBARS and a reduced GSH/GSSG ratio (28). In contrast, the infusion of glutathione diminished the negative effect of the sustained elevation of FFA; although FFA were elevated, the alteration of both oxidative stress and insulin-stimulated glucose uptake were markedly attenuated when glutathione was coinfused with intralipid. In addition, glutathione even improved insulin sensitivity and oxidative stress in the control experiment in which no intralipid was given (28).

Ammon et al. (77) showed that the administration of acetyl-cysteine, a compound that could increase endogenous formation of glutathione, improved glucose disposal in healthy volunteers; this was associated with an improved GSH/GSSG ratio. Furthermore, experimental studies indicate a protective role of glutathione on endothelial function (78).

3. Vitamin E

A large epidemiological study indicates that a low level of vitamin E confers a marked risk for the development of a type 2 diabetes mellitus (26). Low levels of vitamin E are also documented in patients with coronary artery disease (20). A regular intake of higher doses of vitamin E was associated with a marked decline in vascular events in coronary artery disease patients (79). These observations suggest a role for vitamin E and/or oxidative stress in these chronic diseases.

In experimental studies, it was shown that vitamin E has beneficial effects on insulin sensitivity. Fructose feeding induces insulin resistance and hypertension in rats; this is also associated with an increase in radical oxygen species formation (80). Vitamin E administration prevented not only the diet-induced alterations in insulin sensitivity but also reduced oxidative stress. Finally, several clinical studies by Paolisso's group suggest that vitamin E intake improves insulin sensitivity as measured by the glucose clamp technique in healthy and diabetic subjects (81–84).

Vitamin E could also modulate insulin sensitivity by indirect effects because it can improve endothelial function. It was shown that in diabetes mellitus endothelial dysfunction is present (1,4), and it is suggested that oxidative stress reduces vasodilatation (3,85,86). Vitamin E administration restores this defect (3,85,86).

If endothelial dysfunction is involved in modulating insulin's action, a restoration of endothelial function should also augment insulin sensitivity (see III.A and Table 2, Fig. 4). Furthermore, vitamin E improves insulin secretion in experimentally induced (type 1) diabetes mellitus (87). At present, however, there are no data concerning the effect of vitamin E on β-cell function in type 2 diabetes mellitus.

4. *Vitamin C*

There are a few studies indicating a role for vitamin C in modulating insulin sensitivity. Epidemiological data identify low serum levels of the vitamin as a risk factor for the development of type 2 diabetes mellitus (27). Experimental data describe a protective role of vitamin C on the age-associated deterioration of insulin sensitivity (88). Clinical studies describe an enhanced insulin-stimulated glucose uptake in a glucose clamp study after acute vitamin C treatment in healthy subjects and in those with type 2 diabetes (89,90); the beneficial effects on insulin sensitivity were closely associated with the increases in the plasma levels of the vitamin C (90). Experimental studies indicate also a beneficial effect on endothelial function in experimental polyneuropathy (3). Clinical studies also describe an improvement of endothelial dysfunction (91).

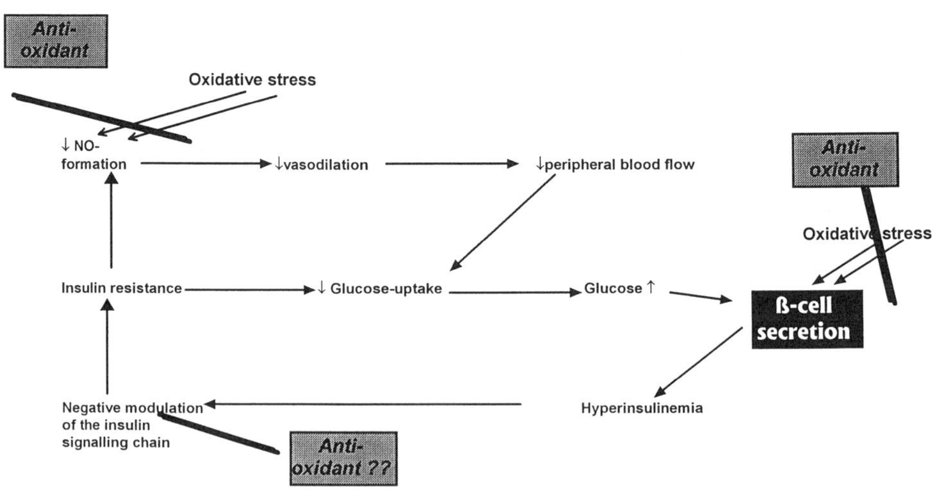

Figure 4 Decrease of insulin resistance by antioxidants (hypothetical mechanisms).

5. α-Lipoic Acid

Thioctic acid, also known as α-lipoic acid, was found to improve insulin action in various experimental models (92–95). Its action seems to involve interaction with the insulin receptor signaling cascade and potentially also insulin-independent steps (see Chaps. 18 and 19). In vivo experimental studies found an improvement of insulin sensitivity and glucose tolerance after the administration of the racemic mixture (95,96).

Clinical pilot trials suggest that this compound might also have beneficial effects in humans, because insulin resistance was improved after acute or chronic intravenous administration of α-lipoic acid (97–99). Recently, a small placebo-controlled pilot trial found an improvement of insulin sensitivity in patients with type 2 diabetes mellitus after oral administration (100). The changes in insulin sensitivity seen after the active treatment was significantly different from that seen in placebo: whereas insulin sensitivity decreased in the control group, it improved after α-lipoic acid. Furthermore, thioctic acid improves endothelial function (101) and microcirculation by reducing adhesion molecules (102) and preserves endothelial structure (103).

6. Other Compounds

There are several other compounds with antioxidant activity also shown to have a beneficial effect on insulin sensitivity. Two groups of antihypertensive agents are known to improve insulin sensitivity and oxidative stress.

Angiotensin-converting enzyme inhibitors increase the availability of kinins by inhibition of kininase II (104) and consequently NO (47). They were shown to augment insulin-stimulated glucose uptake in clinical and experimental studies (104,105). Recent data suggest that treatment with Ramipril has pronounced effects on NO synthase expression and NO formation and a concomitant decrease in superoxide accumulation, which was associated with an extended lifespan in the angiotensin-converting enzyme treated rats (47).

The vasodilating beta-blockers carvedilol and celiprolol have a marked antioxidant capacity (46,106,107) and were found to improve endothelial function (108). In clinical studies they increased insulin sensitivity as documented by the glucose clamp (109–111).

V. CONCLUSION AND OUTLOOK

At present, experimental and clinical data suggest but do not prove an association between insulin sensitivity and oxidative stress. Furthermore, experimental and some clinical studies suggest a beneficial effect on insulin secretion or insulin action after treatment with certain antioxidants. Currently, it is still unknown whether the effects on insulin sensitivity are modulated by direct mechanisms, for instance on the insulin receptor-signal transduction cascade, or whether metabolism improves indirectly such by an improvement of endothelial function.

It is necessary and seems to be promising to analyze further the association between oxidative stress and insulin action (112); this involves both the quantitative assessment of insulin sensitivity and the radical oxygen species respective of the oxidant defense system.

If an antioxidant is supposed to improve insulin sensitivity by decreasing oxidative stress, this should be associated with a decrease in radical oxygen species. Furthermore, it would be important to show a dose-response relationship, that is, the more the oxidative stress is reduced, the better the insulin resistance is improved.

To date, only small clinical trials with a short duration of treatment have been conducted (Table 2). It is absolutely necessary in the near future to conduct larger trials involving intensive assessment of the oxidative stress and antioxidant defense and the exact analysis of insulin sensitivity and metabolic control. Therefore, there is a need for a ''radical initiative'' (113).

REFERENCES

1. Giugliano D, Ceriello A, Paolisso G. Oxidative stress and diabetic vascular complications. Diabetes Care 1996; 19:257–267.
2. Giugliano D, Ceriello A, Paolisso G. Diabetes mellitus, hypertension, and cardiovascular disease: which role for oxidative stress? Metabolism 1995; 44:363–368.
3. Cotter MA, Love A, Watt MJ, Cameron NE, Dines KC. Effects of natural free radical scavengers on peripheral nerve and neurovascular function in diabetic rats. Diabetologia 1995; 38:1285–1294.
4. Brownlee M, Cerami A, Vlassara H. Advanced glycosylation end products in tissue and the biochemical basis of diabetic complications. N Engl J Med 1988; 318:1315–1321.
5. Paolisso G, Giugliano D. Oxidative stress and insulin action: is there a relationship? Diabetologia 1996; 39:357–363.
6. Santini SA, Marra G, Giardina B, Cotroneo P, Mordente A, Martorana GE, et al. Defective plasma antioxidant defenses and enhanced susceptibility to lipid peroxidation in uncomplicated IDDM. Diabetes 1997; 46:1853–1858.
7. Nourooz Zadeh J, Tajaddini Sarmadi J, McCarthy S, Betteridge DJ, Wolff SP.

Elevated levels of authentic plasma hydroperoxides in NIDDM. Diabetes 1995; 44:1054–1058.

8. Ceriello A, Bortolotti N, Falleti E, Taboga C, Tonutti L, Crescentini A, et al. Total radical-trapping antioxidant parameter in NIDDM patients. Diabetes Care 1997; 20:194–197.
9. Peuchant E, Delmas Beauvieux MC, Couchouron A, Dubourg L, Thomas MJ, Perromat A, et al. Short-term insulin therapy and normoglycemia. Effects on erythrocyte lipid peroxidation in NIDDM patients. Diabetes Care 1997; 20: 202–207.
10. Lasker RD. The diabetes control and complications trial. Implications for policy and practice. N Engl J Med 1993; 329:1035–1036.
11. The effect of intensive treatment of diabetes on the development and progression of long-term complications in insulin-dependent diabetes mellitus. The Diabetes Control and Complications Trial Research Group. N Engl J Med 1993; 329:977–986.
12. Implications of the Diabetes Control and Complications Trial. American Diabetes Association. Diabetes 1993; 42:1555–1558.
13. Freitas JP, Filipe PM, Rodrigo FG. Lipid peroxidation in type 2 normolipidemic diabetic patients. Diabetes Res Clin Pract 1997; 36:71–75.
14. Marangon K, Herbeth B, Lecomte E, PaulDauphin A, Grolier P, Chancerelle Y, et al. Diet, antioxidant status, and smoking habits in French men. Am J Clin Nutr 1998; 67:231–239.
15. Paolisso G, Di Maro G, Pizza G, D'Amore A, Sgambato S, Tesauro P, et al. Plasma GSH/GSSG affects glucose homeostasis in healthy subjects and non-insulin-dependent diabetics. Am J Physiol 1992; 263:E435–E440.
16. Paolisso G, D'Amore A, Volpe C, Balbi V, Saccomanno F, Galzerano D, et al. Evidence for a relationship between oxidative stress and insulin action in non-insulin-dependent (type II) diabetic patients. Metabolism 1994; 43:1426–1429.
17. Vijayalingam S, Parthiban A, Shanmugasundaram KR, Mohan V. Abnormal antioxidant status in impaired glucose tolerance and non-insulin-dependent diabetes mellitus. Diabet Med 1996; 13:715–719.
18. Sadasivudu B, Sasikala M, Sailaja V, Reddy SS. Serum malondialdehyde, insulin, glucose and lipid profile in hypertension. Med Sci Res 1997; 25:631–633.
19. Niskanen LK, Salonen JT, Nyyssonen K, Uusitupa MI. Plasma lipid peroxidation and hyperglycaemia: a connection through hyperinsulinaemia? Diabet Med 1995; 12:802–808.
20. Regnstrom J, Nilsson J, Moldeus P, Strom K, Bavenholm P, Tornvall P, et al. Inverse relation between the concentration of low-density-lipoprotein vitamin E and severity of coronary artery disease. Am J Clin Nutr 1996; 63:377–385.
21. DeFronzo RA, Ferrannini E. Insulin resistance. A multifaceted syndrome responsible for NIDDM, obesity, hypertension, dyslipidemia, and atherosclerotic cardiovascular disease. Diabetes Care 1991; 14:173–194.

22. Lind L, Lithell H. Decreased peripheral blood flow in the pathogenesis of the metabolic syndrome comprising hypertension, hyperlipidemia, and hyperinsulinemia. Am Heart J 1993; 125:1494–1497.
23. Eliasson B, Attvall S, Taskinen MR, Smith U. The insulin resistance syndrome in smokers is related to smoking habits. Arterioscler Thromb 1994; 14:1946–1950.
24. Eliasson B, Mero N, Taskinen MR, Smith U. The insulin resistance syndrome and postprandial lipid intolerance in smokers. Atherosclerosis 1997; 129:79–88.
25. Paolisso G, D'Amore A, Di Maro G, Galzerano D, Tesauro P, Varricchio M, et al. Evidence for a relationship between free radicals and insulin action in the elderly. Metabolism 1993; 42:659–663.
26. Salonen JT, Nyyssonen K, Tuomainen TP, Maenpaa PH, Korpela H, Kaplan GA, et al. Increased risk of non-insulin dependent diabetes mellitus at low plasma vitamin E concentrations: a four year follow up study in men. BMJ 1995; 311:1124–1127.
27. Feskens EJ, Virtanen SM, Rasanen L, Tuomilehto J, Stengard J, Pekkanen J, et al. Dietary factors determining diabetes and impaired glucose tolerance. A 20-year follow-up of the Finnish and Dutch cohorts of the Seven Countries Study. Diabetes Care 1995; 18:1104–1112.
28. Paolisso G, Gambardella A, Tagliamonte MR, Saccomanno F, Salvatore T, Gualdiero P, et al. Does free fatty acid infusion impair insulin action also through an increase in oxidative stress? J Clin Endocrinol Metab 1996; 81:4244–4248.
29. DeFronzo RA, Bonadonna RC, Ferrannini E. Pathogenesis of NIDDM. A balanced overview. Diabetes Care 1992; 15:318–368.
30. Häring H-U, Mehnert H. Pathogenesis of type 2 (non-insulin-dependent) diabetes mellitus: candidates for a signal transmitter defect causing insulin resistance of the skeletal muscle. Diabetologia 1993; 36:176–182.
31. Kellerer M, Häring HU. Pathogenesis of insulin resistance: modulation of the insulin signal at receptor level. Diabetes Res Clin Pract 1995; 28(suppl):S173–S177.
32. Baron AD. Hemodynamic actions of insulin. Am J Physiol 1994; 267:E187–E202.
33. Baron AD, Brechtel Hook G, Johnson A, Hardin D. Skeletal muscle blood flow. A possible link between insulin resistance and blood pressure. Hypertension 1993; 21:129–135.
34. Petrie JR, Ueda S, Webb DJ, Elliott HL, Connell JM. Endothelial nitric oxide production and insulin sensitivity. A physiological link with implications for pathogenesis of cardiovascular disease. Circulation 1996; 93:1331–1333.
35. Rocchini AP, Moorehead C, Katch V, Key J, Finta KM. Forearm resistance vessel abnormalities and insulin resistance in obese adolescents. Hypertension 1992; 19:615–620.
36. Rittig K, Balletshofer B, Enderle M, Volk A, Maerker E, Pfohl M, et al. Endo-

thelial dysfunction and intima-media thickness in healthy but insulin-resistant first degree realtives of type 2 diabetics (abstr). Diabetes 1998; 47:A120.
37. Steinberg HO, Brechtel G, Johnson A, Fineberg N, Baron AD. Insulin-mediated skeletal muscle vasodilation is nitric oxide dependent. A novel action of insulin to increase nitric oxide release. J Clin Invest 1994; 94:1172–1179.
38. Kapur S, Bedard S, Marcotte B, Cote CH, Marette A. Expression of nitric oxide synthase in skeletal muscle: a novel role for nitric oxide as a modulator of insulin action. Diabetes 1997; 46:1691–1700.
39. Frandsen U, Lopez Figueroa M, Hellsten Y. Localization of nitric oxide synthase in human skeletal muscle. Biochem Biophys Res Commun 1996; 227: 88–93.
40. Roberts CK, Barnard RJ, Scheck SH, Balon TW. Exercise-stimulated glucose transport in skeletal muscle is nitric oxide dependent. Am J Physiol 1997; 273: E220–E225.
41. Young ME, Leighton B. Evidence for altered sensitivity of the nitric oxide/cGMP signalling cascade in insulin-resistant skeletal muscle. Biochem J 1998; 329:73–79.
42. Balon TW, Nadler JL. Evidence that nitric oxide increases glucose transport in skeletal muscle. J Appl Physiol 1997; 82:359–363.
43. Etgen GJ, Jr., Fryburg DA, Gibbs EM. Nitric oxide stimulates skeletal muscle glucose transport through a calcium/contraction- and phosphatidylinositol-3-kinase-independent pathway. Diabetes 1997; 46:1915–1919.
44. Kusunoki M, Storlien LH, MacDessi J, Oakes ND, Kennedy C, Chisholm DJ, et al. Muscle glucose uptake during and after exercise is normal in insulin-resistant rats. Am J Physiol 1993; 264:E167–E172.
45. Sakamoto S, Minami K, Niwa Y, Ohnaka M, Nakaya Y, Mizuno A, et al. Effect of exercise training and food restriction on endothelium-dependent relaxation in the Otsuka Long-Evans Tokushima fatty rat, a model of spontaneous NIDDM. Diabetes 1998; 47:82–86.
46. Mehta JL, Lopez LM, Chen L, Cox OE. Alterations in nitric oxide synthase activity, superoxide anion generation, and platelet aggregation in systemic hypertension, and effects of celiprolol. Am J Cardiol 1994; 74:901–905.
47. Wiemer G, Linz W, Hatrik S, Scholkens BA, Malinski T. Angiotensin-converting enzyme inhibition alters nitric oxide and superoxide release in normotensive and hypertensive rats. Hypertension 1997; 30:1183–1190.
48. De Angelis KL, Oliveira AR, Werner A, Bock P, Bello Klein A, Fernandes TG, et al. Exercise training in aging: hemodynamic, metabolic, and oxidative stress evaluations. Hypertension 1997; 30:767–771.
49. Paolisso G, Tagliamonte MR, Marfella R, Verrazzo G, D'Onofrio F, Giugliano D. L-Arginine but not D-arginine stimulates insulin-mediated glucose uptake. Metabolism 1997; 46:1068–1073.
50. Welch GN, Upchurch GR, Jr., Loscalzo J. Homocysteine, oxidative stress, and vascular disease. Hosp Pract Off Ed 1997; 32:81-2,85,88–92.
51. Hoogeveen EK, Kostense PJ, Beks PJ, Mackaay AJ, Jakobs C, Bouter LM, et al.

Hyperhomocysteinemia is associated with an increased risk of cardiovascular disease, especially in non-insulin-dependent diabetes mellitus: a population-based study. Arterioscler Thromb Vasc Biol 1998; 18:133–138.
52. Hofmann MA, Kohl B, Zumbach MS, Borcea V, Bierhaus A, Henkels M, et al. Hyperhomocyst(e)inemia and endothelial dysfunction in IDDM. Diabetes Care 1997; 20:1880–1886.
53. Araki A, Sako Y, Ito H. Plasma homocysteine concentrations in Japanese patients with non-insulin-dependent diabetes mellitus: effect of parenteral methylcobalamin treatment. Atherosclerosis 1993; 103:149–157.
54. Stampfer MJ, Malinow MR, Willett WC, Newcomer LM, Upson B, Ullmann D, et al. A prospective study of plasma homocyst(e)ine and risk of myocardial infarction in US physicians. JAMA 1992; 268:877–881.
55. Upchurch GR, Jr., Welch GN, Fabian AJ, Freedman JE, Johnson JL, Keaney JF, Jr., et al. Homocyst(e)ine decreases bioavailable nitric oxide by a mechanism involving glutathione peroxidase. J Biol Chem 1997; 272:17012–17017.
56. O'Dea K. Marked improvement in carbohydrate and lipid metabolism in diabetic Australian aborigines after temporary reversion to traditional lifestyle. Diabetes 1984; 33:596–603.
57. Manson JE, Nathan DM, Krolewski AS, Stampfer MJ, Willett WC, Hennekens CH. A prospective study of exercise and incidence of diabetes among US male physicians. JAMA 1992; 268:63–67.
58. Manson JE, Rimm EB, Stampfer MJ, Colditz GA, Willett WC, Krolewski AS, et al. Physical activity and incidence of non-insulin-dependent diabetes mellitus in women. Lancet 1991; 338:774–778.
59. Lynch J, Helmrich SP, Lakka TA, Kaplan GA, Cohen RD, Salonen R, et al. Moderately intense physical activities and high levels of cardiorespiratory fitness reduce the risk of non-insulin-dependent diabetes mellitus in middle-aged men. Arch Intern Med 1996; 156:1307–1314.
60. Helmrich SP, Ragland DR, Leung RW, Paffenbarger RS Jr. Physical activity and reduced occurrence of non-insulin-dependent diabetes mellitus. N Engl J Med 1991; 325:147–152.
61. Eliasson B, Attvall S, Taskinen MR, Smith U. Smoking cessation improves insulin sensitivity in healthy middle-aged men. Eur J Clin Invest 1997; 27:450–456.
62. Bethge H, Häring HU. The thiazolidinediones—a novel approach for the treatment of type-2 diabetes. Arzneim Forsch Drug Res 1998; 48:97–119.
63. Hofmann CA, Colca JR. New oral thiazolidinedione antidiabetic agents act as insulin sensitizers. Diabetes Care 1992; 15:1075–1078.
64. Inzucchi SE, Maggs DG, Spollett GR, Page SL, Rife FS, Walton V, et al. Efficacy and metabolic effects of metformin and troglitazone in type II diabetes mellitus. N Engl J Med 1998; 338:867–872.
65. Nolan JJ, Ludvik B, Beerdsen P, Joyce M, Olefsky J. Improvement in glucose tolerance and insulin resistance in obese subjects treated with troglitazone. N Engl J Med 1994; 331:1188–1193.

66. Cavaghan MK, Ehrmann DA, Byrne MM, Polonsky KS. Treatment with the oral antidiabetic agent troglitazone improves beta cell responses to glucose in subjects with impaired glucose tolerance. J Clin Invest 1997; 100:530–537.
67. Kellerer M, Kroder G, Tippmer S, Berti L, Kiehn R, Mosthaf L, et al. Troglitazone prevents glucose-induced insulin resistance of insulin receptor in rat-1 fibroblasts. Diabetes 1994; 43:447–453.
68. Peraldi P, Xu M, Spiegelman BM. Thiazolidinediones block tumor necrosis factor-alpha-induced inhibition of insulin signaling. J Clin Invest 1997; 100: 1863–1869.
69. Shimabukuro M, Zhou YT, Lee Y, Unger RH. Troglitazone lowers islet fat and restores beta cell function of Zucker diabetic fatty rats. J Biol Chem 1998; 273: 3547–3550.
70. Cominacini L, Garbin U, Pasini AF, Campagnola M, Davoli A, Foot E, et al. Troglitazone reduces LDL oxidation and lowers plasma E-selectin concentration, in NIDDM patients. Diabetes 1998; 47:130–133.
71. Cominacini L, Garbin U, Pastorino AM, Campagnola M, Fratta Pasini A, Davoli A, et al. Effects of troglitazone on in vitro oxidation of LDL and HDL induced by copper ions and endothelial cells. Diabetologia 1997; 40:165–172.
72. Inoue I, Katayama S, Takahashi K, Negishi K, Miyazaki T, Sonoda M, et al. Troglitazone has a scavenging effect on reactive oxygen species. Biochem Biophys Res Commun 1997; 235:113–116.
73. Paolisso G, Giugliano D, Pizza G, Gambardella A, Tesauro P, Varricchio M, et al. Glutathione infusion potentiates glucose-induced insulin secretion in aged patients with impaired glucose tolerance. Diabetes Care 1992; 15:1–7.
74. Unger RH. Lipotoxicity in the pathogenesis of obesity-dependent NIDDM. Genetic and clinical implications. Diabetes 1995; 44:863–870.
75. Lee Y, Hirose H, Ohneda M, Johnson JH, McGarry JD, Unger RH. Beta-cell lipotoxicity in the pathogenesis of non-insulin-dependent diabetes mellitus of obese rats: impairment in adipocyte-beta-cell relationships. Proc Natl Acad Sci USA 1994; 91:10878–10882.
76. Laurenti O, Bravi MC, Cassone Faldetta M, Ferri C, Bianco G, Armiento A, et al. Glutathione effects on insulin resistance in non-insulin-dependent diabetes mellitus (abstr). Diabetologia 1997; 40:A305.
77. Ammon HP, Muller PH, Eggstein M, Wintermantel C, Aigner B, Safayhi H, et al. Increase in glucose consumption by acetylcysteine during hyperglycemic clamp. A study with healthy volunteers. Arzneim Forsch Drug Res 1992; 42: 642–645.
78. Brigelius Flohe R, Friedrichs B, Maurer S, Schultz M, Streicher R. Interleukin-1-induced nuclear factor kappa B activation is inhibited by overexpression of phospholipid hydroperoxide glutathione peroxidase in a human endothelial cell line. Biochem J 1997; 328:199–203.
79. Stephens NG, Parsons A, Schofield PM, Kelly F, Cheeseman K, Mitchinson MJ. Randomised controlled trial of vitamin E in patients with coronary disease: Cambridge Heart Antioxidant Study (CHAOS). Lancet 1996; 347:781–786.

80. Faure P, Rossini E, Lafond JL, Richard MJ, Favier A, Halimi S. Vitamin E improves the free radical defense system potential and insulin sensitivity of rats fed high fructose diets. J Nutr 1997; 127:103–107.
81. Paolisso G, D'Amore A, Giugliano D, Ceriello A, Varricchio M, D'Onofrio F. Pharmacologic doses of vitamin E improve insulin action in healthy subjects and non-insulin-dependent diabetic patients. Am J Clin Nutr 1993; 57:650–656.
82. Paolisso G, D'Amore A, Galzerano D, Balbi V, Giugliano D, Varricchio M, et al. Daily vitamin E supplements improve metabolic control but not insulin secretion in elderly type II diabetic patients. Diabetes Care 1993; 16:1433–1437.
83. Paolisso G, Di Maro G, Galzerano D, Cacciapuoti F, Varricchio G, Varricchio M, et al. Pharmacological doses of vitamin E and insulin action in elderly subjects. Am J Clin Nutr 1994; 59:1291–1296.
84. Paolisso G, Gambardella A, Giugliano D, Galzerano D, Amato L, Volpe C, et al. Chronic intake of pharmacological doses of vitamin E might be useful in the therapy of elderly patients with coronary heart disease. Am J Clin Nutr 1995; 61:848–852.
85. Rosen P, Ballhausen T, Bloch W, Addicks K. Endothelial relaxation is disturbed by oxidative stress in the diabetic rat heart: influence of tocopherol as antioxidant. Diabetologia 1995; 38:1157–1168.
86. Keegan A, Walbank H, Cotter MA, Cameron NE. Chronic vitamin E treatment prevents defective endothelium-dependent relaxation in diabetic rat aorta. Diabetologia 1995; 38:1475–1478.
87. Beales PE, Williams AJ, Albertini MC, Pozzilli P. Vitamin E delays diabetes onset in the non-obese diabetic mouse. Horm Metab Res 1994; 26:450–452.
88. Moustafa SA, Webster JE, Mattar FE. Effects of aging and antioxidants on glucose transport in rat adipocytes. Gerontology 1995; 41:301–307.
89. Paolisso G, Balbi V, Volpe C, Varricchio G, Gambardella A, Saccomanno F, et al. Metabolic benefits deriving from chronic vitamin C supplementation in aged non-insulin dependent diabetics. J Am Coll Nutr 1995; 14:387–392.
90. Paolisso G, D'Amore A, Balbi V, Volpe C, Galzerano D, Giugliano D, et al. Plasma vitamin C affects glucose homeostasis in healthy subjects and in non-insulin-dependent diabetics. Am J Physiol 1994; 266:E261–E268.
91. Timimi FK, Ting HH, Haley EA, Roddy MA, Ganz P, Creager MA. Vitamin C improves endothelium-dependent vasodilation in patients with insulin-dependent diabetes mellitus. J Am Coll Cardiol 1998; 31:552–557.
92. Streeper RS, Henriksen EJ, Jacob S, Hokama JY, Fogt DL, Tritschler HJ. Differential effects of lipoic acid stereoisomers on glucose metabolism in insulin-resistant skeletal muscle. Am J Physiol 1997; 273:E185–E191.
93. Estrada DE, Ewart HS, Tsakiridis T, Volchuk A, Ramlal T, Tritschler H, et al. Stimulation of glucose uptake by the natural coenzyme alpha-lipoic acid/thioctic acid: participation of elements of the insulin signalling pathway. Diabetes 1996; 45:1798–1804.

94. Strodter D, Lehmann E, Lehmann U, Tritschler HJ, Bretzel RG, Federlin K. The influence of thioctic acid on metabolism and function of the diabetic heart. Diabetes Res Clin Pract 1995; 29:19–26.
95. Khamisi M, Potashnik R, Tirosh A, Demshchak E, Rudich A, Tritschler H, et al. Lipoic acid reduces glycemia and increases muscle GLUT4 content in streptozotocin-diabetic rats. Metabolism 1997; 46:763–768.
96. Jacob S, Streeper RS, Fogt DL, Hokama JY, Tritschler HJ, Dietze GJ, et al. The antioxidant alpha-lipoic acid enhance insulin-stimulated glucose metabolism in insulin-resistant rat skeletal muscle. Diabetes 1996; 45:1024–1029.
97. Jacob S, Henriksen EJ, Tritschler HJ, Augustin JH, Dietze GJ. Improvement of insulin-stimulated glucose-disposal in type 2 diabetes after repeated parenteral administration of thioctic acid. Exp Clin Endocrinol Diabetes 1996; 104:284–288.
98. Jacob S, Henriksen EJ, Schiemann AL, Simon I, Clancy DE, Tritschler HJ, et al. Enhancement of glucose disposal in patients with type 2 diabetes by alpha-lipoic acid. Arzneimittelforschung 1995; 45:872–874.
99. Rett K, Wicklmayr M, Maerker E, Ruus P, Nehrdich D, Herrmann R, et al. Effect of acute infusion of thioctic acid on oxidative and non-oxidative metabolism in obese subjects with NIDDM (abstr). Diabetologia 1995; 38:A41.
100. Jacob S, Ruus P, Rett K, et al. Oral lipoic acid improves insulin sensitivity—results of a placebo controled trial in patients with type 2 diabetes. Free Radic Biol Med 1999; 27(3–4):309–314.
101. Nagamatsu M, Nickander KK, Schmelzer JD, Raya A, Wittrock DA, Tritschler H, et al. Lipoic acid improves nerve blood flow, reduces oxidative stress, and improves distal nerve conduction in experimental diabetic neuropathy. Diabetes Care 1995; 18:1160–1167.
102. Kusterer K, Haak E, Ulrich H, Haak T. Lipoate prevention of diabetic microangiopathy. In: Fuchs J, Packer L, Zimmer G, eds. Lipoic Acid in Health and Disease. New York: Marcel Dekker, 1997:429–434.
103. Hofmann MA, Tritschler HJ, Bierhaus A, Ziegler R, Wahl P, Nawroth PP. Lipoate effects on atherogenesis. In: Fuchs J, Packer L, Zimmer G, eds. Lipoic Acid in Health and Disease. New York: Marcel Dekker, 1997:321–335.
104. Henriksen EJ, Jacob S, Augustin HJ, Dietze GJ. Glucose transport activity in insulin-resistant rat muscle. Effects of angiotensin-converting enzyme inhibitors and bradykinin antagonism. Diabetes 1996; 45(suppl 1):S125–S128.
105. Lithell HO. Effect of antihypertensive drugs on insulin, glucose, and lipid metabolism. Diabetes Care 1991; 14:203–209.
106. Yue TL, Lysko PG, Barone FC, Gu JL, Ruffolo RR Jr, Feuerstein GZ. Carvedilol, a new antihypertensive drug with unique antioxidant activity: potential role in cerebroprotection. Ann NY Acad Sci 1994; 738:230–242.
107. Yue TL, Mckenna PJ, Gu JL, Cheng HY, Ruffolo RR Jr, Feuerstein GZ. Carvedilol, a new antihypertensive agent, prevents lipid peroxidation and oxidative injury to endothelial cells. Hypertension 1993; 22:922–928.
108. Giugliano D, Marfella R, Acampora R, Giunta R, Coppola L, D'Onofrio F.

Effects of perindopril and carvedilol on endothelium-dependent vascular functions in patients with diabetes and hypertension. Diabetes Care 1998; 21:631–636.

109. Jacob S, Rett K, Wicklmayr M, Agrawal B, Augustin HJ, Dietze GJ. Differential effect of chronic treatment with two beta-blocking agents on insulin sensitivity: the carvedilol-metoprolol study. J Hypertens 1996; 14:489–494.
110. Malminiemi K, Lahtela JT, Huupponen R. Effects of celiprolol on insulin sensitivity and glucose tolerance in dyslipidemic hypertension. Int J Clin Pharmacol Ther 1995; 33:156–163.
111. Jacob S, Rett K, Henriksen EJ. Anti-hypertensive therapy and insulin sensitivity-do we have to redefine the role of beta-blocking agents? Am J Hypertension 1998; 11:1258–1265.
112. Rudich A, Kozlovsky N, Potashnik R, Bashan N. Oxidant stress reduces insulin responsiveness in 3T3-L1 adipocytes. Am J Physiol 1997; 35:E935–E940.
113. Cominacini L, Garbin U, Lo Cascio V. The need for a ''free radical initiative.'' Diabetologia 1996; 39:364–366.

Index

Acetylcystein,
  GSH/GSSG, 327
Adaptation,
  defined, 37
Advanced glycation end products (AGEs), 80, 187–190
  diabetes, 188, 189t
  formation, 22–23, 138
  glycation, 285
  production, 206f
  VCAM-1, 212
Advanced glycation end products (AGEs) binding proteins,
  localization, 189t
AGE-RAGE interactions, 188–190
Akt,
  α-lipoic acid, 294
ALADIN study, 176–178
ALADIN 3 study, 180
Aldose reductase, 138
Angiotensin-converting enzyme (ACE) inhibitors, 135
  insulin sensitivity, 326t, 329
Antioxidant enzymes,
  experimental diabetic neuropathy, 122
Antioxidant network, 3–6
  defined, 2
  diabetes, 6–11
Antioxidants,
  atherogenesis, 86
[Antioxidants]
  autoimmune disease, 86
  defined, 203
  essential fatty acid interactions, 140–146
  insulin resistance, 310–313
  plasma ROOH, 59–61
Antioxidant therapy,
  diabetic complications, 191–195
  diabetic polyneuropathy, 129–146
  dose considerations, 135
  neurovascular function, 132–140
  rationale, 86
Apoptosis, 40
  oxidative stress, 267
AR inhibitor (ARI), 95, 138
  NCV, 142
AR pathway,
  activation, 113–114
  mitochondrial dysfunction, 114
Ascorbic acid (AA), 70–71, 284
  NCV, 135
Ascorbyl-6-GLA,
  NCV, 142
Atherogenesis,
  antioxidants, 86
Atherosclerosis, 219
Autoimmune diabetes,
  thioredoxin, 269–270
Autoimmune disease,
  antioxidants, 86
Autooxidative glycosylation, 113

BAPTA, 21
Basic fibroblast growth factor,
  EDN, 156
BIM, 20
Biomarkers (*see* Oxidative stress markers)
β-blockers,
  insulin sensitivity, 326t
Blood flow,
  DAG-PKC activation, 245–247
  neuropathy, 129–130
Blood glucose,
  peripheral nerve, 99
BM 150639,
  NCV, 142
Body weights,
  peripheral nerve, 99
Buthionine sulfoximine-induced catalase,
  α-lipoic acid, 105

Calcium,
  hyperglycemia-mediated, 23–24
Carbonyl assay,
  proteins, 45
Carbonyl compounds,
  detoxification, 84–85
Carbonyl stress, 84–85
Carboxyethyllsysine (CEL), 81
Carboxymethyllysine (CML), 81
Cardillo,
  insulin sensitivity, 329
Cardiovascular autonomic neuropathy (CAN), 174
  α- lipoic acid, 173–182
Caspases, 40
Catalase,
  peripheral nerve, 98, 102–103
CEL, 84
Celiprolol,
  insulin sensitivity, 329
Cell death, 39–40
Cell signaling pathways,
  insulin-dependent, 11
  lipoate, 11
Ciliary neurotrophic factor,
  EDN, 156
Collagen, 248
Cuprozinc superoxide dismutase, 122
Cyclooxygenases, 21

DAG-PKC activation,
  vascular cell alterations, 245–249
Deferoxamine,
  EDN, 135–136
DEKAN study, 178–180
Diabetes,
  oxidative stress, 6–11, 24–26, 77–87
  reactive oxygen species (ROS), 130–132
Diabetes-induced neurovascular dysfunction, 93–94
Diabetes mellitus,
  AGE, 188, 189t
  autoimmune, 269–270
  defined, 303
  free radicals, 205–208
  insulin-dependent, 265–270
  ischemia-reperfusion, 209–211
  oxidative stress, 186–187
  thrombomodulin, 195f
  type 1, 305
  type 2 (*see* type 2 diabetes)
Diabetic complications,
  antioxidant therapy, 191–195
  hyperglycemia, 186
  α-lipoic acid, 192–195
  NF-κB activation, 186
  vitamin C, 192
  vitamin E, 191–192
Diabetic distal symmetric sensorimotor polyneuropathy (DPN), 115
Diabetic microangiopathy, 205–213

Diabetic neuropathy, 173
experimental, 121–127
antioxidant enzymes, 122
glucose-mediated oxidative stress, 111–115
oxidative stress role, 174–175
Diabetic polyneuropathy,
antioxidant therapy, 129–146
diabetes, 11–13
lipoic acid, 11–13
Diene conjugation, 42
Diet,
insulin sensitivity, 326t
ROS, 324–325
Diurnal variation,
plasma ROOHs, 54–55
DNA,
oxidative stress markers, 41–42
DPN,
pathogenesis, 112–113
ROS, 114
DRG,
neuropathology, 125–126
vascular perfusion, 125–126

ELAM-1, 213
Electromobility shift assay (EMSA), 24–25
Endoneurial ischemia/hypoxia,
oxidative stress, 121
Endothelial dysfunction,
glycoxidation, 45
nitric oxide, 322–323
synergistic therapy, 141–142
Endothelial function,
vitamin E, 327
Endothelin-1, 193, 245
Endothelium,
EDN, 132–135
superoxide anions, 20–24
vascular,
experimental diabetes, 132–135
Endothelium-dependent vasodilation, 208–209
Endothelium-derived hyperpolarizing factor (EDHF), 141
Energy metabolism,
EDN, 127
8-epiPGF2a, 42
ESR signal, 4
Essential fatty acids,
antioxidant interactions, 140–146
n-6, 142–146
neurovascular dysfunction, 141
Ethane,
breath excretion, 44
Evening primrose oil,
NCV, 142
Exercise,
insulin sensitivity, 326t
ROS, 325
Experimental diabetic neuropathy (EDN), 121–127
antioxidant dose, 135
antioxidant enzymes, 122
basic fibroblast growth factor, 156
energy metabolism, 127
essential fatty acids, 141
etiology, 155–156
fatty acid/antioxidant interaction, 140–146
glucose uptake, 127
α-lipoic acid, 123–124
nerve growth, 136–138
neuropathology, 125–127
neurotrophic factors, 156–157
neurotrophins, 157–158
neurovascular function, 132–140
NF-κB, 139–140
NGF, 156
PKC, 139–140
polyol pathway, 138–139
sciatic nerve, 175
thioctic acid-γ-linolenic acid, 155–165
transition metal chelators, 135–136
vascular endothelium, 132–135

Extracellular matrix components, 248–249

Fatty acid/antioxidant interaction,
  EDN, 140–146
Fatty acids,
  essential, 141–146
  free, 320
  n-6 essential, 142–146
Ferrous oxidation (FOX) assay, 54
Fibronectin, 248
Free fatty acids (FFA),
  insulin resistance, 281–282
  TBARS, 320
Free radicals,
  diabetes mellitus, 205–208
  generation, 1
Fructose,
  peripheral nerve, 100–101
  sorbitol, 285–287

GLA,
  NCV, 142
GLA-α-lipoic acid,
  NCV, 142–146
Glomerular filtration,
  nitric oxide, 246
Glomerular filtration rate (GFR), 246
Glomerular hyperfiltration, 246
Glucosamine,
  insulin resistance, 282–283, 291
Glucose,
  peripheral nerve, 100–101
Glucose enolization, 285
Glucose levels,
  type 2 diabetes mellitus, 320–321
Glucose-mediated oxidative stress,
  diabetic neuropathy, 111–115
Glucose uptake,
  EDN, 127
  α-lipoic acid, 292–294
  nitric oxide, 323
Glucotoxicity, 284–287
  metabolic initiators, 111–112
  sorbitol pathway, 206
GLUT1, 242
  translocation,
    α-lipoic acid, 293
GLUT4,
  isoform, 276
  translocation, 276–277
    α-lipoic acid, 293
    skeletal muscle glucose transport, 304–305
    type 2 diabetes, 279–280
Glutathione (GSH), 3, 78, 86, 288
  insulin sensitivity, 325–326, 326t
  lipid peroxidation, 106
  peripheral nerve, 97, 102
  streptozotocin-induced diabetic rats, 306
  type 2 diabetes mellitus, 325–327
  xenobiotics, 36
Glutathione (GSH)-containing enzymes, 122
Glutathione (GSH)/GSSG,
  acetylcystein, 327
  obese Zucker rat, 307–308
  streptozotocin-induced diabetic rats, 306
Glutathione peroxidase (GSH-Px), 122
  α-lipoic acid, 105
  peripheral nerve, 102–103
Glycoxidation,
  vascular endothelial dysfunction, 45
GSSG, 86, 95
GSSGR,
  peripheral nerve, 102–103

Homocysteine,
  insulin sensitivity, 324
Human umbilical vein endothelial cells (HUVECs),
  ROIs, 20
Hydroperoxide (ROOH),
  antioxidant treatment, 59–61

[Hydroperoxide (ROOH)]
diurnal variation, 54–55
glycemic control, 59
insulin therapy, 59
NIDDM, 58
plasma levels, 55–58
4-hydroxyalkenal,
peripheral nerve, 97–98, 101
8-hydroxydeoxyguanosine (8OHdG0), 41
Hyperglycemia, 284–287
diabetic complications, 186
insulin resistance, 291
microvasculature, 209
NF-κB, 24–26, 196f
oxidative stress, 6–7
ROS, 17–27
sorbitol pathway, 207f
Hyperglycemia-induced protein kinase C (PKC) activation, 243–245
Hyperglycemia-mediated intracellular calcium, 23–24
Hyperglycemic autooxidation,
oxidative stress, 122
Hyperglycemic glycation,
oxidative stress, 122
Hyperglycemic pseudohypoxia,
sorbitol oxidation, 207f
Hyperinsulinemia, 287
insulin resistance, 321f
Hypoxia,
endoneurial,
oxidative stress, 121

ICAM-1, 211–213, 212, 213
Imidazolones, 80
Insulin,
3T3-L1 adipocytes, 290
Insulin-dependent cell signaling pathways, 11
Insulin-dependent diabetes mellitus (IDDM),
oxidative stress, 266–267
[Insulin-dependent diabetes mellitus (IDDM)]
pancreatic β—cell destruction, 265–270
pathogenesis, 266
Insulin-mediated glucose transport,
obese Zucker rat, 310
Insulin receptor substrate-1 (IRS-1), 304
Insulin resistance,
antioxidants, 310–313
defined, 305
glucosamine, 291
hyperglycemia, 291
hyperinsulinemia, 321f
α-lipoic acid, 292–293
molecular basis, 276–280
oxidative stress, 275–294, 288–292
ROS, 319–320
3T3-L1 adipocytes, 291–292
triggers, 280–283
type 2 diabetes, 275–283
in vitro, 290–292
in vivo, 288–290
Insulin sensitivity,
ACE inhibitors, 329
carvedilol, 329
celiprolol, 329
clinical observations, 320
glutathione, 325–326
homocysteine, 324
interventions, 326t
α-lipoic acid, 328–329
nitric oxide, 322–324, 324
pharmacological intervention, 325–329
vitamin C, 328
vitamin E, 327–328
Insulin signaling,
type 2 diabetes, 279–280
Insulin signaling cascade,
α-lipoic acid, 313
Insulin signaling pathway,
α-lipoic acid, 292–293

Insulin therapy,
plasma ROOH, 59
Intracellular calcium,
hyperglycemia-mediated, 23–24
Intracellular signaling,
thioredoxin, 269
IRS proteins, 11
Ischemia,
endoneurial
oxidative stress, 121
Ischemia-reperfusion,
diabetes mellitus, 209–211
α-lipoic acid, 124–125
Isoprostanes,
measurement, 44

JNK, 163

Laminin, 248
Lifestyle,
ROS, 324–325
Lipid hydroperoxide,
vitamin E, 53–61
Lipid peroxidation,
diabetes relevance, 43
GSH, 106
induction, 208
measurement, 43–44
oxidative stress markers, 42–44
TA, 159
Lipoate,
cell signaling pathways, 11
Lipoic acid (*see also* α-Lipoic acid)
diabetes, 11–13
diabetic polyneuropathy, 11–13
hypoglycemic effects, 12
ischemia-reperfusion, 211
$NADH/NAD^+$, 7
redox potential, 4
therapeutic aspects, 86
therapeutic effects, 7–9
α-Lipoic acid, 159, 160, 288
Akt, 294
[α-Lipoic acid]
buthionine sulfoximine-induced catalase, 105
CAN, 178–180
clinical trials, 173–182
diabetic complications, 192–195
diabetic neuropathy, 176–178
EDN, 123–124
efficacy, 177
glucose uptake, 292–294
GLUT1 translocation, 293
GLUT4 translocation, 293
GSH-Px, 105
insulin resistance, 292–293
insulin sensitivity, 326t, 328–329
insulin signaling cascade, 313
insulin signaling pathway, 292–293
ischemia reperfusion injury, 124–125
lipid peroxidation, 159
neurovascular function, 132–133
NF-κB DNA binding, 193–194
obese Zucker rat, 308–310
polyneuropathy, 180
safety, 178
streptozotocin-induced diabetic rats, 293, 306–307
therapeutic aspects, 292
Lipoproteins,
low-density,
oxidation, 26
Lipoxygenases, 21
Low-density lipoprotein (LDL), 53
oxidation, 26
vitamin E, 66–68

Maillard reaction, 187
MDA,
peripheral nerve, 97–98, 101
MDA-Lys, 81
Metabolic initiators,
glucose toxicity, 111–112
Metal chelators, 135–136

Metatyrosines, 45
Methionine sulfoxide, 80
Methionine sulfoxide reductase, 2
Microangiopathy, 210, 210f
Microvascular dysfunction,
  streptozotocin diabetic rats, 209
Mitochondrial dysfunction,
  AR pathway, 114
Mitogen-activated protein (MAP) kinases, 163
25 mM ryanodine, 10–11
MOLD, 84
Muscle glucose transport,
  regulation, 304–305

N-acetylcysteine,
  therapeutic aspects, 86, 137
NADH/NAD$^+$,
  lipoic acid, 7
Na^+-K^+ATPase, 248
Natural oxidants, 287–288
Necrosis, 40
Neovascularization,
  PKC, 247
Nerve blood flow,
  neuropathy, 129–130
Nerve function, 132–135
Nerve growth, 136–138
Nerve regeneration,
  antioxidant therapy, 136–138
N-6 essential fatty acids, 142–146
Neurological Assessment of Thioctic Acid in Diabetic Neuropathy, 181
Neuropathy,
  nerve blood flow, 129–130
Neuropeptide Y (NPY), 160–161
Neurotrophic factors,
  EDN, 156–157
Neurotrophic growth factor (NGF),
  EDN, 156
  oxidative stress, 158
  sciatic nerve, 157–158
Neurotrophins,
  EDN, 157–158
  oxidative stress, 158
Neurovascular dysfunction, 138–139, 141
  diabetes-induced, 93–94
  ROS-induced, 94–95
Neurovascular function,
  oxidative stress and antioxidant therapy, 132–140
NF-κB,
  EDN, 139–140
  hyperglycemia, 24–25
NF-κB activation, 190–191
  diabetic complications, 186
  hyperglycemia, 196f
NF-κB DNA binding,
  α-lipoic acid, 193–194
Nitric oxide (NO), 130–132
  calcium, 208–209
  endothelial dysfunction, 322–323
  glomerular filtration, 246
  glucose uptake, 323
  insulin sensitivity, 322–324, 324
  radical scavenger, 323–324
  reactive oxygen species (ROS), 130–132
Noninsulin-dependent diabetes mellitus (NIDDM)
  complications, 53
  ROOH, 58
Nonobese diabetic (NOD) mice,
  pancreatic β-cell destruction, 265–270
  pathogenesis, 266
Normoglycemia, 173
NT-3 mRNA,
  leg muscle, 157–158

Obese Zucker rat,
  characteristics of, 306
  GSH/GSSG, 307–308
  insulin-mediated glucose transport, 310
  α-lipoic acid, 308–310

Orthotyrosines, 45
Overadaptation, 39
Oxidants,
  natural, 287–288
Oxidative damage, 79–81
  secondary, 80–81
Oxidative stress,
  apoptosis, 267
  defined, 1–2, 34–36, 77
  detection, 283–284
  diabetes, 6–11, 77–87
  diabetes consequences, 24–26
  disease, 34–40
  endoneurial ischemia/hypoxia, 121
  factors affecting, 78–79
  glucose-mediated,
    diabetic neuropathy, 111–115
  hyperglycemia, 6–7
  hyperglycemic glycation and autooxidation, 122
  increased, 82
  insulin-dependent diabetes mellitus, 266–267
  insulin resistance, 275–294, 288–292
  measurement, 78–79
  mechanisms, 36–37, 121–122
  neurotrophins, 158
  neurovascular function, 132–140
  NGF, 158
  parameters, 39t
  peripheral nerve, 158–159
  polyol pathway, 138–139
  tissue injury, 33–34
Oxidative stress markers, 33–46, 38f, 80t, 82–83
  DNA, 41–42
  lipid peroxidation, 42–44
  need for, 40
  protein damage, 44–45
  ROS/RNS/RCS, 40
Oxygen,
  ROS/RNS/RCS, 36
P38, 163
Pancreatic β-cells,
  endogenous thioredoxin, 269
  insulin-dependent diabetes mellitus, 265–270
PDTC, 10
Pentane,
  breath excretion, 44
Pentosidine, 81
Peripheral nerve,
  MDA, 97–98, 101
  oxidative stress, 158–159
Peripheral nerve studies, 93–107
  animals, 95–96
  autooxidative defense enzyme measurement, 98–99
  biochemical measurements, 96–99
  experimental procedure, 96
  GSH measurement, 97
  4-hydroxyalkenal measurement, 97–98, 101
  materials and methods, 95–99
  reagents, 96
  results, 99–104
  sorbitol pathway intermediates measurement, 96–97
  statistical analysis, 99
  total MDA measurement, 97–98
Peroxynitrite, 22
  diabetic vascular complications, 26
Physical activity,
  ROS, 325
Pioglitazone, 325
PKC isoforms in A7r5 smc,
  α-tocopherol, 226–227
Polyol pathway,
  EDN, 138–139
  oxidative stress, 138–139
PP_2A,
  α-tocopherol, 236
  β-tocopherol, 236
Primaquine, 133
Probucol, 133

Protein kinase C (PKC),
EDN, 139–140
inhibitors, 20
α-tocopherol, 220–221
vitamin E, 249–251
Protein kinase C (PKC) activation, hyperglycemia-induced, 243–245
Protein kinase C (PKC) α inhibition, α-tocopherol, 227–228, 232–233
Protein kinase C (PKC) β-isoform inhibition, 249
Protein kinase C (PKC) isoforms, 242
α-tocopherol, 229–231
Protein kinases,
stress-activated
thioctyl-γ-linolenic acid, 163–164
Protein phosphatase PP2A,
α-tocopherol, 233–235
Proteins,
carbonyl assay, 45
diabetes relevance, 45–46
oxidative stress markers, 44–45
ROS/RNS/RCS, 44–45
Proteoglycans, 248
P-selectin, 212
Pseudohypoxia, 107
Pyrraline, 80

Reactive oxygen intermediates (ROI),
generation, 22–23
HUVEC, 20
hyperglycemia, 20–24
streptozotocin diabetic rats, 19–20
vasculature source, 18–20
vitamin E, 18–19
Reactive oxygen species (ROS), 37t
alterations, 324–329
diabetes, NO, and vasorelaxation, 130–132
diet, 324–325
DPN, 114
exercise, 325
hyperglycemia, 17–27
[Reactive oxygen species (ROS)]
insulin resistance, 319–320
lifestyle, 324–325
sources, 130–132
Reactive oxygen species (ROS)-induced neurovascular dysfunction, 94–95
Receptor for AGE (RAGE), 188–189, 206
R-lipoic acid, 7, 11–12
Rochester Diabetic Neuropathy Study, 180–181
ROS/RNS/RCS,
oxidative stress markers, 40
oxygen, 36
proteins, 44–45
RRR-α-tocopherol (*see* Vitamin E)

Sciatic nerve,
EDN, 125
nerve conduction studies, 126
Skeletal muscle glucose transport,
GLUT4 translocation, 304–305
regulation, 304–305
Smoking cessation,
insulin sensitivity, 326t
Smooth muscle cell proliferation,
α-tocopherol, 220
Smooth muscle cells (smc), 219
SNAP23, 277
Sorbitol,
fructose levels, 285–287
peripheral nerve, 100–101
Sorbitol oxidation,
hyperglycemic pseudohypoxia, 207f
Sorbitol pathway,
glucotoxicity, 206
hyperglycemia, 207f
Sorbitol pathway intermediates,
peripheral nerve, 96–97
Stauroporine, 20
Streptozotocin diabetic rats,
ROIs, 19–20

Streptozotocin-induced diabetic rats,
  characteristics of, 305
  glutathione, 306
  GSSG/GSH, 306
  α-lipoic acid, 293, 306–307
  microvascular dysfunction, 209
  sciatic nerve blood flow, 129–130
Stress-activated protein kinases (SAPKs),
  thioctyl-γ-linolenic acid, 163–164
Suicide mechanism, 40
Suicide response, 40
Superoxide anions,
  endothelial formation, 20–24
Superoxide dismutase (SOD), 2
  peripheral nerve, 98, 102–103
Syntaxin 4, 277

TBA-reactive substances (TBARS), 43
TBA test, 42
Thiobarbituric acid reactive substances (TBARS), 53–54
  free fatty acids, 320
Thioctic acid-γ-linolenic acid,
  EDN, 155–165
Thioctyl-γ-linolenic acid,
  stress-activated protein kinases, 163–164
  in vivo studies, 160–163
Thiol antioxidants, 10
Thioredoxin (TRX),
  antioxidative effects, 267–269
  autoimmune diabetes, 269–270
  intracellular signaling, 269
  pancreatic β-cells, 269
Thiotic acid (*see* α-Lipoic acid)
Thrombomodulin,
  diabetes mellitus, 195f
Tissue injury, 39
  oxidative stress, 33–34
3T3-L1 adipocytes,
  insulin, 290
  insulin resistance, 291–292
Tocopherol (*see* α-Tocopherol; β-Tocopherol)
α-tocopherol,
  cell proliferation inhibition, 226
  molecular basis, 219–237
  PKC inhibition, 226–235
  PKC α inhibition, 227–228, 232–233
  PKC isoforms autophosphorylation, 229–231
  PKC isoforms in A7r5 smc, 226–227
  plasma levels, 36, 58–59
  PP_2A, 236
  protein phosphatase PP2A, 233–235
  smooth muscle cell proliferation, 220
β-Tocopherol,
  PP_2A, 236
α-Tocopherol studies, 219–237
  animals, 219
  cell cultures, 219
  cell proliferation, 219
  immunoprecipitated PKCα, 224
  methods, 219–225
  PKC activity, 219–220
  PKC isoform autophosphorylation, 223–224
  PKC isoform immunoprecipitation, 223
  PKCα/protein phosphatase assay, 225
  protein phosphatase activity assay, 225
  in vivo cell labeling, 224
  Western blot analyses, 223
Torglitazone,
  insulin sensitivity, 325
Transition metal chelators, 135–136
Transretinol, 69–70
Trientine,
  EDN, 135–136
Triphenylphosphine (TPP), 54

Troglitazone,
insulin sensitivity, 326t
Trytophan,
hydroxylation, 45
Tumor necrosis factor-α,
insulin resistance, 281
Type 1 diabetes,
animal models, 305
Type 2 diabetes,
animal models, 3–6, 305
glutathione, 325–327
insulin resistance, 275–283
metabolic alterations, 321t
oxidative stress origin, 284–288
plasma glucose levels, 320–321
vitamin E, 289–290, 327
Tyrosine, 80

Van der Waerden rest, 99
Vascular cell adhesion molecule (VCAM)-1, 212, 213
Vascular endothelial growth factor (VEGF), 246
formation, 23–24
Vascular endothelium, 132–135
Vascular permeability,
PKC, 247
Vasorelaxation,
reactive oxygen species (ROS), 130–132
Vesperlysine, 81
Vitamin A, 69–70
plasma, 69–70
Vitamin B,
diabetic neuropathy, 176–178
Vitamin C, 3, 70–71, 288
diabetic complications, 192
insulin sensitivity, 326t, 328
NCV, 135
plasma, 70–71
Vitamin E, 3, 66–68, 288
diabetic complications, 191–192
endothelial function, 327
insulin sensitivity, 326t, 327–328
LDL, 66–68
PKC inhibition, 249–251
plasma, 36, 58–59, 66–68
plasma lipid hydroperoxide, 53–61
ROI, 18–19
standardization, 68–69
type 2 diabetes, 289–290
type 2 diabetes mellitus, 327
Vitamin E deficiency,
premature cell aging, 220
Vitamin E radical, 5

Wistar rats, 95–96

Xenobiotics,
GSH, 36